D1543248

Medizinische Hochschule Hannover
Anaesthesiologie I - 8056
Interdisziplinäre Intensivstation
Prof. Dr. S. Piepenbrock
Carl-Neuberg-Str. 1 • 30625 Hannover
Tel. (05 11) 5 32-22 47

European Resuscitation Council Guidelines for Resuscitation

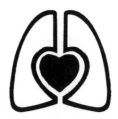

European Resuscitation Council Guidelines for Resuscitation

Edited by:

Leo Bossaert
University of Antwerp
Antwerp, Belgium

for the

European Resuscitation Council

1998

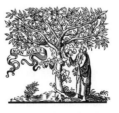

Elsevier

Amsterdam - Lausanne - New York - Oxford - Shannon - Singapore - Tokyo

Published by
ELSEVIER SCIENCE B.V.
Sara Burgerhartstraat 25
P.O. Box 211, 1000 AE Amsterdam, The Netherlands

Library of Congress Cataloging in Publication Data
A catalog record from the Library of Congress has been applied for.

ISBN 0-444-82957-1

©1998 European Resuscitation Council. All rights reserved.

No part of this publication may be reproduced, stored in a retrieval system or transmitted in any form or by any means, electronic, mechanical, photocopying or otherwise, without the prior written permission of the European Resuscitation Council, c/o ERC Secretariat, P.O. Box 113, 2610 Antwerp, Belgium.

Ch 4.3, Figs. 10, 11; Ch. 6, Figs 2, 3, 5-15. Copyright ©1997 Bunge (Elsevier's Bedrijfsinformatie).

No responsibility is assumed by the European Resuscitation Council or the Publisher for any injury and/or damage to persons or property as a matter of products liability, negligence or otherwise, or from any use or operation of any methods, products, instructions or ideas contained in the material herein. Because of rapid advances in the medical sciences, the Publisher recommends that independent verification of diagnosis and drug dosages should be made.

⊗ The paper used in this publication meets the requirements of ANSI/NISO Z39.48-1992 (Permanence of Paper).
Printed in The Netherlands

Preface

The European Resuscitation Council (ERC) was established in 1989 as an interdisciplinary council for resuscitation medicine and emergency medical care.

The objectives of the ERC are to preserve life by improving standards of resuscitation in Europe and to co-ordinate the activities of European organisations with a major interest in Cardiopulmonary Resuscitation (CPR).

The ERC pursues its objectives by

- producing guidelines and recommendations appropriate to Europe for the practice of Cardiopulmonary and Cerebral Resuscitation;
- updating these guidelines in the light of critical review of CPR practice;
- promoting audit of resuscitation practice including standardisation of records of resuscitation attempts;
- designing standardised teaching programmes suitable for all trainees in Europe ranging from the lay public to the qualified physician;
- promoting and co-ordinating appropriate research;
- organising relevant congresses and other scientific meetings in Europe;
- promoting political and public awareness of resuscitation requirements and practice in Europe.

In 1992, the European Resuscitation Council has presented *Guidelines for Basic Life Support and Advanced Life Support* at the first Scientific Congress of the ERC in Brighton. In 1994, *Guidelines for Paediatric Life Support* and *Guidelines for the Management of Periarrest Arrhythmias* were presented at the second Congress in Mainz. In 1996,

Guidelines for the Basic and Advanced Management of the Airway and Ventilation during Resuscitation were presented at the third Congress in Sevilla.

The guidelines were published in Resuscitation, which is the official journal of the ERC. Eventually, they were translated in many European languages and received wide acceptance and distribution throughout Europe.

In 1992 the *International Liaison Committee on Resuscitation*, ILCOR, was founded with the following mission: *"To provide a consensus mechanism by which the international science and knowledge relevant to emergency cardiac care can be identified and reviewed. This consensus mechanism will be used to provide consistent international guidelines for basic life support, paediatric life support and advanced life support. These international guidelines will aim for a commonality supported by science for BLS, PLS and ALS."*

The constituent organisations agreed to make use of this resource so that all future guidelines will reflect the commonality of opinion that has evolved during the process.

The first ILCOR advisory statements were presented at the Congress CPR'97 in Brighton, UK, and were first published in the April 1997 issues of the journals Resuscitation and Circulation.

As a consequence, the European Resuscitation Council has decided to update the 1992 Guidelines and to adjust them to the Advisory Statements of ILCOR.

In the time period after the publication of the ILCOR statements, the ERC Working Groups on Basic Life Support, Paediatric Life Support and Advanced Life Support of the ERC have prepared the new 1998 ERC Guidelines for Resuscitation and they were field-tested in late 1997 and early 1998. This field test was most essential since it provided important feedback for the final adjustment of the Guidelines.

Because of the rapidly growing use of Automated External Defibrillators (AED) by ambulance personnel and by first responders, guidelines for the use of AEDs were also developed.

The ERC Working Group on Training and Education has further prepared the materials that support the ERC Guidelines: the publication of the Guidelines book, the production of educational wall posters and the supporting course materials.

The Guidelines were carefully reviewed by the members of the Executive Committee of the ERC and they were endorsed by the Board of the ERC in March 1998.

This 1998 edition of the ERC Guidelines for Resuscitation brings together all new and revised Guidelines for Resuscitation that were produced in accordance with ILCOR, and they are presented at the 4th Scientific Congress of the ERC in Copenhagen in June 1998.

The book is the great merit of the many contributors, but in the first place of the chairmen and members of the Working Groups. The names of all contributors are included in the beginning of the book.

For the illustration of the Guidelines and the supporting materials, drawings were made by Diane Bruyninckx. Some of her drawings, namely those relating to the management of Airway and Ventilation, were initially made for the book "Reanimatie" that was edited by B.T.J. Meursing and R.G. van Kesteren, and published by Bunge-Elsevier publishers in 1997. They have kindly given the ERC permission to use these drawings.

For the publication of this book, educational grants were received from Aurum Pharmaceutical Ltd, Laerdal Medical Corporation and Laerdal Foundation for Acute Medicine, Heartstream Company, Marquette Medical Systems, Physio Control, Zoll Medical Corporation.

Additional copies of this publication are available via booksellers and on application at the ERC Secretariat.

Prof. Dr. Leo Bossaert
Hon. Secretary of the European Resuscitation Council
Editor

For information relating to ERC, its membership, publications and activities, write to:

ERC Secretariat
P.O. Box 113
2610 Antwerp, Belgium
Fax +32-3-8284882

Contents

List of Contributors

Jennifer Adgey (Belfast, UK)
Richard Arntz (Berlin, Germany)
Jan Bahr (Göttingen, Germany)
Peter Baskett (Bristol, UK)
Michael Baubin (Innsbruck, Austria)
Tom Beattie (Edinburgh, UK)
Robert Bingham (London, UK)
Jonathan Bland (Stavanger, Norway)
Leo Bossaert (Antwerp, Belgium)
Marieta Bruins-Stassen (Huizen, The Netherlands)
Pierre Carli (Paris, France)
Pascal Cassan (Lyon, France)
Luis G. Castrillo (Spain)
Erga Cerchiari (Milano, Italy)
Douglas Chamberlain (Brighton, UK)
Francisco De Latorre (Barcelona, Spain)
Wolfgang Dick (Mainz, Germany)
Lars Ekström (Göteborg, Sweden)
Franz Frei (Basel, Switzerland)
Harold Gamsu (London, UK)
Patricia Hamilton (London, UK)
Anthony Handley (Colchester, UK)
Svein A. Hapnes (Stavanger, Norway)
Stig Holmberg (Göteborg, Sweden)
Rudolph Juchems (Aschaffenburg, Germany)
Fulvio Kette (Trieste, Italy)
Dietrich Kettler (Göttingen, Germany)
Rudy Koster (Amsterdam, The Netherlands)
Karl Lindner (Innsbruck, Austria)
Andrew Marsden (Edinburgh, UK)

Dietmar Mauer (Mainz, Germany)
Anthony Milner (London, UK)
Olivier Moeschler (Lausanne, Switzerland)
Michael Mohr (Göttingen, Germany)
Koen Monsieurs (Antwerp, Belgium)
Jerry Nolan (Bristol, UK)
Michael Parr (Bristol, UK)
Jacques Peper (Amsterdam, The Netherlands)
Paul Petit (Lyon, France)
Barbara Phillips (London, UK)
Colin Robertson (Edinburgh, UK)
Miguel Ruano (Valencia, Spain)
Tom Silfvast (Helsinki, Finland)
Christian Speer (Tübingen, Germany)
Petter Steen (Oslo, Norway)
Ank van Drenth (The Hague, The Netherlands)
Patrick Van Reempts (Antwerp, Belgium)
Richard Vincent (Brighton, UK)
David Zideman (London, UK)

WITH CONTRIBUTION FROM:

Raul Alasino (Consejo Latino Americano de Resucitacion)
Vic Callanan (Australian Resuscitation Council)
Jim Christensen (Heart and Stroke Foundation of Canada)
Richard Cummins (American Heart Association)
Walter Kloeck (Resuscitation Council of Southern Africa)

List of Abbreviations

ACD	Active Compression Decompression
AED	Automated External Defibrillator
AHA	American Heart Association
ALS	Advanced Life Support
ARC	Australian Resuscitation Council
ATN	Acute Tubular Necrosis
BLS	Basic Life Support
CCU	Cardiac (Coronary) Care Unit
CDC	Centers for Disease Control
CLAR	Consejo Latino Americano de Resucitacion
CNS	Central Nervous System
COPD	Chronic Obstructive Pulmonary Disease
CPAP	Continuous Positive Airway Pressure
CPR	Cardio Pulmonary Resuscitation
CRS	Comprehensive Resuscitation Scenario
DNR	Do Not Resuscitate
DNAR	Do Not Attempt Resuscitation
ECG	Electrocardiogram
ED	Emergency Department
EMS	Emergency Medical System
EMT	Emergency Medical Technician
EMT(D)	Emergency Medical Technician (Defibrillation)
ERC	European Resuscitation Council
ESC	European Society of Cardiology
GCS	Glasgow Coma Score
HBV	Hepatitis B virus
HIV	Human Immunodeficiency Virus
HSFC	Heart and Stroke Foundation of Canada
ICU	Intensive Care Unit
ILCOR	International Liaison Committee on Resuscitation
LMA	Laryngeal Mask Airway
mcg	Microgram
MCQ	Multiple Choise Questions
OPA	Oro Pharyngeal Airway
PAP	Positive Airway Pressure
PEEP	Positive End Expiratory Pressure
PLS	Paediatric Life Support
RCSA	Resuscitation Council of Southern Africa
ROSC	Restoration of Spontaneous Circulation
VF	Ventricular Fibrillation
VT	Ventricular Tachycardia

1. Introduction: From ILCOR Policy Statements to ERC Model Guidelines

In 1973 the AHA first published the "Standards for Cardiopulmonary Resuscitation and Emergency Cardiac Care". At that time, only a few of the recommended measures were based on scientific evidence, but the medical world accepted them as international precepts that formed the gold standard for resuscitation care. Although they had been evolved only on the basis of national experience and requirements within the United States, they quickly acquired medicolegal significance both within and beyond the borders of that country. Moreover, manufacturers of manikins, ventilation bags, and airway adjuncts developed devices strictly in accordance with these new standards.

Since then, many additional national and supranational guidelines have been developed and published to replace or complement the 1973 Standards. They include publications from the AHA in 1980, 1986 and 1992; from the ERC in 1992; and material from smaller councils such as those from Australia and Southern Africa.

In the absence of any new scientific base, all the new guidelines have included detailed advice that remains scientifically unproven but which has been justified only on the basis of clinical experience and precedent. Lack of certainty can lead to tension when experience and precedent in one area are at variance with those in others. Difficulties have arisen in relation to medical considerations (examples being disparate opinions on mouth-to-nose ventilation, ventilation volumes, pulse check, the Heimlich maneuver, and availability of drugs); to medicolegal issues (for example, the role in resuscitation of nonphysicians); to ethical and religious matters (notable in relation to DNAR orders); and to linguistic problems (especially in Europe where more than 50 different languages are spoken).

Against this background, the International Liaison Committee on Resuscitation (ILCOR) has worked in recent years to produce agreed policy statements on CPR based as far as possible on scientifically proven material and attentive to educational aspects that demanded simplification of algorithms. ILCOR comprises the AHA, the ERC, the Australian Resuscitation Council, the Resuscitation Council of Southern Africa and the Resuscitation Council of Latin America. The policy statements have therefore been published in several journals and languages, and are intended as a resource for the production of more detailed supranational and national guidelines.

The ERC has closely followed the ILCOR statements in the 1998 "Model Guidelines" which offer an authoritative supranational European model. These in turn may be adopted in toto by European national councils or adapted as necessary for specific national guidelines where medicolegal, ethical, religious or medical considerations make it necessary to have local variations. These variations must, however, be approved by the ERC in order to carry its logo and name.

The Model Guidelines themselves have been issued by the respective ERC Working Groups (BLS, ALS, PLS). In order to promote their distribution and clinical acceptance, the Working Group on Training and Education has put together a Guideline Book, slide sets, and videos.

The policy of the ERC is not to run its own courses but rather to provide national councils and other organizations in Europe with appropriate material for National CPR Courses based on the ERC Model Guidelines.

The material includes:

- Guidelines for Basic Life Support
- Guidelines for Advanced Life Support
- Guidelines for the Use of Automated External Defibrillators
- Guidelines for Paediatric Life Support
- Guidelines for Management of Airway and Ventilation
- Guidelines for Resuscitation of Babies at Birth

- Guidelines of Management of Periarrest Arrhythmias (updated)
- Guidelines for Early Management of Heart Attack (produced as a cooperative effort between European Resuscitation Council and European Society for Cardiology)
- Considerations on Ethics of Resuscitation

Prof. Dr. W.F. Dick, FRCA
Chairman European Resuscitation Council
June 1998

2. Adult Basic Life Support

CONTENTS

2.1. Introduction

The term basic life support (BLS) refers to maintaining airway patency and supporting breathing and the circulation without the use of equipment other than a protective shield [1]. It comprises the elements: initial assessment; airway maintenance; expired air ventilation (rescue breathing); and chest compression. When all three are combined the term cardiopulmonary resuscitation (CPR) is used. Basic life support implies that no equipment is employed; when a simple airway, or face mask for mouth-to-mask resuscitation is used, this is defined as "basic life support with airway adjunct". The development of automated defibrillation (AED) has allowed minimally trained persons to extend their BLS skills.

The purpose of BLS is to maintain adequate ventilation and circulation until means can be obtained to reverse the underlying cause of the arrest. It is therefore a "holding operation", although on occasions, particularly when the primary pathology is respiratory failure, it may itself reverse the cause and allow full recovery.

Failure of the circulation for 3 to 4 minutes (less if the patient is initially hypoxaemic) will lead to irreversible cerebral damage. Delay, even within that time, will lessen the eventual chances of a successful outcome. Emphasis must therefore be placed on rapid institution of basic life support by a rescuer, who nonetheless should follow the recommended sequence of action.

History

The earliest reference to mouth-to-mouth ventilation is considered to be in the Bible, when the prophet Elisha revived an apparently dead child. The first medical report of success was by Tossach in 1744. Following this report, however, there was no further progress with the technique, and attention was turned towards the manual methods such as those described by Silvester, Schaefer, and Nielsen. It was not until the 1950s that mouth-to-mouth ventilation was rediscovered by Safar and Ruben and became accepted universally as the method of choice. The inefficiency of the manual methods has led to them being abandoned.

Closed chest cardiac massage was first described in 1878 by Boehm and successfully applied in a few cases of cardiac arrest over the next 10 years or so. After that, however, open chest massage became the standard management for cardiac arrest until 1960, when the classic paper by Kouwenhoven, Jude and Knickerbocker was published [2], showing the effectiveness of closed chest massage. As this coincided with the rebirth of mouth-to-mouth ventilation, 1960 could be considered the year in which modern cardiopulmonary resuscitation was born.

Theory of chest compression

The original term "cardiac massage" and its successor "external cardiac compression" reflect the initial theory as to how chest compressions achieve an artificial circulation – namely, by squeezing the heart. This "heart pump theory" was criticized in the mid-1970s, firstly because echocardiography demonstrated that the cardiac valves became incompetent during resuscitation; secondly, because coughing alone was shown to produce a life-sustaining circulation. The alternative "thoracic pump" theory proposes that chest compression, by increasing intrathoracic pressure, propels blood out of the thorax, forward flow occurring because veins at the thoracic inlet collapse while the arteries remain patent.

An extension of the controversy raised by these conflicting theories is the argument whether the rate of chest compression during resuscitation should be fast or slow. However, the current recommendation is for a rate of 100/min, and this has been shown to be effective in practice.

It is important to recognize that even when performed optimally chest compressions do not achieve more than 30% of the normal cardiac output.

2.2. The 1998 European Resuscitation Council Guidelines for Adult Basic Life Support

In producing guidelines on basic life support (BLS) the BLS Group of the European Resuscitation Council (ERC) studied the "Advisory Statements" of the International Liaison Committee on Resuscitation (ILCOR), and received feedback on their use during 1997 from a number of training organizations in Europe. The Training & Education Group of the ERC advised on the educational aspects. These resulting ERC Guidelines are consistent with the ILCOR Advisory Statements, with minor variations to make them suitable for general use in Europe.

2.2.1. ILCOR ADVISORY STATEMENTS

The original papers were published in *Resuscitation* in 1997 [3]. The following edited extract gives the background to the new ERC BLS Guidelines.

"These "advisory statements" represent the consensus view of the Basic Life Support (BLS) Working Group of the International Liaison Committee on Resuscitation (ILCOR), which itself represents the world's major resuscitation organisations (including the American Heart Association, Australian Resuscitation Council, European Resuscitation Council, Heart and Stroke Foundation of Canada, and Resuscitation Council of Southern Africa).

The scientific basis for the treatment of cardiac arrest has an active international literature [4]. The purpose of creating these advisory statements is to take full advantage of international perspective and experience in the basic management of cardiac arrest. It is hoped that the "Sequence of Action" can be used as a template

by individual national resuscitation organisations. This template should not, however, be considered a rigid standard. It is intended primarily to remove the many minor international differences in BLS education that have developed over the last 30 years, often without any basis in science. For example, when the existing BLS guidelines of the European Resuscitation Council (ERC) and the American Heart Association (AHA) were compared, most of the differences existed without any particular rationale and were simply based on quirks of historical practice. It is hoped that by removing these, BLS training can become as uniform as possible throughout the world.

The process for the development of the advisory statements involved:

1. Identification of major and minor differences between existing BLS guidelines [5,6]. Minor differences mostly involved the use of words, rather than any real difference of opinion regarding scientific content. They were resolved by arriving at a consensus.

2. Presentation of formal position papers on areas of major difference, with an emphasis on available scientific evidence. The committee attempted to reach consensus on items of controversy, but sometimes the resulting statements reflect a majority opinion.

3. Presentation of the newly developed guidelines to the ILCOR Advanced Life Support and Paediatric Working Groups with incorporation of the comments received.

4. Feedback from the individual national BLS Committees of the member resuscitation organizations.

5. Preparation of the final Sequence of Action.

Modification of the ILCOR BLS Template

The BLS template is not intended to restrict national resuscitation organizations or prevent them from making modifications when valid concerns (or future studies) support these. It is fully anticipated that the significant differences in culture and emergency facilities that exist between communities will result in modification of these statements by national resuscitation organisations in order to meet specific local or regional needs. For example, decisions on when to call for help or whether to perform a pulse check may vary depending on local epidemiology, EMS technology, or public CPR education. Therefore this template should be used as a basic resource from which to develop appropriate local BLS guidelines.

Lay Rescuer Training

Readers familiar with CPR guidelines from other sources will note that there are some differences between these statements and prior publications. A central concern was to ensure that guidelines are as simple as possible. The reason for a "movement towards simplicity" comes from a critical examination of the successes and failures of public sector CPR education. There is no question that CPR saves lives, yet after 30 years of attempts at public CPR education most communities still do not train a sufficiently high proportion of the public to perform basic CPR; rates of community CPR have not increased significantly since the 1970s in the USA and Europe. Paradoxically, in some higher risk populations, the rate of bystander CPR is particularly poor [7,8]. Therefore, the ILCOR BLS Working Group recognize that a redoubling of efforts to teach CPR to the public is a vital priority for nearly all communities.

There are many possible obstacles to lay person CPR training, the reasons for which are multifactorial. It has been noted by some investigators that the psychomotor skills required to perform CPR are relatively difficult for the lay public. Moreover, even when they are taught to professionals their retention by people who do not use them regularly has been disappointing [9–11]. In addition, in some communities there is a reluctance to perform rescue breathing on a "stranger" due to a concern over disease transmission (for example fear of contracting HIV) [12,13].

There is scientific uncertainty within the literature regarding how "good" CPR has to be in order to save a life [14]. Do victims who receive perfectly performed compressions and rescue breathing (so-called "good CPR") fare better than victims who get less effective CPR? A definitive answer is still awaited, but the clear conclusion from many studies is that the lowest survival rates occur when there is no attempt at CPR [15]. Any CPR is clearly better than no CPR. Therefore a simple, basic, approach that can be effectively taught to the largest number of people should help to increase the pool of individuals willing to attempt basic life support.

It is possible to imagine a wide spectrum of BLS instruction from simple to very complex. For example, some have suggested that CPR instruction for lay persons be as simple as "pump and blow". By contrast, far more complicated protocols than those currently available could be developed and recommended for public education by addition of more medical assessment steps to the various manoeuvres. The recipe for the most "simple CPR", while maintaining effectiveness for survival, has not been adequately addressed.

Circulatory Assessment

It has been traditional when checking for cardiac arrest in a nonresponsive (unconscious) adult victim to palpate the carotid artery. To date, all resuscitation councils world-wide require this single determination of carotid pulselessness as the diagnostic step which immediately leads to the initiation of chest compression. The time allowed to feel for the existence of a pulse differs between resuscitation councils [5,6,16] but no council advocates more than 10 s for a nor-mothermic victim as time is taught to be critical when initiating CPR.

Should the "carotid pulse check" still be taught to lay persons as the sole criterion for the initiation of chest compression?

Many emergency medical service despatch centres now offer telephonic CPR instruction to callers reporting victims who have collapsed. The criteria for the initiation of CPR are normally a combination of unresponsiveness and lack of breathing [17]. It is not normal practice for the dispatcher to ask for a carotid pulse check prior to advising chest compression, mainly because of the perceived difficulty in describing the tech-nique over the telephone. Is the carotid pulse check in fact difficult, particularly for lay per-sons?

Recent studies [18–22] have strongly sug-gested that the time needed to diagnose with confidence the presence or absence of a carotid pulse is far greater than the 5–10 s normally recommended, with times in excess of 30 s being needed to achieve a diagnostic accuracy of 95%. Even with prolonged palpation, 45% of carotid pulses may be pronounced absent even when present [21]. It should also be borne in mind that most of these studies were undertaken using normotensive volunteers, a situation far different from finding a collapsed and cyanosed victim in the street who is likely to be hypotensive, vaso-constricted, or worse.

As a result of these studies, the BLS Group considered that the carotid pulse check should be "de-emphasized" and that other criteria should be used to determine the need for chest compression in an unresponsive, apnoeic, adult, patient. It was therefore decided to use the expression: "Look for signs of a circulation" which includes seeing movement as well as checking the carotid pulse. It has also been made clear that the rescuer should limit the time taken for this check to no more than 10

s. Therefore, the absence of any obvious signs of life, not necessarily the absence of the carotid pulse, should be sufficient indication to initiate chest compression.

It should be emphasized that this departure from current teaching is aimed, at least for now, only at the lay rescuer; checking for a pulse remains an important part of advanced life support.

Volume and Rate of Ventilation

Rescue breathing (expired air ventilation; mouth-to-mouth ventilation) has been a well-accepted technique of airway management in BLS since the early 1960s [23]. The volume of air required to be given with each inflation is normally quoted as 800–1200 cc, with each breath taking 1–1.5 s. The BLS Group questioned the validity of these figures.

Artificial ventilation without airway protection (such as tracheal intubation) carries a high risk of gastric inflation, regurgitation, and pulmonary aspiration [5]. The risk of gastric inflation depends upon: (a) the proximal airway pressure, which is determined by tidal volume and infla-tion rate; (b) the alignment of the head and neck, and degree of patency of the airway; (c) the opening pressure of the lower oesophageal sphincter (approximately 20 cmH_2O). It has recently been shown that a tidal volume of 400–500 cc is sufficient to give adequate venti-lation in adult basic life support because CO_2 production during cardiac arrest is very low [24]. This recommendation overrules earlier guidelines [5] and makes it necessary to recali-brate adult training manikins [25]. It is, however, consistent with the accepted teaching that the tidal volume should be that which causes the chest to rise.

During combined rescue breathing and chest compression the rate of ventilation is dependent both on the ventilation volume and the compres-sion rate. An inflation time of 1½–2 s diminishes the risk of exceeding the oesophageal opening pressure [5] and results in an inflation/exhalation cycle of about 3 s [25]. To obtain optimum perfusion of vital organs a chest compression rate of about 100/min is recommended. It therefore takes 12 s to perform 15 cardiac compressions [25]. Allowing 6 s for the two rescue breaths, single-rescuer CPR should result in eight breaths and 60 chest compressions per minute.

Call First — Call Fast

The first link in the Chain of Survival [26] is to gain access to the emergency medical services. Advice as to the optimum time during a resuscitation attempt at which to leave the victim to go for help will depend on several factors: whether the rescuer is alone; whether the victim has a primary respiratory or primary cardiac arrest; the distance to the nearest point of aid (for example a telephone); the facilities offered by the emergency services.

The importance of early defibrillation in the treatment of sudden cardiac death is now accepted, and major initiatives are moving forward in the world to deliver a defibrillator and the first shock at the earliest possible moment [27]. The 1992 AHA Guidelines [5] emphasized that the rescuer should, if no other help is available, leave an adult victim immediately after establishing unresponsiveness in order to call an ambulance or emergency medical service system ("phone first"). The 1992 ERC Guidelines [6] advise that a shout for assistance should be made as soon as the victim is found to be unconscious, but that the lone rescuer should not leave to go for help until cardiac arrest is diagnosed by means of a pulse check ("phone fast"). Both the AHA and the ERC Guidelines seek to ensure that a defibrillator reaches the victim at the earliest appropriate opportunity. Both agree that if the victim is a child, the rescuer should provide rescue support (ventilatory or circulatory or both) for about 1 min before leaving the victim and calling the rescue team [28].

The rationale for phoning first (rather than fast) is based on several factors [29]. Clearly defibrillation is the key to survival from sudden cardiac death. However, it has been documented that rescuers finding unconscious victims frequently encounter psychological blocks that prevent them starting CPR or even calling for help. Valuable minutes are lost because of this inactivity, resulting in less chance of survival for the victim. Other rescuers can become so consumed with providing CPR that they persist far too long before summoning the EMS system.

In children the aetiology of cardiopulmonary arrest is different from that of the adult [30]. Respiratory arrest is far more common than cardiac arrest which, if it occurs, is usually secondary to respiratory arrest. The outcome of attempts at resuscitation from cardiac arrest in children is dismal at best, with a high chance of poor neurological status afterwards [31]. Survival following cardiopulmonary arrest in children is dependent mainly upon the immediate provision of effective rescue breathing [32], hence the recommendation of 1 min rescue support before leaving and phoning for help.

There has recently been interesting data to suggest that ventricular fibrillation is relatively rare in individuals up to the age of 30 years [33,34] and that perhaps a similar strategy to that of the management of childhood cardiac arrest would be prudent up until this age.

The EMS system in the USA responds in a way that uses the AHA Guidelines, but also considers other causes of collapse with separate protocols to manage them. It is recognized that the result of the "call first vs. call fast" debate will vary in different parts of the world because of the different ways in which EMS systems are composed and staffed, as well as their different approaches to first aid. For this reason these advisory statements include two possible points in time when the loan rescuers may need to leave the victim to get help — after responsiveness is established, or after the airway has been opened but breathing has not resumed. In order to try and identify cases of primary respiratory arrest, "one min of resuscitation" is advised when dealing with children and victims of trauma and near drowning.

Recovery Position

The airway of an unconscious victim who is

breathing spontaneously is at risk of obstruction by the tongue and from inhalation of mucus and vomit. Placing the victim on the side helps to prevent these problems, and allows fluid to drain easily from the mouth. This lateral, coma, side, or recovery position has been advocated in anaesthesia for over 100 years [35] and is still standard practice today. It is surprising, therefore, that its introduction into first aid practice was within the last 50 years [36]. Perhaps even more surprising is that in 1992 there was no mention of any recovery position in the AHA Guidelines [5].

Some compromise is needed when positioning the victim; a true lateral posture tends to be unstable, involves excessive lateral flexion of the cervical spine, and results in less free drainage from the mouth. A near-prone position, on the other hand, can result in under-ventilation because of splinting of the diaphragm and reduction in pulmonary and thoracic compliance [37].

Potential injury to the victim has also to be considered [38]. There have been a number of recent reports of potential interference with upper limb blood flow association with the recovery position advocated by the ERC [39,40]. This involves the lowermost arm being brought into a ventral position with the uppermost arm crossing it and producing a pressure effect on the blood vessels and, possibly, the nerve supply. Placing the lowermost arm in a dorsal position may not necessarily be the answer, as this involves movement that could, at least theoretically, injury the shoulder joint. There is inadequate published evidence to come to definite conclusions but the recognition of the potential for harm as well as for benefit from placing the victim on the side has been highlighted.

The BLS Group of ILCOR agreed on six principles that should be followed when managing the unconscious, spontaneously breathing victim:

1. The victim should be in as near a true lateral position as possible with the head dependent to allow free drainage of fluid

2. The position should be stable

3. Any pressure on the chest that impairs breathing should be avoided

4. It should be possible to turn the victim onto the side and return to the back easily and safely, having particular regard to the possibility of cervical spine injury

5. Good observation of and access to the airway should be possible

6. The position itself should not give rise to any injury to the victim

Health Care Providers

Health care providers and emergency personnel are likely to possess extended resuscitation skills, and the situations in which they are called upon to use them may require more complicated BLS guidelines. These requirements have not been addressed in the current advisory statements, which are aimed predominately at lay persons. They are, however, planned as the subject of a future ILCOR publication.

Automated External Defibrillators

The use of an automated external defibrillator (AED) should now be considered to be within the domain of BLS [41]. In fact, learning to use an AED may be easier than learning the skills required to perform CPR. Most investigators believe that these devices should be distributed as widely as possible. Over the last 5 years the use of AEDs has been extended to include EMTs, fire fighters, police, airline personnel, hospital personnel, and lay citizens [42]. The AHA statement on "Public Access Defibrillation" lays down scientific evidence for the widest practical distribution of these devices throughout all communities [41]. However, there is not yet sufficient world-wide experience, nor is there sufficient world-wide availability of AEDs to warrant inclusion of training in their use in the current BLS

Sequence of Action. Nevertheless, it should be noted that many resuscitation organisations are already adding training in the use of an AED to their BLS programmes, in the hope of saving more lives.

Early CPR coupled with early defibrillation is a very powerful combination that improves survi-val from cardiac arrest. The expansion of early defibrillation into BLS is expected to continue in the future. Resuscitation organisations would do well to consider this when customizing the ILCOR BLS template to serve the particular needs of their region.''

2.2.2. SEQUENCE OF ACTIONS

The following is the agreed sequence of actions that constitute the European Resuscitation Council Guidelines for Adult Basic Life Support. In the text, use of the masculine includes the feminine.

1. Ensure safety of rescuer and victim

2. Check the victim and see whether he responds:

   * Gently shake his shoulders and ask loudly: "Are you all right?" (Fig. 1)

3. <u>A</u> If he responds by answering or moving:

   * Leave him in the position in which you find him (provided he is not in further danger), check his condition and get help if needed

   * Reassess him regularly

   <u>B</u> If he does <u>not</u> respond:

   * Shout for help

   * Open his airway by tilting his head and lifting his chin: (Fig. 2)

ADULT BASIC LIFE SUPPORT

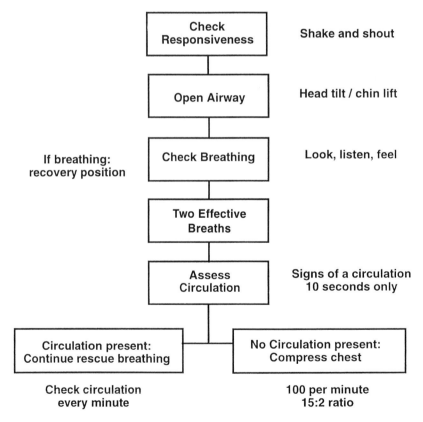

Check Responsiveness	**Shake and shout**
Open Airway	**Head tilt / chin lift**
Check Breathing	**Look, listen, feel**
Two Effective Breaths	
Assess Circulation	**Signs of a circulation 10 seconds only**

If breathing: recovery position

Circulation present: Continue rescue breathing   **No Circulation present: Compress chest**

Check circulation every minute   100 per minute 15:2 ratio

Send or go for help as soon as possible according to guidelines

TABLE I. The Algorithm for Adult Basic Life Support. The sequence of actions is aimed primarily at the single lay rescuer dealing with an adult victim.

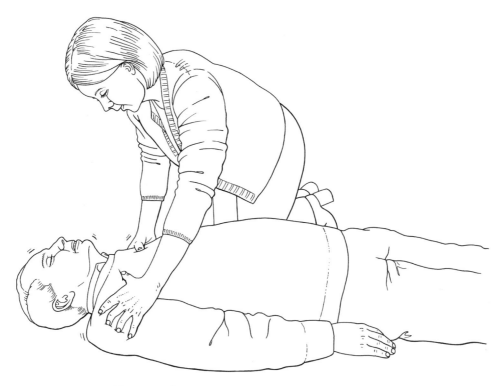

FIG. 1. Check the victim and see if he responds.

— If possible with the victim in the position in which you find him, place your hand on his forehead and gently tilt his head back keeping your thumb and index finger free to close his nose if rescue breathing is required

— At the same time, with your fingertip(s) under the point of the victim's chin, lift the chin to open the airway

— If you have any difficulty, turn the victim on to his back and then open the airway as described

Try to avoid head tilt if trauma (injury) to the neck is suspected

4. Keeping the airway open, look, listen, and feel for breathing (more than an occasional gasp):

— Look for chest movements (Fig. 3)
— Listen at the victim's mouth for breath sounds

— Feel for air on your cheek

* Look, listen, and feel for **10 s** before deciding that breathing is absent

5. A If he is breathing (other than an occasional gasp):

* Turn him into the recovery position (*see below*)

* Check for continued breathing

B If he is not breathing:

* Send someone for help or, if you are on your own, leave the victim and go for help; return and start rescue breathing as below

* Turn the victim onto his back if he is not already in this position

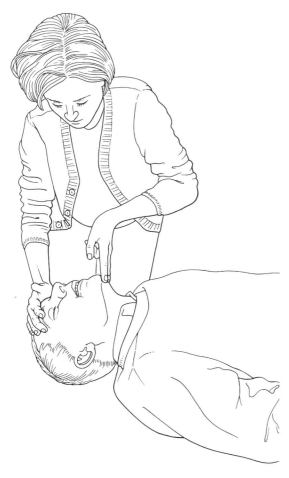

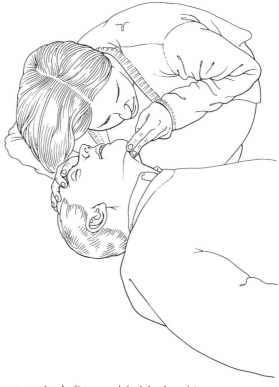

FIG. 3. Look, listen and feel for breathing.

FIG. 2. Open his airway by tilting his head and lifting his chin.

* Remove any visible obstruction from the victim's mouth, including dislodged dentures, but leave well fitting dentures in place

* Give two **effective** rescue breaths, each of which makes the chest rise and fall
— Ensure head tilt and chin lift
— Pinch the soft part of his nose closed with the index finger and thumb of your hand on his forehead
— Open his mouth a little, but maintain chin lift (Fig. 4)
— Take a breath and place your lips around his mouth, making sure that you have a good seal

— Blow steadily into his mouth over about 1.5–2 s watching for his chest to rise as in normal breathing (In an adult this usually requires 400–600 mls air) (Fig. 5)
— Maintaining head tilt and chin lift, take your mouth away from the victim and watch for his chest to fall as air comes out (Fig. 6)

* Take another breath and repeat the sequence as above to give two effective rescue breaths in all

* If you have difficulty achieving an effective breath:
— Recheck the victim's mouth and remove any obstruction (Fig. 7)
— Recheck that there is adequate head tilt and chin lift
— Make up to five attempts in all to achieve two effective breaths

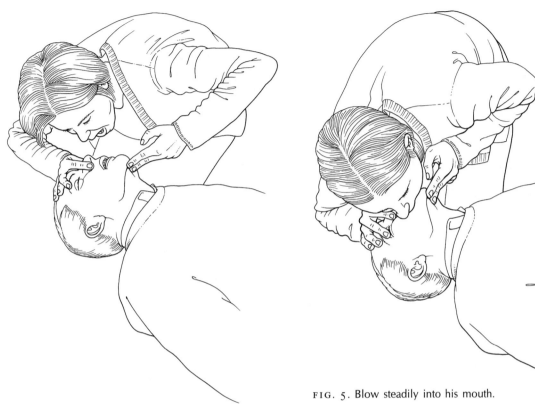

FIG. 5. Blow steadily into his mouth.

FIG. 4. Open his airway, pinch his nose, open his mouth, but maintain chin lift.

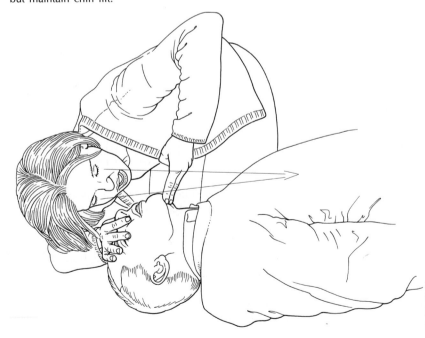

FIG. 6. Maintaining head tilt and chin lift, take your mouth away from the victim and watch for his chest to fall as air comes out.

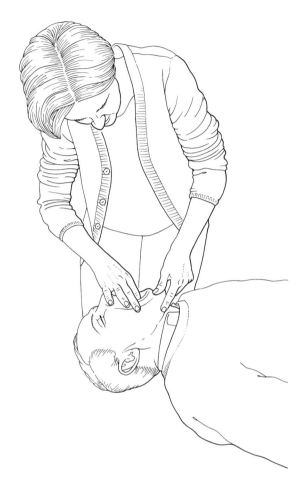

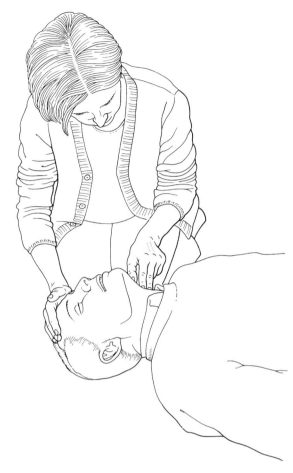

FIG. 7. Recheck the victim's mouth and remove any obstruction.

FIG. 8. Check the carotid pulse.

— Even if unsuccessful, move on to assessment of circulation

6. Assess the victim for signs of a circulation:

* Look for any movement, including swallowing or breathing (more than an occasional gasp)

* Check the carotid pulse (Fig. 8)

* Take **no more than 10 s** to do this

7. <u>A</u> If you are <u>confident</u> that you can detect signs of a circulation within 10 s:

* Continue rescue breathing, if necessary, until the victim starts breathing on his own

* About every 10 breaths (or about every minute) recheck for signs of a circulation; take no more than 10 s each time

* If the victim starts to breathe on his own but remains unconscious, turn him into the recovery

position. Check his condition and be ready to turn him onto his back and restart rescue breathing if he stops breathing

B If there are <u>no</u> signs of a circulation, or you are at all unsure start chest compression:

* Locate the lower half of the sternum:
– Using your index and middle fingers, identify the lower rib margins (Fig. 9a). Keeping your fingers together, slide them upwards to the point where the ribs join the sternum. With your middle finger on this point, place your index finger on the sternum (Fig. 9b)
– Slide the heel of your other hand down the sternum until it reaches your index finger; this should be the middle of the lower half of the sternum (Fig. 9c)
– Place the heel of one hand there, with the other hand on top of the first
– Interlock the fingers of both hands and lift them to ensure that pressure is not applied over the victim's ribs. Do not apply any pressure over the upper abdomen or bottom tip of the sternum (Fig. 10)

– Position yourself vertically above the victim's chest, and with your arms straight, press down on the sternum to depress it between 4–5 cm (Fig. 11)
– Release the pressure, without losing contact between the hand and sternum, then repeat at a rate of about 100 times a minute (a little less than two compressions a second). Compression and release should take an equal amount of time

* Combine rescue breathing and compression:
– After 15 compressions tilt the head, lift the chin and give two effective breaths (Fig. 12)
– Return your hands without delay to the correct position on the sternum and give 15 further compressions, continuing compressions and breaths in a ratio of 15:2

8. Continue resuscitation until:

– Qualified help arrives
– The victim shows signs of life
– You become exhausted

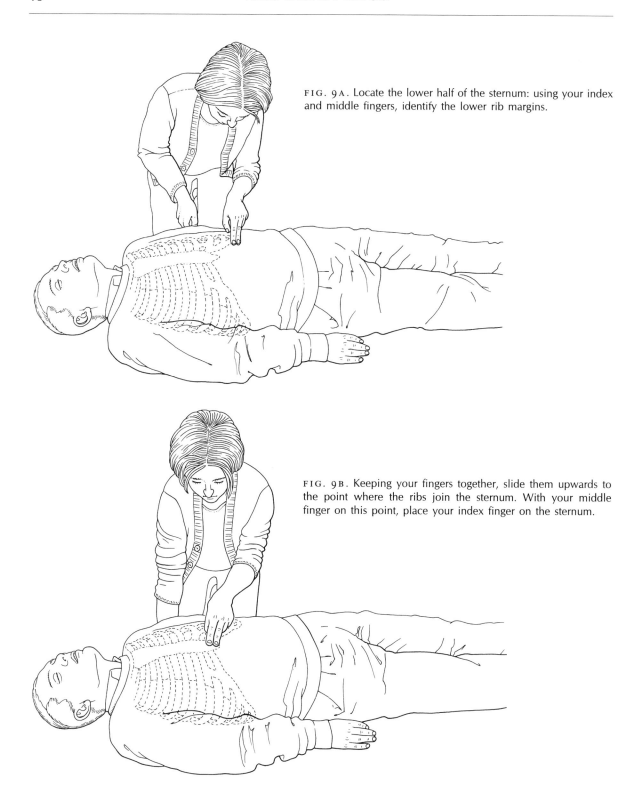

FIG. 9A. Locate the lower half of the sternum: using your index and middle fingers, identify the lower rib margins.

FIG. 9B. Keeping your fingers together, slide them upwards to the point where the ribs join the sternum. With your middle finger on this point, place your index finger on the sternum.

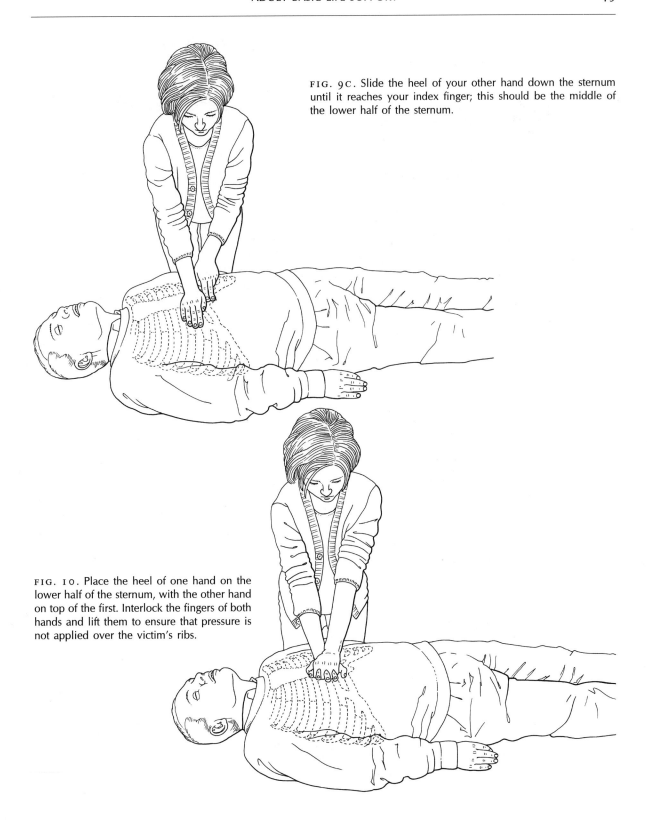

FIG. 9C. Slide the heel of your other hand down the sternum until it reaches your index finger; this should be the middle of the lower half of the sternum.

FIG. 10. Place the heel of one hand on the lower half of the sternum, with the other hand on top of the first. Interlock the fingers of both hands and lift them to ensure that pressure is not applied over the victim's ribs.

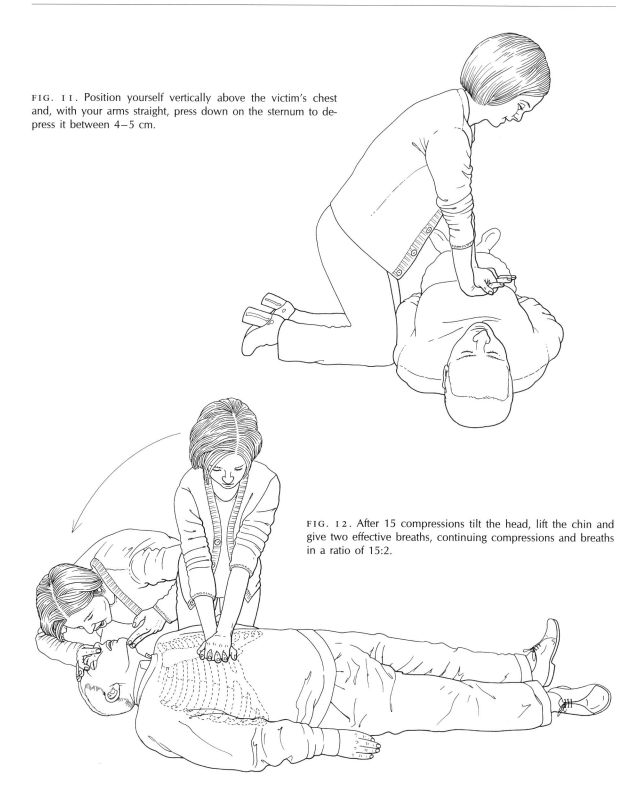

FIG. 11. Position yourself vertically above the victim's chest and, with your arms straight, press down on the sternum to depress it between 4–5 cm.

FIG. 12. After 15 compressions tilt the head, lift the chin and give two effective breaths, continuing compressions and breaths in a ratio of 15:2.

RECOVERY POSITION

There are a number of different recovery positions which fulfil most or all of the criteria recommended by ILCOR, each of which has its advocates. National resuscitation councils and other major organisations should consider adopting one of the several available options so that training and practice can be consistent.

The Training & Education Group of the ERC recommends that the recovery position described in the 1992 Guidelines [3] be used for training purposes, but that particular care is taken to ensure that a conscious volunteer is not left in this position for more than a few minutes. If this recovery position is used for a patient, care should be taken to monitor the peripheral circulation of the lower arm, and steps taken to ensure that the duration for which there is pressure on this arm is kept to a minimum. A description of this position follows.

* Remove the victim's spectacles

* Kneel beside the victim and make sure that both his legs are straight

* Open the airway by tilting the head and lifting the chin

* Place the arm nearest to you out at right angles to his body, elbow bent with the hand palm uppermost (Fig. 13)

* Bring his far arm across the chest, and hold the back of the hand against the victim's nearest cheek (Fig. 14)

* With your other hand, grasp the far leg just above the knee and pull it up, keeping the foot on the ground (Fig. 15)

* Keeping his hand pressed against his cheek, pull on the leg to roll the victim towards you onto his side

* Adjust the upper leg so that both the hip and knee are bent at right angles (Fig. 16)

* Tilt the head back to make sure the airway remains open

* Adjust the hand under the cheek, if necessary, to keep the head tilted

* Check breathing regularly

Finally, it must be emphasized that in spite of possible problems during training and in use, it remains above doubt that placing the unconscious, breathing victim into the recovery position can be life-saving.

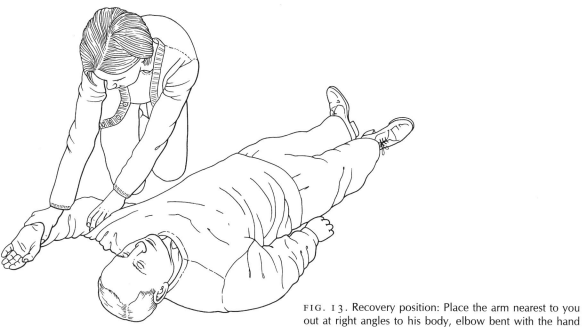

FIG. 13. Recovery position: Place the arm nearest to you out at right angles to his body, elbow bent with the hand palm uppermost.

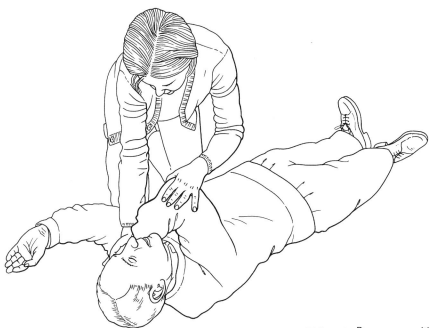

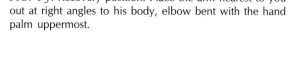

FIG. 14. Recovery position: Bring his far arm across the chest, and hold the back of the hand against the victim's nearest cheek.

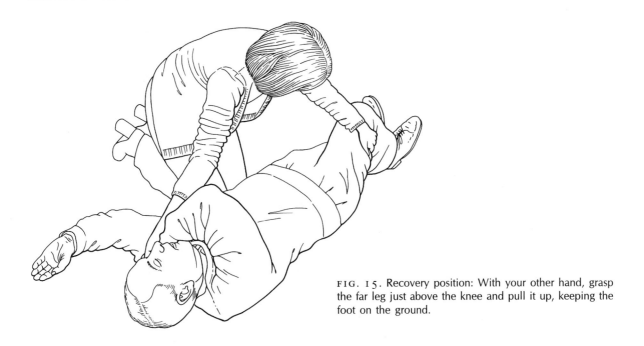

FIG. 15. Recovery position: With your other hand, grasp the far leg just above the knee and pull it up, keeping the foot on the ground.

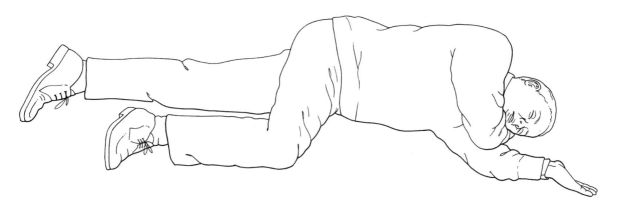

FIG. 16. Recovery position: Keeping his hand pressed against his cheek, pull on the leg to roll the victim towards you onto his side. Adjust the upper leg so that both the hip and knee are bent at right angles.

WHEN TO GET HELP

It is vital for rescuers to get help as quickly as possible.

* When more than one rescuer is available, one should start resuscitation while another rescuer goes for help

* A lone rescuer will have to decide whether to start resuscitation or to go for help first. This decision will be influenced by the availability of emergency medical services and local practice.

However, if the likely cause of unconsciousness is:
  trauma (injury)
  drowning
  or if the victim is an infant or a child

the rescuer should perform resuscitation for **about 1 min** before going for help.

If the victim is an **adult**, and the cause of unconsciousness is **not** trauma (injury) or drowning, the rescuer should assume that the victim has a heart problem and go for help immediately it has been established that the victim is not breathing.

RESUSCITATION WITH TWO PERSONS

Two-person CPR is less tiring than single-person CPR. However, it is important that both rescuers are proficient and practised in the technique. The following points should be noted:

1. The first priority is to summon help. This may mean that one rescuer has to start CPR alone whilst the other leaves to find a telephone.

2. When changing from single-person to two-person CPR, the second rescuer should take over chest compressions after the first rescuer has given two ventilations. During these ventilations, the incoming rescuer should determine the correct position on the sternum and should be ready to start compressions immediately after the second inflation has been given. It is preferable that the rescuers work from opposite sides of the victim.

3. A ratio of five compressions to one inflation should be used. By the end of each series of five compressions, the rescuer responsible for ventilation should be positioned ready to give an inflation with the least possible delay. It is helpful if the rescuer giving compressions counts out aloud: "1 − 2 − 3 − 4 − 5".

4. Chin lift and head tilt should be maintained at all times. Ventilation should take the usual 1.5 − 2 s during which chest compressions should cease; they should be resumed immediately after inflation of the chest, waiting only for the rescuer to remove his or her lips from the victim's face.

5. If the rescuers wish to change places, usually because the one giving compressions becomes tired, this should be undertaken as quickly and smoothly as possible. The rescuer responsible for compressions should announce the change, and at the end of a series of five compressions, move rapidly to the victim's head, obtain an open airway, and give a single inflation. During this manoeuvre the second rescuer should position him or herself to commence compressions as soon as the inflation has been completed.

CHOKING

If blockage of the airway is only partial the victim will usually be able to dislodge it by coughing, but if there is complete obstruction to flow of air, this may not be possible.

Diagnosis

* The victim may have been seen to be eating, or a child may have put an object into his mouth

* A victim who is choking often grips his throat with his hand

* **With partial airway obstruction** the victim will be distressed and coughing. There may be inspiratory wheeze.

* **With complete airway obstruction** the victim will be unable to speak, breathe or cough, and will eventually lose consciousness.

Treatment (Table 2)

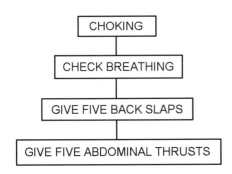

TABLE 2. The algorithm for management of choking of an adult victim.

1. If the victim is breathing, encourage him to continue coughing, but do nothing else

2. If the victim shows signs of becoming weak or stops breathing or coughing:

* Leave him in the position in which you find him, remove any obvious debris or loose false teeth from the mouth and carry out back slapping:

* If he is standing or sitting

– Stand to the side and slightly behind him
– Support his chest with one hand and lean him well forwards so that when the obstructing object is dislodged it comes out of the mouth rather than goes further down the airway
– Give **up to five** sharp slaps between his shoulder blades with the heel of your other hand (Fig. 17)

* If he is lying

– Kneel beside him and roll him on to his side facing you
– Support his chest with your thigh
– Give **up to five** sharp slaps between his shoulder blades with the heel of your other hand

With back slaps the aim should be to relieve the obstruction with each slap rather than necessarily to give all five.

3. If back slapping fails, try giving abdominal thrusts:

* If the victim is standing or sitting

– Stand behind the victim and put both arms round the upper part of his abdomen
– Make sure the victim is bending well forwards so that when the obstructing object is dislodged it comes out of the mouth rather than goes further down the airway
– Clench your fist and place it between the umbilicus and xiphisternum (Fig. 18). Grasp it with your other hand (Fig. 19)
– Pull sharply inwards and upwards; the obstructing object should be dislodged and fly out of the mouth

* If he is lying on the ground

– Turn him onto his back if necessary
– Kneel astride the victim
– Place the heel of one hand in the upper part

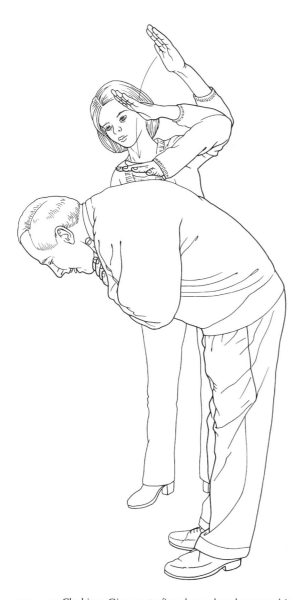

FIG. 17. Choking: Give up to five sharp slaps between his shoulder blades with the heel of your hand.

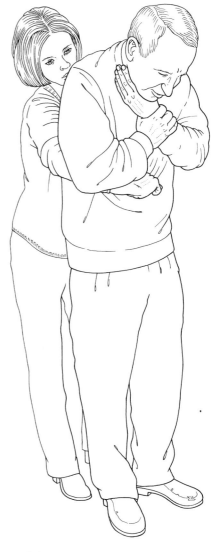

FIG. 18. Choking: Stand behind the victim and put your arms round the upper part of his abdomen. Clench your fist and place it between the umbilicus and xiphisternum.

of his abdomen between the umbilicus and xiphisternum; take care to avoid any pressure on the ribs themselves

– Place the other hand on top of the first and thrust sharply downwards and towards his head. If the obstruction is not relieved, repeat the action, giving **up to five** thrusts if necessary

– If the obstruction is still not relieved, recheck the mouth for any obstruction that can be reached with a finger, and continue alternating five back slaps with five abdominal thrusts

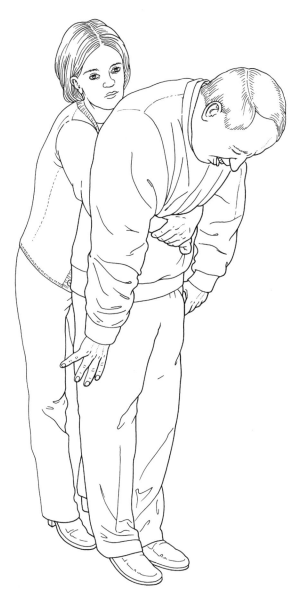

FIG. 19. Grasp your fist with your other hand. Pull sharply inwards and upwards; the obstructing object should be dislodged and fly out of the mouth.

4. If the victim at any time becomes unconscious

Loss of consciousness may result in relaxation of the muscles around the larynx and allow air to pass down into the lungs. If at any time the choking victim loses consciousness follow the sequence of life support.

In summary:

* Open his airway by lifting his chin and tilting his head

* Check for breathing by looking, listening, and feeling

* Remove any visible obstruction from the mouth

* Attempt to give two effective rescue breaths

  – If effective breaths **can** be achieved: Continue life support as appropriate

  – If effective breaths **cannot** be achieved: Continue to alternate five backslaps with five abdominal thrusts. Attempt rescue breaths at the end of each series of backslaps and abdominal thrusts

2.2.3. REFERENCES

1. Recommended guidelines for uniform reporting of data from out-of-hospital cardiac arrest: the Utstein style. Prepared by a task force of representatives from the European Resuscitation Council, American Heart Association, Heart and Stroke Foundation of Canada, and Australian Resuscitation Council. Resuscitation 1991;22:1–26.
2. Kouwenhoven WB, Jude JR, Knickerbocker GG. Closed-chest cardiac massage. J Am Med Ass 1960;173:1064–1067.
3. Handley A, Becker L, Allen M, Van Drenth A, Kramer E, Montgomery W. Single rescuer adult basic life support. An advisory statement by the Basic Life Support Working Group of the International Liaison Committee on Resuscitation. Resuscitation 1997;34:101–108.
4. Chamberlain D, Cummins RO. International emergency cardiac care: support, science, and universal guidelines. Ann Emerg Med 1993;22:508–511.
5. Emergency Cardiac Care Committee and Subcommittees, American Heart Association. Guidelines for cardiopulmonary resuscitation and emergency cardiac care. J Am Med Ass 1992;268:2171–2295.
6. Basic Life Support Working Party of the European Resuscitation Council. Guidelines for basic life support. Resuscitation 1992;24:103–110.
7. Becker LB, Han BH, Meyer PM, Wright FA, Rhodes KV, Smith DW, Barrett J, and CPR Chicago. Racial differences in the incidence of cardiac arrest and subsequent survival. N Engl J Med 1993;329:600–606.

8. Eisenberg MS, Horwood BT, Cummins RO, Reynolds-Haertle R, Herne TR. Cardiac arrest and resuscitation: A tale of 29 cities. Ann Emerg Med 1990;19: 179–186.

9. Bell JH, Harrison DA, Carr B Resuscitation skills of trainee anaesthetists. Anaesthesia 1995;50:692–694.

10. Broomfield R. A quasi-experimental research to investigate the retention of basic cardiopulmonary resuscitation skills and knowledge by qualified nurses following a course in professional development. J Adv Nursing 1996;23:1016–1023.

11. Quiney NF, Gardner J, Brampton W. Resuscitation skills amongst anaesthetists. Resuscitation 1995;29: 215–218.

12. Brenner DE, Kauffman J. Reluctance of internists and medical nurses to perform mouth-to-mouth resuscitation. Arch Intern Med 1993;153:1763–1769.

13. Ornato JP, Hallagan L, McMahan SB, Peeples EH, Rostafuiski AG. Attitudes of BCLS instructors about mouth-to-mouth resuscitation. Ann Emerg Med 1990; 19:151–156.

14. Lombardi G, Gallager J, Gennis P. Outcome of out-of-hospital cardiac arrest in New York City. J Am Med Assoc 1994;271:678–683.

15. Bossaert L, Van Hoeyweghen R and the Cerebral Resuscitation Study Group. Bystander cardiopulmonary resuscitation: CPR in out-of-hospital arrest. Resuscitation 1989;17(Suppl):S99–S109.

16. Kloeck WGJ. New recommendations for basic support in adults, children and infants. Trauma Emerg Med 1993;10:738–748.

17. Medical Priority Consultants Inc. Pre-arrival instructions from the Advanced Medical Priority Dispatch System, version 10.2.

18. Mather C, O'Kelly S. The palpation of pulses. Anaesthesia 1996;51:189–191.

19. Flesche CW, Tucker TP, Lorenz C, Nerudo B, Tarnow J. The carotid pulse check as a diagnostic tool to assess pulselessness during adult basic life support. Euroanaesthesia '95 (Abstract).

20. Flesche CW, Brewer S, Mandel LP, Brevik H, Tarnow J. The ability of health professionals to check the carotid pulse. Circulation 1994;90:1–288.

21. Bahr J, Klingler H, Panzer W, Rode H, Kettler D. Skills of lay people in checking the carotid pulse. Resuscitation 1997;35:23–26.

22. Eberle B, Dick WF, Schneider T, Wisser G, Doetsch S, Tzanova I. Checking the carotid pulse check: Diagnostic accuracy of first responders in patients with or without a pulse. Resuscitation 1996;33:107–116.

23. Safar P, Aguto Escarrage L, Elam JO. A comparison of the mouth-to-mouth and mouth-to-airway methods of artificial respiration with the chest-pressure arm-lift methods. New Engl J Med 1958;258:671–677.

24. Baskett P, Nolan J, Parr M. Tidal volumes which are perceived to be adequate for resuscitation. Resuscitation 1996;3:231–234.

25. Baskett P, Bossaert L, Carli P, Chamberlain D, Dick W, Nolan JP, Parr MJA, Scheidegger D, Zideman D. Guidelines for the basic management of the airway and ventilation during resuscitation. A statement by the Airway and ventilation Management Working Group of the European Resuscitation Council. Resuscitation 1996;31:187–200.

26. Cummins RO, Ornato JP, Thies WH, Pepe PE. Improving survival from sudden cardiac arrest: The "Chain of Survival" concept. A statement for health professionals from the Advanced Cardiac Life Support Subcommittee and the Emergency Cardiac Care Committee, American Heart Association. Circulation 1991;83:1832–1847.

27. Eisenberg MS, Copass MK, Hallstrom AP, Blake B, Bergner L, Short FA, Cobb LA. Treatment of out-of-hospital cardiac arrests with rapid defibrillation by emergency medical technicians. N Engl J Med 1980; 302:1379–1383.

28. Montgomery W, Brown DD, Hazinski MF, Clawse J, Newell LD, Flint. Citizen response to cardiopulmonary emergencies. Ann Emerg Med 1993;22:428–434.

29. Stults KR, Brown DD, Schug VL, Bean JA. Prehospsital defibrillation performed by emergency medical technicians in rural communities. N Engl J Med 1984;310: 219–223.

30. Hazinski MF. Is paediatric resuscitation unique? Relative merits of early CPR and ventilation versus early defibrillation for young victims of cardiac arrest. Ann Emerg Med 1995;25:540–543.

31. Schindler MB, Bohn D, Cox P, McCrindle BW, Jarvis A, Edmonds J, Barker G. Outcome of out-of-hospital cardiac or respiratory arrest in children. N Engl J Med 1996;35:1473–1479.

32. Friesen RM, Duncan P, Tweed W, Bristow G. Appraisal of pediatric cardiopulmonary resuscitation. Can Med Assoc J 1982;126:1055–1058.

33. Appleton GO, Cummins RO, Larson MP, Graves JR. CPR and the single rescuer: At what age should you "call first" rather than "call fast"? Ann Emerg Med 1995;25:492–494.

34. Mogayzel C, Quan L, Graves JR, Tiedeman D, Fahrenbruch C, Herndon P. Out-of-hospital ventricular fibrillation in children and adolescents: Causes and outcome. Ann Emerg Med 1995;25:484–491.

35. Bowles RL. On stertor, apoplexy, and the management of the apoplectic state. London: Bailliere, Tindall and Cox, 1891;26–28.

36. St John Ambulance Association. First aid to the injured. 39th edn. London: St John Ambulance Association, 1937;134.

37. Safar P, Escarrage LA. Compliance in apneic anesthetized adults. Anesthesiology 1959;20:283–289.

38. Baker JHE. The first aid management of spinal cord injury. Semin Orthopaedics 1989;4:2−14.

39. Fulstow R, Smith GB. The new recovery position. A cautionary tale. Resuscitation 1993;26:89−91.

40. Handley AJ. Recovery position. Resuscitation 1993; 26:93−95.

41. Weisfeldt ML, Kerber RE, McGoldrick RP, Moss AJ, Nichol G, Ornato JP, Palmer DG, Riegel B, Smith SC Jr. Public access defibrillation. A statement for health-care professionals from the American Heart Association Task Force on Automated External Defibrillation. Circulation 1995;92:2763.

42. Kaye W, Mancini ME, Guiliano KK, Richards N, Nagid DM, Marler CA, Sawyer-Silva S. Strengthening the in-hospital chain of survival with rapid defibrillation by first responders using automated external defibrillators: training and retention issues. Ann Emerg Med 1995;25:163−168.

2.3. Course Content

2.3.1. OBJECTIVES

To teach recognition of cardiopulmonary arrest, activation of the emergency medical services, and the techniques of basic life support (BLS) to as great a proportion of the population as possible.

2.3.2. TARGET GROUPS

Training in basic life support is applicable to all age groups from school age upwards.

It is incumbent upon all healthcare providers to become proficient in, and maintain practice in BLS as a basis for additional skills as appropriate.

Certain professional groups such as police, fire fighter, and ambulance personnel will need these skills as part of their training, as will all those whose occupation is associated with a high risk of cardiac arrest (e.g., electricity workers).

The larger the proportion of the general public who are trained in BLS and are willing to apply the techniques, the greater is the likelihood of survival of a victim of out of hospital cardiac arrest. For this reason all efforts must be made to reach as large a proportion of the public as possible.

2.3.3. PREREQUISITES

No previous knowledge or experience is required although this is, of course, always desirable.

2.3.4. COURSE

Where possible each instructor should have no more than six trainees. The course should be designed to take from 2 to 3 h. The content should be based on the ERC BLS Guidelines and instructors are recommended to refer to the ERC CPR Instructors Guide:

* Determination of responsiveness
* Airway:
  – Head Tilt – Chin Lift
* Breathing:
  – Assessment of breathing
  – Rescue breathing – mouth-to-mouth
* Circulation:
  – Determination of the need for chest compressions: Signs of a circulation
  – Chest Compressions:
    – Compression landmarks
    – Compression technique
    – Compression depth
    – Compression rate
    – Compression/ventilation ratio
* Activation of Emergency Medical Services
* Recovery position

The following is a model course programme:

1. Introduction (10 min)

Define the incidence of cardiopulmonary arrest in the community. Introduce the Chain of Survival. Emphasize the importance of alerting the emergency services. Define place of BLS in improving outlook for victims before arrival of Emergency Services. Discuss possible risks to rescuer and trainee.

2. Video (20 min)

An appropriate video may be shown at this stage.

3. Demonstration of techniques (5 min)

The instructor demonstrates the full sequence of basic life support.

4. Practical training (90–120 min)

Individual instructors will have their own methods of teaching but demonstration of each step within the Sequence of Actions followed by practice by the trainees is likely to be the most satisfactory.

Practice by trainees, with two to each manikin, probably provides the most effective and time efficient method.

Once all the steps in the Sequence of Actions have been demonstrated and practised, the whole sequence should be combined.

5. Retraining (5 min)

Information should be given to the trainees about skill decay and the need for repeated practice and refresher courses.

6. Evaluation

Where trainees are lay members of the public, formal evaluation of skills is usually inappropriate and a Course Attendance Certificate may be offered. For healthcare professionals, those requiring the skills for professional use, and lay-persons specifically requesting evaluation, this should take place according to the following Evaluation Protocol (Table 1).

2.3.5. ADDITIONAL SKILLS

According to the requirements of the trainees, the following additional skills may be added if additional time is available:
1. Two rescuer CPR
2. Management of upper airway obstruction
3. Simple adjuncts to basic airway management
4. Automated external defibrillation.

TABLE I. BASIC LIFE SUPPORT EVALUATION PROTOCOL
Tick boxes according to performance.

	STEPS	A	B	C	D	E	F
1	Assessment of responsiveness						
2	**Assessment of breathing**						
3	Mouth-to-mouth breathing: 2 breaths of 0.4 - 0.6 litres, inspired slowly						
4	Assessment of circulation						
5	Call appropriate emergency telephone number for help						
6	Mouth-to-mouth breathing: at least 50% of breaths 0.4 - 0.6 litres, inspired slowly						
7	Compression area: no gross errors						
8	Compression depth: at least 50% of compressions 4-5 cm						
9	Compression rate: 80-120 per minute						
10	Ratio approximately 15:2						

2.4. Risks to the Rescuer

2.4.1. INTRODUCTION

A rescuer should never place himself or others at more risk than the victim. Unfortunately, the need for resuscitation is often allowed to override all other considerations, and danger to the rescuer may be ignored in an effort to reach and administer care to the victim. Before starting a resuscitation attempt, the rescuer must rapidly and correctly assess the risks; traffic, falling masonry, toxic fumes, and gas are obvious factors. In many cases proper assessment, a little care, and full co-operation with the rescue services can provide a safe environment. For example, a strategically placed vehicle will shield the victim and rescuer from oncoming traffic. Hazard triangles, hazard warning lights, and high visibility clothing will alert other road users. After a car accident, switching off the ignition will stop the fuel supply and lessen the risk of fire. Hazchem notices alert the rescuer to the risk of contact with hazardous chemicals.

2.4.2. POISONING

Victims of poisoning may require basic or advanced life support, which should follow standard guidelines. If the poison can be identified, where possible advice should be sought from poisons information centres. In most cases there is little risk to the resuscitation team. Exceptions include incidents involving hydrogen cyanide and hydrogen sulphide gas poisoning.

Hydrogen cyanide impairs cellular oxygen usage. Early signs of cyanide poisoning are hyperventilation and tachycardia, followed by coma, cyanosis, and convulsions. Immediate treatment with oxygen at a high inspired concen-

tration is indicated, but if assisted ventilation is required it should be performed only with a mask and non-return valve system, so that the rescuer is not exposed to exhaled air. Fixed dilated pupils should not preclude resuscitation; high success rates have been reported in such patients. On confirmation of the diagnosis an antidote (hydroxocobalamin, or sodium thiosulphate) can be given.

Other cases of poisoning may involve corrosive chemicals (such as strong acids, alkalis, or paraquat), or substances, such as organophosphates, that are easily absorbed through the rescuer's skin or respiratory tract. In such cases, care must be taken when handling the victim's clothes or any of the victim's body fluids, especially vomit. Correct protective clothing, including gloves, should be worn to protect against direct skin contact and the inhalation of toxic fumes.

2.4.3. INFECTION

The possibility of transmission of infection between a victim and a rescuer has caused much concern, especially more recently with the heightened anxiety over hepatitis and AIDS. To date there have been only anecdotal reports of isolated incidents. A small number of publications have indicated transmission of infection to the rescuer from mouth-to-mouth resuscitation. These have been concerned with the transmission of cutaneous tuberculosis, shigellosis, meningococcal meningitis, herpes simplex virus, and, most recently, salmonella. To put these reports into perspective, not a single case of transmission of an infectious disease by mouth-to-mouth ventilation was recorded in New York City firemen over a 22-year period.

Hepatitis B and HIV

Hepatitis B virus (HBV) and human immunodeficiency virus (HIV) have recently given rise to concern, although there has been no reported case of transmission of either virus through mouth-to-mouth ventilation. Nevertheless a recent report from the Centers for Disease Control (CDC) in the United States advises universal precautions against mucous membrane, parenteral, or nonintact skin exposures to HBV and HIV. This report emphasizes that blood is the single most important source of these viruses but recommends precautions against contact with semen; vaginal secretions; cerebrospinal, pleural, peritoneal, pericardial, and amniotic fluids; together with any body fluid containing visible blood. Precautions are not considered necessary against contact with sputum, nasal secretions, faeces, sweat, tears, urine, or vomit.

Transmission of HBV in humans through mouth-to-mouth ventilation involving contact with HBV antigen-positive saliva only is unlikely. However, it is possible that infection could be transmitted by saliva contaminated with HBV positive blood penetrating small cracks in the oral mucosa. The only report of HIV transmission through saliva has been in laboratory animals that have received direct intravenous injections of HIV positive saliva. In addition, there have been many studies of occupational and social exposure to patients with HIV infection which have included direct exposure of mucous membranes or nonintact skin to infected body fluids. In those studies, which included needlestick injuries, seroconversion has been less than one percent. Mucous membrane exposure must be considered less of a risk than needlestick exposure, thus the chance of infection from mouth-to-mouth ventilation must be negligible.

2.4.4. PRECAUTIONS

Although mouth-to-mouth ventilation seems to be safe, some health care workers may feel the need to use an interpositional airway device, particularly if the saliva of trauma victims has been contaminated with blood. Before selecting such a device, the user must be satisfied that it will function effectively in both its resuscitation and protective roles. There must be proper training in its use, cleaning and disposal. Most importantly, the selected device must be immediately available at all times. A pocket handkerchief is ineffective as protection, and may enhance the passage of virus material.

There is a small, but quantifiable risk of infection by direct needlestick injury. Care must be taken over needles and other 'sharps' and a sharps disposal box must be included in every advanced resuscitation pack. Blood is the infectious medium, and particular care must be taken where there is obvious spillage of blood or staining of body fluids with blood. Rescuers should wear plastic or rubber gloves, and eye protection if an aerosol of blood particles is likely.

2.4.5. MANIKINS

Resuscitation practice is essential. Resuscitation manikins have been shown not to be a source of infection. Nevertheless, sensible precautions must be taken to minimize the potential for cross-infection. Manikins should be regularly cleaned and disinfected after use, according to the manufacturers recommendations. Some of the more modern manikins have disposable face pieces and airways to simplify these procedures.

2.4.6. FURTHER READING

1. Blenkharn JL, Buckingham SE, Zideman DA. Prevention of transmission of infection during mouth-to-mouth resuscitation. Resuscitation 1990;19:151−157.
2. Cardiopulmonary resuscitation, AIDS, and public panic. Lancet 1992;340:456−457.
3. Memon A, Salzer J, Hillman E, Marshall C. Fatal myocardial infarction following CPR training: the question of risk. Ann Emerg Med 1982;11:322−323.
4. Safar P, Bircher N. Infection risk of mouth-to-mouth ventilation. Ann Emerg Med 1990;19:(letter).
5. Van Hoeyweghen R, Bossaert L, Rademakers F, Verbruggen G. Physiologic response of training CPR. Ann Emerg Med 1991;20:279−282.

3. Adult Advanced Life Support

CONTENTS:

3.1. The 1998 European Resuscitation Council Guidelines for Adult Advanced Life Support

3.1.1. INTRODUCTION

The publication of Guidelines for Advanced Life Support (ALS) by the European Resuscitation Council (ERC) in 1992 was a landmark in international co-operation and co-ordination [1]. Previously, individual countries or groups had produced guidelines [2,3] but for the first time an international group of experts produced consensus views based on the best available information. Since 1992, even wider international collaboration and support has occurred. In particular, the establishment of the International Liaison Committee on Resuscitation (ILCOR) has facilitated global co-operation and discussion between representatives from North America, Europe, Southern Africa, Australia, and most recently, Latin America.

The 1992 ERC Guideline documents indicated that review would occur on a regular basis. Change is not advocated for its own sake, and is not warranted without convincing scientific or educational reasons. Education and its organisation is a process with a long latency, and it can be confusing and distracting for trainers and trainees if the message lacks consistency.

The ERC ALS working group recognised that the previous guidelines necessitated a level of rhythm recognition, interpretation and subsequent decision-making that some users found difficult. While automated external defibrillators (AEDs) ease some of these problems, the 1992 guidelines were not specifically designed for these devices. These new guidelines are applicable to manual and automated external defibrillators. Decision-making has been reduced to a minimum whenever possible. This increases clarity, while still allowing individuals with specialist knowledge to apply their expertise.

Changes in guidelines are only the first step in the process of care. Their implementation necessitates considerable effort. Training materials and methods may require modification, information must be disseminated and, perhaps most importantly, evaluation of efficacy is needed. For these purposes, reporting and publication of out-of-hospital and in-hospital cardiac arrest events using the Utstein templates [4,5] is strongly advised to provide objective outcome assessment.

The limitations of guidelines must be recognised. As always in the practice of medicine, words and flow charts must be interpreted with common sense and an appreciation of their intent. While much is known about the theory and practice of resuscitation, in many areas our ignorance is profound. Resuscitation practice remains as much an art as a science. Further, the interpretation of guidelines may differ according to the environment in which they are employed. We acknowledge that individual resuscitation councils may wish to customise the details while accepting that the guiding principles are universal. Any such changes must be approved by the ERC if they are to be regarded by this organisation as their official guidelines.

3.1.2. PRECURSOR TO CARDIAC ARREST

In the so-called industrialised world, the most common cause of adult sudden cardiac death is ischaemic heart disease [6–9]. Prevention of cardiac arrest is to be greatly preferred to *post hoc* treatment. The "Management of periarrest arrhythmias" produced by the ERC in 1994 and updated in 1996 and 1998 provides guidance for treatment of arrhythmias which may lead to the development and recurrence of cardiac arrest in critical situations[10].

Small, but important, subgroups of patients sustain cardiac arrest in certain special circumstances other than ischaemic heart disease. These include trauma, drug overdose, hypothermia, immersion, anaphylaxis, pregnancy, hypovolaemia. While this ALS algorithm is universally applicable, specific modifications may be required to maximise the likelihood of success in these circumstances.

3.1.3. SPECIFIC ALS INTERVENTIONS AND THEIR USE IN THE ALS ALGORITHM (Fig. 1)

3.1.3.1. Defibrillation

In adults, the most common primary arrhythmia at the onset of cardiac arrest is ventricular fibrillation (VF) or pulseless ventricular tachycardia (VT) [11–14]. The overwhelming majority of eventual survivors come from this group [15–18]. If the definitive therapy for these arrhythmias – defibrillation – can be implemented promptly, a perfusing cardiac rhythm may be restored and lead to ultimate survival. The *only* interventions which have been shown unequivocally to improve long-term survival are basic life support and defibrillation. VF is an eminently treatable rhythm, but the chances of successful defibrillation decline substantially with the passage of each minute [19,20]. The amplitude and waveform of VF deteriorate rapidly reflecting the depletion of myocardial high energy phosphate stores [21,22]. The rate of decline in success depends in part upon the provision and adequacy of BLS [23]. As a result, the priority is to minimise any delay between the onset of cardiac arrest and the administration of defibrillating shocks.

At present, the most commonly used transthoracic defibrillation waveform has a damped sinusoidal pattern. Newer techniques such as biphasic waveforms, or sequentially overlapping shocks producing a rapidly shifting electrical vector during a multipulse shock, may reduce the energy requirements for successful defibrillation [24–26]. Automated defibrillators which can deliver a current-based shock appropriate to the measured transthoracic impedance are available and are being evaluated. Their use may increase the efficacy of individual shocks, while reducing myocardial injury in patients with unusually high, or low, transthoracic impedance [27,28].

The use of groups of three shocks is retained, the initial sequence having energies of 200 J, 200 J and 360 J. The reasons for choosing 200 J as the energy for the first two shocks of conventional waveform defibrillation have been presented [29]. Subsequent shocks, if required, should have energies of 360 J. If a co-ordinated rhythm has supervened for a limited interval, there is no strong scientific basis for deciding whether one should revert to 200 J or continue at 360 J. There is evidence that myocardial injury, both functionally and morphologically, is greater with increasing energies, but the comparative success rates for defibrillation attempts at this point with 200 J vs. 360 J are unknown. Both strategies are therefore acceptable. Most AEDs have an algorithm that does not revert to 200 J after a short period of non-VF/VT. In this case, defibrillation should continue with 360 J instead of restarting the AED to allow a 200 J shock to be given.

Alternative waveforms and energy levels are acceptable if demonstrated to be of equal or greater net clinical benefit in terms of safety and efficacy. A pulse check is required after a shock (and should be prompted by an AED), only if a change in waveform to one compatible with cardiac output is produced. Thus if VF, or VT with an identical waveform, persists after the first 200 J shock, the second shock at 200 J is given without a pulse check being performed. If, in turn, this shock is unsuccessful, the third shock – this time at 360 J – is given.

With modern defibrillators, charging times are sufficiently short for three shocks to be administered within 1 min.

Only a very small proportion of the delivered electrical energy traverses the myocardium during transthoracic defibrillation [30] and efforts to maximise this proportion are important. The most common defects are inadequate contact with the chest wall, failure or poor use of couplants to aid

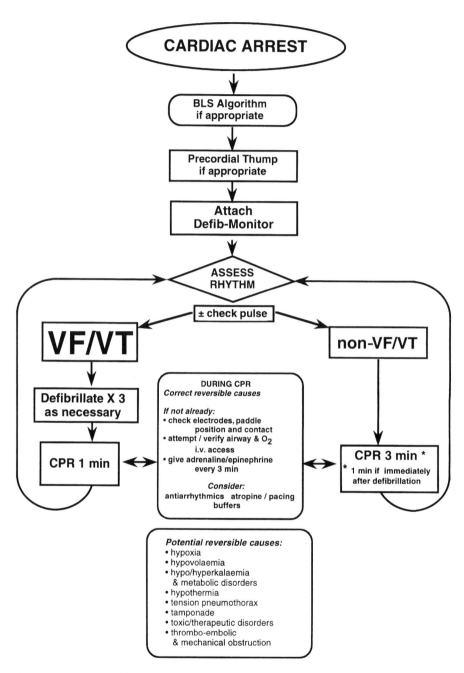

FIG. I. The algorithm for advanced life support.

the passage of current at the interface between the paddles and the chest wall, and faulty paddle positioning or size [31−34]. One paddle should be placed below the right clavicle in the mid-clavicular line and the other over the lower left ribs in the mid/anterior axillary line (just outside the position of the normal cardiac apex). In female patients the second pad/paddle should be placed firmly on the chest wall just outside the position of the normal cardiac apex avoiding the breast tissue [35].

If unsuccessful, other positions such as Apex-Posterior can be considered [36,37]. Although the polarity of the electrodes affects success with internal techniques such as implantable defibrillators, during transthoracic defibrillation the polarity of the paddles seems unimportant [38–40].

3.1.3.2. Airway management and ventilation

In 1996, guidelines for the advanced management of the airway and ventilation during resuscitation were published by a working group of the ERC [41]. These guidelines outline basic and advanced approaches to airway management together with their separate indications, contraindications and descriptions of the procedures. Further reviews have been published in 1997 [42,43].

While recognising that tracheal intubation remains the optimal procedure, these guidelines acknowledge that the technique can be difficult and sometimes hazardous and that regular experience and refresher training are required. The laryngeal mask airway (LMA) offers an alternative to tracheal intubation and although it does not guarantee absolutely against aspiration, the incidence in reported series is low [44,45]. The pharyngotracheal lumen airway and the oesophageal/tracheal Combitube are alternatives but require more training and have their own specific problems in use [41].

During cardiac arrest and CPR, lung characteristics change because of an increase in dead space while the development of pulmonary oedema reduces lung compliance [46,47]. Oxygenation of the patient is the primary objective of ventilation and the aim should be to provide inspired oxygen concentrations (FiO_2) of 1.0. Carbon dioxide production and delivery to the lungs is limited during the initial period of cardiac arrest. Tidal volumes of 400–600 ml are adequate to make the chest rise [48]. Adequate minute ventilation is necessary to facilitate carbon dioxide elimination and prevent the potential development of hypercarbic acidosis following the administration of carbon dioxide-producing buffers such as sodium bicarbonate.

Ventilation techniques vary from simple bag valve devices to the most sophisticated automatic ventilators which can provide an FiO_2 of 1.0, consistent tidal volumes, inspiratory flow rates and respiratory frequencies that are adjustable on demand.

3.1.3.3. CPR techniques

The only change recommended in the technique of closed chest compression is that the rate should be 100/min. There have been and are ongoing trials of new techniques, most notably with active compression-decompression (ACD) CPR, but there are, at present, no clinical data showing unequivocal improvement in outcomes [49–52]. To improve the scientific basis for future recommendations, the use of new techniques should be carefully evaluated by clinical trials before implementation into prehospital and in-hospital practice.

3.1.3.4. Drug delivery

The venous route remains the optimal method of drug administration during cardiopulmonary resuscitation. The previous guidance with regard to venous cannulation is unchanged [53]. If already in situ, central venous cannulae can deliver agents rapidly to the central circulation. If a central line is not present, the risks associated with the technique – which can themselves be life-threatening – mean that for an individual patient the decision as to peripheral versus central cannulation will depend upon the skill of the operator, the nature of the surrounding events, and available equipment. If a decision is made to attempt central venous cannulation, this must not delay defibrillation attempts, CPR, or airway security. When peripheral venous cannulation and drug delivery is performed, a flush of 20 ml of 0.9% saline is advised to expedite entry to the circulation.

The administration of drugs via a tracheal tube remains only a second line approach because of

impaired absorption and unpredictable pharmacodynamics. The agents which can be given by
this route are limited to adrenaline/epinephrine,
lidocaine, and atropine. Doses of 2–3 times the
standard i.v. dose diluted up to a total volume of
at least 10 ml of 0.9% saline are currently recommended. Following administration, five ventilations are given to increase dispersion to the distal
bronchial tree thus maximising absorption.

3.1.3.5. Specific drug therapy

Vasopressors

Experimentally adrenaline/epinephrine improves
myocardial and cerebral blood flow and resuscitation rates in animals, and higher doses are more
effective than the "standard" dose of 1 mg
[54,55]. There is no clinical evidence that adrena-
line/epinephrine improves survival or neurological recovery in humans irrespective of whether
standard or high dose is used [56,57]. Some clinical trials have reported slightly increased rates of
spontaneous circulation with high dose adrena-
line/epinephrine but without improvement in
overall survival rate [58–62]. The reasons for
the difference between experimental and clinical
results are likely to reflect differences in underlying pathology and the relatively long periods of
arrest before the ALS team is able to give adrena-
line/epinephrine in the out of hospital clinical
setting. It is also possible that higher doses of
adrenaline/epinephrine may be detrimental in
the postresuscitation period [63,64]. Pending definitive placebo-controlled trials the indications,
dosage, and time interval between doses for adre-
naline/epinephrine are unchanged. In practical
terms for non-VF/VT rhythms each loop of the
algorithm lasts 3 min and therefore adrenaline/
epinephrine is given with every loop. For VF/VT
rhythms, the process of rhythm assessment, three
defibrillatory shocks followed by 1 min of CPR
will take 2–3 min. Thus, adrenaline/epinephrine
should generally be given with each loop if precise timing of administration is impractical.

Considerable caution should be employed
before routinely administering adrenaline/epi-

nephrine in patients whose arrest is associated
with solvent abuse, cocaine, and other sympatho-
mimetic drugs [65–68].

The evidence with regard to other adrenergic
and nonadrenergic vasopressors is limited.
Experimentally, vasopressin leads to significantly
higher coronary perfusion pressures and preliminary data in relation to ROSC rates may be
encouraging [69,70], but at present, no pressor
agent other than adrenaline/epinephrine can be
recommended.

Antiarrhythmic agents

There is incomplete evidence to make firm recommendations on the use of *any* antiarrhythmic
agent, although our knowledge of lidocaine is
greater than for the others. Early studies suggested
that lidocaine increased the ventricular defibrillation threshold in animals [71–74], but this may
have been influenced by experimental techniques
[75]. In humans, the administration of lidocaine
prior to defibrillation may not increase the energy
requirements for defibrillation [76,77]. In one randomised placebo-controlled trial there was a beneficial effect on the threshold in the special circum-
stance of patients undergoing myocardial reperfusion after coronary artery bypass grafting [78].

For these reasons and pending the results of
trials, it is recommended that no change is
made in the previous recommendations with
regard to lidocaine, bretylium and other antiarrhythmic agents [79].

Atropine has a well established role in the
treatment of haemodynamically compromising
bradyarrhythmias and some forms of heart block
[10]. It was advocated for asystole in the 1992
guidelines on the basis that increased vagal tone
could contribute to the development or unresponsiveness of this arrhythmia. Evidence of
value in this condition is equivocal and limited
to small series and case reports [80–83]. Since
any adverse effect is unlikely in this situation its
use can still be considered in a single dose of 3
mg i.v. This dose is known to be sufficient to
block vagal activity effectively in fit adults with
a cardiac output [84].

Buffer agents

In previously healthy individuals, arterial blood gas analysis does not show a rapid or severe development of acidosis during cardiorespiratory arrest provided effective BLS is performed [85−87]. Simply measuring arterial (or even mixed venous blood) gas tensions may, however, be misleading and bear little relationship to the internal milieu of myocardial or cerebral intracellular values [88−92].

With this background, the role of buffers in CPR is still uncertain. Much of the evidence against the routine use of bicarbonate is based on animal studies, and may have limited applicability to the human situation as the doses of bicarbonate used have often been high [93−95]. One prospective randomised controlled trial has been reported on the use of buffers in patients with out-of-hospital cardiac arrest [96]. The buffer used was Tribonat (a mixture of sodium bicarbonate, trometamol, disodium phosphate and acetate). There was no improvement in hospital admission or discharge rates. In this study the dispatch-response time interval was short, and the confidence interval with the odds ratio was wide [97].

Pending further studies, it is suggested that the judicious use of buffers is limited to severe acidosis as defined in the previous guidelines (arterial pH < 7.1 and base excess < -10) and to certain special situations, such as cardiac arrest associated with hyperkalaemia or following tricyclic antidepressant overdose. For sodium bicarbonate, a dose of 50 mmol (50 ml of an 8.4% solution) is appropriate, with further administration dependent upon the clinical situation and repeat arterial blood gas analysis.

3.1.3.6. Using the Universal Algorithm

Each step that follows in the ALS algorithm (Fig. 1) assumes that the preceding one has been unsuccessful.

A precordial thump may, in certain situations such as a witnessed event, precede (albeit by a few seconds only) the attachment of a monitor/ defibrillator [98,99].

ECG monitoring then provides the link between BLS and ALS procedures. Electrocardiographic rhythm assessment must be always interpreted within the clinical context as movement artefact, lead disconnection, and electrical interference can mimic rhythms associated with cardiac arrest.

Following this assessment, the algorithm splits into two pathways − VF/VT and other rhythms.

VF/VT rhythms

The first defibrillating shock must be given without any delay. If unsuccessful it is repeated once and if necessary, twice. This initial group of three shocks should occur with successive energies of 200 J, 200 J, and 360 J. If VF/VT persists, further shocks are given with 360 J energies or the biphasic equivalent. A pulse check is performed, and should be prompted by an AED if, following a defibrillating shock a change in waveform is produced which is compatible with output. If the monitor/defibrillator indicates that VF/VT persists, then further DC shocks are administered without a further pulse check.

It is important to note that after a shock the ECG monitor screen will often show an isoelectric line for several seconds. This is commonly due to a transient period of electrical and/or myocardial "stunning", and does not necessarily mean that the rhythm has converted to asystole, as a co-ordinated rhythm or return of VF/VT may supervene subsequently. If the monitor screen of a manual defibrillator shows a "straight" line for more than one sweep immediately after a shock, 1 min of CPR should be given without a new dose of adrenaline/epinephrine, and the patient reassessed. Only if the result of this reassessment is a non-VF/VT rhythm without a pulse should a new dose of adrenaline/epinephrine be administered and CPR given for a further 2 min before the patient is assessed again. Algorithms of AEDs should also take account of this phenomenon.

Emphasis must be placed on the correct performance of defibrillation including the use of couplants. The safety of the resuscitation team is paramount. During defibrillation, no-one must be in contact with the patient. Liquids, wet clothing or the spreading of excess electrode gel can cause problems. Transdermal patches should be removed to prevent the possibility of electrical arcing [100]. Paddle/pads should be kept 12–15 cm away from implanted pacemakers. During manual defibrillation, the operator must give a command e.g., ''Stand clear!'', and check that this is obeyed before the shock is given. With automated systems an audio command is given, and all team members must comply with this command.

Over 80% of individuals who will be successfully defibrillated have this achieved by one of the first three shocks [17,19,20,101]. Subsequently, the best prospects for restoring a perfusing rhythm still remain with defibrillation, but at this stage the search for and correction of potentially reversible causes or aggravating factors is indicated, together with an opportunity to maintain myocardial and cerebral viability with chest compressions and ventilation. During CPR attempts can be made to institute advanced airway management and ventilation, venous access, and to administer drugs if appropriate to do so.

The time interval between the third and fourth shocks should not exceed 2 min. Although the interventions which can be performed during this period may improve the prospects for successful defibrillation, this is unproven, while it is well-established that with the passage of time the chances of success for defibrillating shocks lessen.

"Looping" the Algorithm

For the patient with persistent VF/VT, potential causes or aggravating factors may include electrolyte imbalance, hypothermia, and drugs and toxic agents for which specific treatment may be indicated. Where it is appropriate to continue resuscitation, successive loops of the algorithm are followed, allowing further sequences of shocks, basic life support, and the ability to perform and secure advanced airway and ventilation techniques, oxygenation and drug delivery. Antiar-

rhythmic drugs may be considered after the first two sets of three shocks, though maintaining the previous policy of deferring this treatment until four sets would be acceptable.

Non-VF/VT rhythms

If VF/VT can be positively excluded, defibrillation is not indicated as a primary intervention, (although it may be required later if ventricular fibrillation develops), and the right-sided path of the algorithm is followed.

For patients in cardiac arrest with non-VF/VT rhythms, the prognosis is in general much less favourable. The overall survival rate with these rhythms is approximately 10–15% of the survival rate with VF/VT rhythms, but the possibility of survival should not be disregarded. In some series, approximately 20% of eventual survivors present with a non-VF/VT rhythm [102–105].

With the passage of time, all electrical rhythms associated with cardiac arrest deteriorate with the eventual production of asystole. The abysmal prognosis of this degenerated rhythm is well justified. There are, nevertheless, some situations where a non-VF/VT rhythm may be caused or aggravated by remediable conditions, especially if this was the *primary* rhythm. As a consequence the detection and treatment of reversible causes become relatively more important.

During the search for and correction of these causes, CPR together with advanced airway management, oxygenation and ventilation, and any necessary attempts to secure venous access should occur, with adrenaline/epinephrine administered every 3 min.

The use of atropine for asystole has been discussed above. Atropine 3 mg i.v. is given once, along with adrenaline/epinephrine 1 mg for asystole on the first loop. Pacing may play a valuable role in patients with extreme bradyarrhythmias, but its value in asystole is questionable, except in cases of trifascicular block where P waves are seen. In patients where pacing is to be performed, but a delay occurs before it can be achieved, external cardiac percussion (also known as 'fist' or 'thump' pacing) may generate

QRS complexes with an effective cardiac output, particularly in cases where myocardial contractility is not critically compromised [106–108]. External cardiac percussion is performed with blows at a rate of 100/min, given with less force than a precordial thump and delivered over the heart, not the sternum. Conventional CPR should be substituted immediately if QRS complexes with a discernable output are not being achieved.

After 3 min of CPR, the patient's electrical rhythm is reassessed. If VF/VT has supervened, the left-sided path of the algorithm is followed, otherwise loops of the right-sided path of the algorithm will continue for as long as it is considered appropriate for resuscitation to continue. Resuscitation should generally continue for at least 20–30 min from the time of collapse unless there are overwhelming reasons to believe that resuscitation is likely to be futile.

Postresuscitation care

There are no changes in the recommendations for postresuscitation care. The most vulnerable organ for the ischaemic/hypoxic damage occurring in association with cardiac arrest is the central nervous system (CNS). Approximately 1/3 of the patients who have return of spontaneous circulation die a neurologic death, with 1/3 of long-term survivors having recognisable motor or cognitive deficits [109–111]. Fortunately only 1–2% of these individuals do not achieve an independent existence [112].

Intensive research efforts are rapidly increasing our knowledge about the pathophysiology of CNS ischaemia/hypoxia, but there are no new clinically validated treatment strategies for the cerebral damage sustained with cardiac arrest. Efforts should be directed to the avoidance and/or correction of hypotension, hypoxia, hypercarbia, electrolyte imbalance, and hypo- or hyperglycaemia [113–116].

Many victims of cardiac arrest have features indicating that the event was precipitated by acute myocardial infarction [117]. In these patients, there is an urgent need for appropriate management including such aspects as thrombolysis or other methods for obtaining coronary reperfusion and maintaining electrical stability to reduce the chances of further episodes of cardiac arrest and to improve the overall prognosis. These aspects are covered by the publications on the Management of Acute Myocardial Infarction of the European Society of Cardiology and the ESC/ERC Task force on the prehospital management of Myocardial Infarction [118–120].

3.1.4. REFERENCES

1. Guidelines for advanced life support. A statement by the advanced life support working party of the European Resuscitation Council, 1992. Resuscitation 1992;24:111–121.
2. Standards and guidelines for cardiopulmonary resuscitation (CPR) and emergency cardiac care (ECC). J Am Med Assoc 1986;255:2905–2989.
3. Evans T. Editor on behalf of The Resuscitation Council (UK). In ABC of Resuscitation. London Br Med J 1986.
4. Chamberlain DA, Cummins RO, Eisenberg M et al. Resuscitation. Recommended guidelines for uniform reporting of data from out-of-hospital cardiac arrest: the Utstein Style. Resuscitation 1991;22(August): 1–26.
5. Cummins RO, Chamberlain DA et al. Recommended guidelines for uniform reporting of data from in-hospital resuscitation: the in-hospital "Utstein style". Resuscitation 1997;34:151–183.
6. Spain D, Bradess V, Mohr C. Coronary atherosclerosis as a cause of unexpected and unexplained death. JAMA 1960;174:384–388.
7. Schatzkin A, Cupples LA, Fisher R, Heeren T, Morelock S, Mucatel M, Kannel WB. The epidemiology of sudden unexpected death: risk factors for men and women in the Framingham heart study. Am Heart J 1984;107:1300–1306.
8. Holmes DR, Davis K, Gersh BJ, Mock MB, Pettinger MB. Risk factor profiles of patients with sudden cardiac death and death from other cardiac causes: a report from the Coronary Artery Surgery Study (CASS). J Am Coll Cardiol 1989;13:524–530.
9. Myerburg RJ, Kessler KM, Bassett AL, Castellanos A. A biological approach to sudden cardiac death: structure, function and cause. Am J Cardiol 1989;63: 1512–1516.
10. Chamberlain D. Periarrest arrhythmias. Br J Anaesth 1997;79:198–202.
11. Surawicz B. Ventricular fibrillation. J Am Coll Cardiol 1985;5:438–548.
12. Sedgwick ML, Dalziel K, Watson J, Carrington DJ,

Cobbe SM. The causative rhythm in out-of-hospital cardiac arrests witnessed by the emergency medical services in the Heartstart Scotland project. Resuscitation 1994;27:55–59.

13. Deluna AB, Courrel P, Ledercq JF. Ambulatory sudden cardiac death: mechanisms of production of fatal arrhythmia on the basis of data from 157 cases. Am Heart J 1989;117:151–159.

14. Adgey AAJ, Devlin JE, Webb SW, Mulholland H. Initiation of ventricular fibrillation outside hospital in patients with acute ischaemic heart disease. Br. Heart J. 1982;47:55–61.

15. Roth R, Stewart RD, Rogers K, Cannon GM. Out-of-hospital cardiac arrest: factors associated with survival. Ann Emerg Med 1984;13:237–243.

16. Ekstrom L, Herlitz J, Wennerblom B, Axelsson A, Bang A, Holmberg S. Survival after cardiac arrest outside hospital over a 12-year period in Gothenburg. Resuscitation 1994;27:181–188.

17. Tunstall-Pedoe H, Bailey L, Chamberlain D, Marsden A, Ward M, Zideman D. Survey of 3765 cardiopulmonary resuscitations in British hospitals (the BRESUS Study). Br Med J 1992;304:1347–1351.

18. Tortolani AJ, Risucci DA, Rosati RJ, Dixon R. In-hospital cardiopulmonary resuscitation: patient, arrest and resuscitation factors associated with survival. Resuscitation 1990;20:115–128.

19. Hargarten KM, Steuven HA, Waite EM et al. Prehospital experience with defibrillation of coarse ventricular fibrillation: a ten-year review. Ann Emerg Med 1990;19:157–162.

20. Cobbe SM, Redmond MJ, Watson JM, Hollingsworth J, Carrington DJ. "Heartstart Scotland" – initial experience of a national scheme for out of hospital defibrillation. Br Med J 1991;302:1517–1520.

21. Neumar RW, Brown CG, Robitaille PL et al. Myocardial high energy phosphate metabolism during ventricular fibrillation with total circulatory arrest. Resuscitation 1990;19:199–226.

22. Mapin DR, Brown CG, Dzuonczyk R. Frequency analysis of the human and swine electrocardiogram during ventricular fibrillation. Resuscitation 1991;22:85–91.

23. Larsen MP, Eisenberg MS, Cummins RO, Hallstrom AP. Predicting survival from out-of-hospital cardiac arrest: a graphic model. Ann Emerg Med 1993;22:1652–1658.

24. Greene HL, Dimarco JP, Kudenchuk PJ et al. Comparison of monoplasic and biphasic defibrillating pulse waveforms for transthoracic cardioversion. Am J Cardiol 1995;75:1135–1139.

25. Bardy GH, Gliner BE, Kudenchuk PJ et al. Truncated biphasic pulses for transthoracic defibrillation. Circulation 1995;91:1768–1774.

26. Kerber RE, Spencer KT, Kallock M et al. Overlapping sequential pulses: a new waveform for transthoracic defibrillation. Circulation 1994;89:2369–2379.

27. Kerber RE, Kouba C, Martins JB et al. Advance prediction of transthoracic impedence in human defibrillation and cardioversion: importance of impedence in determining the success of low energy shocks. Circulation 1984;70:303–308.

28. Kerber RE, Martins JB, Kienzle MG et al. Energy, current and success in defibrillation and cardioversion: Clinical studies using an automated, impedence-based energy adjustment method. Circulation 1988;77:1038–1046.

29. Bossaert L, Koster R. Defibrillation: methods and strategies. A statement for the Advanced Life Support Working Party of the European Resuscitation Council. Resuscitation 1992;24:211–225.

30. Lermann BB, Deale OC. Relation between transcardiac and tranthoracic current during defibrillation in humans. Circ Res 1990;67:1420–1426.

31. Adgey AAJ, Dalzell GNW. Paddle/pad placement for defibrillation in adults. Br J Int Care 1994;(Suppl): 14–16.

32. Sirna SJ, Ferguson DW, Charbonnier F, Kerber RE. Electrical cardioversion in humans: factors affecting transthoracic impedence. Am J Cardiol 1988;62:1048–1052.

33. Kerber RE. Electrical treatment of cardiac arrhythmias: defibrillation and cardioversion. Ann Emerg Med 1993;27:296–301.

34. Alyward PE, Keiso R, Hite P, Charbonnier F, Kerber RE. Defibrillator electrode-chest wall coupling agents: Influence on transthoracic impedence and shock success. J Am Coll Cardiol 1985;6:682–686.

35. Pagan-Carlo LA, Spencer KT, Robertson CE et al. Transthoracic defibrillation: Importance of avoiding electrode placement directly on the female breast. J Am Coll Cardiol 1996;27:449–452.

36. Kerber RE, Grayzel J, Kennedy J, Jensen SR. Elective cardioversion: influence of paddle electrode location and size on success rates and energy requirements. N Eng J Med 1981;305:658–662.

37. Kerber RE, Martins JB, Kelly J et al. Self-adhesive pre-applied electrode pads for defibrillation and cardioversion: experimental and clinical studies. J Am Coll Cardiol 1984;3:815–820.

38. Bardy GH, Ivey TD, Allen MD, Johnson G, Greene HL. Evaluation of electrode polarity on defibrillation efficacy. Am J Cardiol 1989;63:433–437.

39. Strickberger SD, Hummel JD, Horwood LE et al. Effect of shock polarity on ventricular defibrillation threshold using a transvenous system. J Am Coll Cardiol 1994; 24:1069–1072.

40. Weaver WD, Martin JS, Wirkus MJ et al. Influence of external defibrillator electrode polarity on cardiac resuscitation. Pace 1993;16:285–290.

41. Baskett PJF, Bossaert L, Carli P et al. Guidelines for the advanced management of the airway and ventilation during resuscitation. A statement by the Airway and Ventilation Management Group of the ERC. Resuscitation 1996;31:201–230.
42. Gabbott DA, Baskett PJF. Management of the airway and ventilation during resuscitation. Br J Anaesth 1997;79:159–171.
43. Nolan JP, Parr MJA. Aspects of resuscitation in trauma. Br J Anaesth 1997;79:226–240.
44. Brimacombe JR, Berry A. The incidence of aspiration associated with the Laryngeal mask Airway:a meta-analysis of published literature. J Clin Anaesth 1995; 7:297–305.
45. Owens TM, Robertson P, Twomey C et al. The incidence of gastro oesophageal reflux with the laryngeal mask. Anesth Analg 1995;80:980–984.
46. Davis K, Johannigman JA, Johnson RC, Branson RD. Lung compliance following Cardiac arrest. Acad Emerg Med 1995;2:874–878.
47. Ornato JP, Bryson BL, Donovan PJ et al. Measurement of ventilation during CPR. Crit Care Med 1983;11: 79–82.
48. Baskett PJF, Nolan J, Parr MJA. Tidal volumes which are perceived to be adequate for resuscitation. Resuscitation 1996;31:231–234.
49. Cohen TJ, Tucker KJ, Lurie KG et al. Active compression-decompression. A new method of cardiopulmonary resuscitation. J Am Med Ass 1992;267: 2916–2923.
50. Schwab TM, Callaham ML, Madsen CD, Utecht TA. A randomised clinical trial of active compression-decompression CPR vs. standard CPR in out of hospital cardiac arrest in two cities. J Am Med Ass 1995; 273:1261–1268.
51. Steill IG, Hebert PC, Wells GA et al. The Ontario trial of active compression-decompression cardiopulmonary resuscitation for in-hospital and prehospital cardiac arrest. J Am Med Ass 1996;275:1417–1423.
52. Plaisance P, Adnui F, Viuuni E, et al. Benefit of active compression decompression CPR as a prehospital advanced cardiac life support. Circulation 1997;95: 955–961.
53. Hapnes S, Robertson C. CPR – drug delivery routes and systems. Resuscitation 1992;24:137–142.
54. Redding JS, Pearson JW. Evaluation of drugs for cardiac resuscitation. Anaesthesiology 1963;24:203–207.
55. Redding JS, Pearson JW. Adrenaline in cardiac resuscitation. Am Heart J 1963;66:210–214.
56. Woodhouse SP, Cox S, Boyd P, Case C, Weber M. High-dose and standard-dose adrenaline do not alter survival compared with placebo, in cardiac arrest. Resuscitation 1995;30:243–249.
57. Herlitz J, Ekstrom L, Wennerblom B, Axelsson A, Bang A, Holmberg S. Adrenaline In Out of hospital ventricular fibrillation. Does it make any difference. Resuscitation 1995;29:195–201.
58. Callaham ML, Modsen CD, Barton CW, Saunders CE, Pointer J. A randomised clinical trial of high-dose epinephrine and noradrenaline vs. standard dose epinephrine in prehospital cardiac arrest. J Am Med Ass 1992;268:2667–2672.
59. Abramson NS, Safar P, Sutton-Tyrrel K. A randomised clinical trial of escalating doses of high dose epinephrine during cardiac resuscitation [Abstract]. Crit Care Med 1995;23:A178.
60. Lindner KH, Ahnefeld FW, Prengel AW. Comparison of standard and high-dose adrenaline in the resuscitation of asystole and electromechanical dissociation. Acta Anaesthesiol Scand 1991;35:253–256.
61. Steill IG, Hebert PC, Weitzman BW et al. High dose epinephrine in adult cardiac arrest. N Eng J Med 1992;327:1045–1050.
62. Brown CG, Martin DR, Pepe PE et al. A comparison of standard-dose and high-dose epinephrine in cardiac arrest outside the hospital. The Multicenter High-dose Epinephrine Study Group. N Eng J Med 1992;327:1051–1055.
63. Rivers EP, Wortsnan J, Rady MY et al. The effect of total cumulative epinephrine dose adminstered during human CPR on haemodynamic, oxygen transport and utilisation variables in the postresuscitation period. Chest 1994;5:1315–1316.
64. Tang W, Weil MH, Sun S, Noc M, Yang L, Gasmuri RJ. Epinephrine increases the severity of postresuscitation myocardial dysfunction. Circulation 1995;92: 3089–3093.
65. Lathers CM, Tyau LSY, Spino MM et al. Cocaine-induced seizures, arrhythmias and sudden death. J Clin Pharmacol 1988;28:584–593.
66. Lange RA, Cigarroa RG, Yancy CW et al. Cocaine-induced coronary artery vasoconstriction. N Eng J Med 1989;321:1557–1562.
67. Sheperd RT. Mechanism of sudden death associated with volatile substance abuse. Hum Toxicol 1989;8: 287–292.
68. Boon NA. Solvent abuse and the heart (Editorial). Br Med J 1987;294:722.
69. Lindner KH, Prengel AW, Pfenninger EG et al. Vasopressin improves vital organ blood flow during closed-chest cardiopulmonary resuscitation in pigs. Circulation 1995;91:215–221.
70. Lindner KH, Prengel AW, Brinkmann A et al. Vasopressin administration in refractory cardiac arrest. Ann Intern Med 1996;124:1061–1064.
71. Babbs CF, Yim GKW, Whistler SJ, Tacker WA, Geddes LA. Elevation of ventricular defibrillation threshold in dogs by antiarrhythmic drugs. Am Heart J 1979;98:345–350.
72. Chow MSS, Kluger J, Lawrence R, Fieldman A. The

effect of lidocaine and bretylium on the defibrillation threshold during cardiac arrest and cardiopulmonary resuscitation. Proc Soc Exper Biol Med 1986;182: 63–67.

73. Dorian P, Fain ES, Davy JM, Winkle RA. Lidocaine causes a reversible, concentration-dependent increase in defibrillation energy requirements. J Am Coll Card 1986;8:327–332.

74. Echt DS, Black JN, Barbey JT, Coxe DR, Cato E. Evaluation of antiarrhythmic drugs on defibrillation energy requirements in dogs. Sodium channel block and action potential prolongation. Circulation 1989; 79:1106–1117.

75. Natale A, Jones DL, Kim Y-H, Klein GJ. Effects of lidocaine on defibrillation threshold in the pig: Evidence of Anesthesia Related Increase. PACE 1991; 14:1239–1244.

76. Kerber RE, Pandian NG, Jensen SR et al. Effect of lidocaine and bretylium on energy requirements for transthoracic defibrillation; Experiemental studies. J Am Coll Cardiol 1986;7:397–405.

77. Kerber RE, Jensen SR, Gascho JA, Grayzel J, Hoyt R, Kennedy J. Determinants of defibrillation: prospective analysis of 183 patients. Am J Cardiol 1983;52: 739–745.

78. Lake CL, Kron IL, Mentzer RM, Crampton RS. Lidocaine enhances intraoperative ventricular defibrillation. Anesth Analg 1986;65:337–340.

79. von Planta M, Chamberlain D. Drug treatment of arrhythmias during cardiopulmonary resuscitation. Resuscitation 1992;24:227–232.

80. Brown DC, Lewis AJ, Criley JM. Asystole and its treatment: The possible role of the parasympathetic nervous system in cardiac arrest. J.A.C.E.P. 1979;8: 448–452.

81. Iseri LT, Humphrey SB, Sirer EJ. Prehospital bradyasystolic cardiac arrest. Ann Intern Med 1978;88: 741–745.

82. Coon GC, Clinton JE, Ruiz E. Use of atropine for bradyasystolic prehospital cardiac arrest. Ann Emerg Med 1981;10:462–467.

83. Steuven HA, Tonsfeldt DJ, Thomson BM. Atropine in asystole: Human studies. Ann Emerg Med 1984;13: 815–817.

84. Chamberlain DA, Turner P, Sneddon JM. Effects of atropine on heart-rate in healthy man. Lancet 1967; ii:12–15.

85. Steedman DJ, Robertson CE. Acid base changes in arterial and central venous blood during cardiopulmonary resuscitation. Arch Emerg Med 1992;9: 169–176.

86. Henreman PL, Ember JE, Marx JA. Development of acidosis in human beings during closed chest and open chest CPR. Ann Emerg Med 1988;17:672–675.

87. Gilston A. Clinical and biochemical aspects of cardiac

resuscitation. Lancet 1965;2:1039–1043.

88. von Planta J, Weil MH, Gazmuri RJ, Bisera J, Rackow EC. Myocardial acidosis associated with CO_2 production during cardiac arrest and resuscitation. Circulation 1989;80:684–692.

89. Capparelli EV, Chow MSS, Kluger J, Fieldman A. Difference in systemic and myocardial blood acid-base status during cardiopulmonary resuscitation. Crit Care Med 1989;17:442–446.

90. Gudipati CV, Neil MH, Gazmuri RJ et al. Increases in coronary vein CO_2 during cardiac resuscitation. J Appl Physiol 1990;68:1405–1408.

91. Kette F, Weil MH, Gazmuri RJ, Bisera J, Rackow EC. Intramyocardial hypercarbic acidosis during cardiac arrest and resuscitation. Crit Care Med 1993;21: 901–906.

92. Javaheri S, Clendending A, Papadakos N et al. pH changes in the surface of brain and in cisternal fluid in dogs in cardiac arrest Stroke 1984;15:553–558.

93. Kette F, Weil MH, Gazmuri RJ. Buffer solutions may compromise cardiac resuscitation by reducing coronary perfusion pressure. J Am Med Ass 1991;266: 2121–2126.

94. Gazmuri RJ, von Planta M, Weil MH, Rackow EC. Cardiac effects of carbon dioxide-consuming and carbon dioxide-generating buffers during cardiopulmonary resuscitation. J Am Coll Card 1990;15:482–449.

95. Bleske BE, Rice TL, Warren EW et al. The effect of sodium bicarbonate administration on the vasopressor effect of high-dose epinephrine during cardiopulmonary resuscitation in Swine. Am J Emerg Med 1993; 11:439–443.

96. Dybvik T, Strand T, Steen PA. Buffer therapy during out-of-hospital cardiopulmonary resuscitation. Resuscitation 1995;29:89–95.

97. Koster RW. Correction of acidosis during cardio-pulmonary resuscitation. Resuscitation 1995;29:87–88.

98. Caldwell G, Millar G, Quinn E, Vincent R, Chamberlain DA. Simple mechanical methods for cardioversion: defence of the precordial thump. Br Med J 1985;291:627–630.

99. Robertson C. The precordial thump and cough techniques in advanced life support. Resuscitation 1992; 24:133–135.

100. Paracek EA, Munger MA, Rutherford WF, Gardner SF. Report of nitropatch explosions complicating defibrillation. Am J Emerg Med 1992;10:128–129.

101. Adgey AAJ. The Belfast experience with resuscitation ambulances. Am J Emerg Med 1984;2:193–209.

102. Sedgwick ML, Dalziel K, Watson J, Carrington DJ, Cobbe SM. Performance of an established system of first responder out of hospital defibrillation. Resuscitation 1993;26:75–88.

103. Myerburg RJ, Conde CA, Sing RJ et al. Clinical, electrophysiological and haemodynamic profile of patients

resuscitated from prehospital cardiac arrest. Am J Med 1980;68:568–576.

104. Isen LT, Humphrey SB, Sirer EJ. Prehospital bradya-systolic cardiac arrest. Ann Entern Med 1978;88:741–745.

105. Herlitz J, Ekstrom L, Wennerblom B, Axelsson A, Bang A, Holmberg S. Survival among patients with out-of-hospital cardiac arrest found in electromechanical dissociation. Resuscitation 1995;29:97–106.

106. Sandoe E. Ventricular standstill and percussion. (Editorial). Resuscitation 1996;32:3–4.

107. Dowdle JR. Ventricular standstill and cardiac percussion. Resuscitation 1996;32:31–32.

108. Scherf D, Bornemann C. Thumping of the precordium in ventricular standstill. Am J Cardiol 1960;5:30–40.

109. Edgren E, Hedstrand N, Kelsey S, Sutton-Tyrrell K, Safar P and the BRCT 1 Study Group. Assessment of neurological prognosis in comatose survivors of cardiac arrest. Lancet 1994;343:1055–1059.

110. Roine RO, Kaste M, Kinnunen A, Nikki P, Sarna S, Kajaste S. Nimodipine after resuscitation from out-of-hospital ventricular fibrillation. A placebo controlled, double blind, randomized trial. J Am Med Ass 1990;264:3171–3177.

111. Brain Resuscitation Clinical Trial II Study Group. A randomized study of calcium entry blocker (lidoflazine) administration in the treatment of comatose survivors of cardiac arrest. N Engl J Med 1991;324:1225–1231.

112. Graves JR, Herlitz J, Axelsson A, Ekstrom L, Holmberg M, Lidquist J, Sunnerhagen K, Holmberg S. Survivors of out of hospital cardiac arrest: their prognosis, long-evity and functional status. Resuscitation 1997;35:117–122.

113. Cantu RC, Ames A, Digancinto G et al. Hypotension: a major factor limiting recovery from cerebral ischaemia. J Surg Res 1969;9:525–529.

114. Sieber FE, Traystman RJ. Special issues, glucose and the brain. Crit Care Med 1991;20:104–114.

115. Longstreth WT, Inin TS. High blood glucose level on hospital admission and poor neurological recovery after cardiac arrest. Ann Neurol 1984;15:59–63.

116. Buylaert WA, Calle PA, Honbreckts HN. The cerebral resuscitation study group. Serum electrolyte disturbances in the postresuscitation period. Resuscitation 1989;17:S189–S196.

117. Cobb LA, Werner J, Trobough G. Sudden cardiac death: a decade's experience with out of hospital resuscitation. Mod Concepts Cardiovasc Dis 1980;49:31–39.

118. The task force on the management of acute myocardial infarction of the European Society of Cardiology Acute Myocardial Infarction: prehospital and in-hospital management. Eur Heart J 1996;17:43–63.

119. Guidelines for the early management of patients with acute myocardial infarction. A report of the ACC/AHA task force on assessment of diagnostic and therapeutic cardiovascular procedures. J Am Coll Cardiol 1996;16:249–292.

120. Arntz HR, Bossaert L, Carli P, Chamberlain D, Davies M, Dellborg M et al. The Prehospital management of Acute Heart attacks: Report of a task force of ESC/ERC. Resuscitation 1998;(In press).

3.2. ERC ALS Model Course Proposal

3.2.1. INTRODUCTION

Following the principles of the current ERC Guidelines and the ILCOR advisory statements for Universal ALS algorithm, valid scientific evidence only supports three interventions as unequivocally effective in adult cardiac Resuscitation:
- Basic CPR
- Defibrillation (if the rhythm is VF or pulseless VT (VF/VT))
- Tracheal Intubation and oxygenation.

Performance guidelines should be as simple as possible and can be summarised as follows:
- Perform CPR at all times for pulseless patients, except during rhythm analysis and defibrillation shocks
- Defibrillate VF/VT as long as VF/VT is present
- Gain control of the airway with tracheal intubation if possible, and provide adequate oxygenation and ventilation
- Give intravenous boluses of epinephrine
- Correct reversible causes.

The ALS course will provide the appropriate background knowledge. By the end of the course participants should be able to rapidly and efficiently perform these procedures, while conforming to the ERC algorithms for ALS.

3.2.2. TARGET POPULATION

ALS courses are directed at individuals who are legally assigned to perform ALS in and outside the hospital.

The contents and organisation of the course should be adapted to the different types of personnel involved in ALS in the different European countries. According to the legislation of each country, this course can be supplemented by additional training that makes it possible for non-physicians to perform specific procedures (e.g., tracheal intubation, drug administration, defibrillation, etc.).

3.2.3. BASIC COURSE CONTENTS

The course should include a common core in order to be approved by the ERC. Additional modules (e.g. trauma life support, paediatric life support) can be added to this common core to suit the specific characteristics of the students as well as the different health care systems across Europe.

1. Basic CPR with adjuncts

Performance of basic life support with two rescuers if appropriate, including the use of ventilation with bag-valve-mask and oxygen supply.

2. Precordial thump

Recognition of the indications for and the adequate performance of the precordial thump.

3. Rhythm and defibrillation

Cardiac rhythm monitoring techniques. Recognition of cardiac arrest rhythms and rhythms associated with cardiac arrest. Pacing. Defibrillation.

4. Airway management

Control of the airway by means of orotracheal intubation and use of alternative techniques when tracheal intubation is not possible, such as the laryngeal mask airway and/or Combitube.

5. Intravascular access

Performance of intravascular access. Use of the tracheal tube as an alternative.

6. Drug administration

Administration of adrenaline/epinephrine and other drugs used during the management of a cardiac arrest.

7. Correct reversible causes

Identification and immediate management of the potentially reversible causes of cardiac arrest.

8. Universal algorithm and action plan in different situations

Competence in applying the ERC Universal ALS algorithm to deal with a wide range of cardiac arrest scenarios.

9. Cardiac arrest ethical aspects

An ALS course should also include ethical concepts to help students to solve real problems in their practice with confidence.

3.2.4. COURSE ORGANISATION

The core course lasts between 16 and 20 h and can be done in 2 full days (morning and afternoon sessions, or in four consecutive morning or afternoon sessions).

The course comprises lectures, skills stations and Comprehensive Resuscitation Scenarios (CRS). The duration of the lectures, skills stations and CRSs is usually between 30 and 60 min.

The ERC model course comprises ±7 h of lectures, ±5 skills stations and ±4 CRSs. The description of the ERC model course is given in Appendix 1.

The application of the universal ALS algorithm should be practised in CRSs. In these sessions at least the following scenarios should be practised:

—witnessed VF (e.g., electrocution victim in an emergency department)
—VT without a palpable pulse (e.g., cardiac arrest in the CCU)
—respiratory arrest with a pulse (e.g., drug overdose)
—asystole (e.g., cardiac arrest at home in a possible AMI)
—EMD (e.g., penetrating knife injury).

All skills stations and CRSs should be done with suitable material to realistically simulate the clinical situation (see Appendix 2).

For skills stations and CRSs the student to faculty ratio should not exceed 8:1. Theoretical sessions can be given by one instructor to the whole group. The skills stations and CRSs should be given in separate rooms.

All instructors should be experienced in treating cardiac arrest. The majority of the instructors should hold an ALS instructors certificate which has been issued by an ERC approved CPR school. Lectures are given only by instructors with experience in treating cardiac arrest. The director or codirector of the training programme should be a medically qualified instructor, certified by an ERC approved CPR school.

The ERC ALS course manual should be distributed to the students at least one month before the course (the cost of this manual may be included in the course fee). Students are strongly encouraged to read the manual before attending.

The ERC publication "Guidelines for Resuscitation 1998" will provide the optional additional background information.

3.2.5. EVALUATION

Evaluation is an essential component of the course to test its efficacy. An initial evaluation could be organised (MCQ precourse test) to encourage students to read the manual before attending the course.

The final evaluation should include both theory and practice.

Practical skills are evaluated in skills stations which should include CPR with equipment, tracheal intubation, arrhythmias management and defibrillation, and Comprehensive Resuscitation Scenarios. To evaluate the theoretical knowledge, evaluation should be done by means of an MCQ test.

3.2.6. RETRAINING

Ideally, health care personnel working in an emergency care setting, should recertify in ALS within 3 years by attending a refresher course.

The duration of this refresher course will usually be of 4–5 h and aims at revising the essential theoretical knowledge and practical skills. This number of hours may increase if new guidelines have to be included. Optimally, this refresher course should include a theoretical pretest.

ALS providers who infrequently attend cardiac arrest should be reminded that without clinical practice, they will loose their skills rapidly.

3.2.7. CERTIFICATION OF ATTENDANCE

Participants in the course have been taught current principles and skills in cardiac arrest treatment. Competence will not be certified either by the ERC or the National Resuscitation Councils. ERC will issue only certificates of successful completion of the course. Competence will only be achieved through clinical experience gained during the management of cardiac arrest.

Appendix 1: Examples of timetable for implementing the ERC model course

MODULE 1: Basic Life Support Testing and Basic Life Support with equipment

Theoretical sessions (Main room):

Introduction to Chain of Survival and ALS (15 min)

Pre-course test (MCQ) (30 min)

Risk to the rescuer (15 min)

Basic Life Support Revision and Basic Life Support with equipment (suction, oropharyngeal and nasopharyngeal airways, ventilation with pocked mask and bag-valve-mask and oxygen supply) (45 min)

Break (15 min)

Skill Station A	Skill Station B	Skill Station C
Basic Life Support Testing (60 min) (Group 1)	Basic Life Support Testing (60 min) (Group 2)	Basic Life Support Testing (60 min) (Group 3)
Basic Life Support with equipment (60 min) (Group 1)	Basic Life Support with equipment (60 min) (Group 2)	Basic Life Support with equipment (60 min) (Group 3)

MODULE 2: Defibrillation

Theoretical sessions (Main room):

Causes of cardiac arrest. AMI and prevention (30 min)

Cardiac monitoring and rhythms associated with cardiac arrest recognition Peri-arrest arrhythmias (45 min)

Defibrillation (manual and automatic) Pacing (30 min)

ERC Algorithm for ALS: VF and VT without pulse (Initial actions: precordial thump and first three DC shocks) (15 min)

Break (15 min)

Skill Station A	Skill Station B	Skill Station C
Rhythm recognition skill station (60 min) (Group 1)	Rhythm recognition skill station (60 min) (Group 2)	Rhythm recognition skill station (60 min) (Group 3)
Defibrillation skill station (manual and automatic) and pacing (60 min) (Group 1)	Defibrillation skill station (manual and automatic) and pacing (60 min) (Group 2)	Defibrillation skill station (manual and automatic) and pacing (60 min) (Group 3)

MODULE 3: Advance Life Support (I)

Theoretical sessions (Main room):

Advanced airway management (tracheal intubation, laryngeal mask airway and cricothyroidotomy by puncture) (30 min)

Drugs delivery routes and basic drugs (adrenaline/epinephrine, lidocaine, sodium bicarbonate, atropine) (30 min)

ERC Algorithm for ALS: VF and VT without pulse (Final actions) and No VF and VT without pulse (asystole and electromechanical dissociation) (30 min)

Bereavement and cardiac arrest ethics aspects (30 min)

Break (15 min)

Skill Station A	Skill Station B	Skill Station C
Advanced airway management skill station (60 min) (Group 1)	Drugs delivery routes skill station (60 min) (Group 2)	Cardiac arrest team organisation Practical scenarios (CRS) (60 min) (Group 3)
Advanced airway management skill station (60 min) (Group 2)	Drugs delivery routes skill station (60 min) (Group 3)	Cardiac arrest team organisation Practical scenarios (CRS) (60 min) (Group 1)
Advanced airway management skill station (60 min) (Group 3)	Drugs delivery routes skill station (60 min) (Group 1)	Cardiac arrest team organisation Practical scenarios (CRS) (60 min) (Group 2)

MODULE 4: Advance Life Support (II)

Theoretical sessions (Main room):

Cardiac arrest in special situations (Traumatic and pediatric patients) (45 min)

Postresuscitation care with drugs in peri-arrest arrhythmias (45 min)

Break (15 min)

Skill Station A	Skill Station B	Skill Station C
Advanced airway management skill testing station (60 min) (Group 1)	Rhythm recognition and defibrillation testing skill station (60 min) (Group 2)	Practical scenarios (CRS) (Testing) (60 min) (Group 3)
Advanced airway management skill testing station (60 min) (Group 2)	Rhythm recognition and defibrillation testing skill station (60 min) (Group 3)	Practical scenarios (CRS) (Testing) (60 min) (Group 1)
Advanced airway management skill testing station (60 min) (Group 3)	Rhythm recognition and defibrillation testing skill station (60 min) (Group 1)	Practical scenarios (CRS) (Testing) (60 min) (Group 2)

Evaluation (MCQ) (Main room) (30 min)

Appendix 2: List of materials for implementing the ERC model course

Teaching materials list for theoretical sessions:

1 (2) slides projector
One video reproducer and TV screen
Overhead projector

Skill trainer equipment list

9 BLS manikins trainers (optional)
3 BLS manikins for testing

Oropharyngeal and nasopharyngeal airways
3 pocket resuscitation masks
3 bag-valve-masks with reservoirs

Oxygen supplies
1–2 airway management trainers

1–2 laryngoscopes
1–2 stethoscopes

3 Arrhythmia simulators
3 Defibrillators (automatic and manual) with screen monitor
3 Defibrillation manikins or 3 BLS manikins with a conductive band

Manikin with or without arms for peripheral cannulation (Central venous cannulation manikin?)

1 ALS trainer with arrhythmia simulator
Drugs or drugs delivery simulator (?)
Miscellaneous material such as i.v. catheter, endotracheal tubes, laryngeal mask airways, etc.

Appendix 3: Requirements for the approval of an ALS course as ERC approved ALS course

Only ERC approved CPR schools can organise ERC approved ALS courses.

The ERC approved CPR schools will be set up in a national network. The National Resuscitation Councils, or the national organisations in the countries where the National Resuscitation Countries do not exist, have the primary responsibility in the management of ERC approved CPR schools, in order to guarantee the standards and quality of the ERC ALS courses.

Situation A: Countries without a network of ALS schools.

The ERC, by means of the Training and Education Working Group can provide support in setting up a training network of ERC approved schools, providing the first ERC ALS instructor courses. Later on, the ERC ALS instructor courses will be run under the responsibility of the National Resuscitation Councils or the ERC-approved national organisations, and will be given by the instructors previously trained by the ERC, in a cascade form of teaching.

Situation B: Countries with a network of ALS schools.

The ERC will approve the already established network of ALS schools in those countries which accept the ERC regulations for ERC approved CPR schools and after checking their competence in ALS teaching.

The multilingual material for an ERC approved course will be copyrighted material by the ERC. The translation to the different European languages of the ERC ALS course materials will be done by the National Resuscitation Councils or the ERC approved national organisations. These translations will need the approval of the ERC. It could be possible to adapt these materials in each country by adding some topics to the ERC approved ALS model course, e.g., AMI prevention, bereavement, etc. These adaptations will need the ERC approval to be used as ERC copyrighted ALS course material. The ERC and the National Resuscitation Councils or the ERC approved national organisations will share out the profits of the sale of the material.

Therefore, for an ALS course to be approved as an ERC ALS course, it must follow the following regulations:

1. It must be approved by the National Resuscitation Council or national organisation with ERC approved responsibility in dealing with the ERC approved CPR schools in this country.
2. The content (programme) and schedule of the course will follow that of the ERC approved ALS model course.
3. At least 60% of the course instructors will be ERC approved ALS instructors. One of them will act as Director or Co-director of the course.
4. The course materials will be ERC copyrighted materials in the language of the country, if a translation is available (manual, slides, MCQ tests, skill stations tests).
5. These materials could be used in several courses by the instructors of the same ERC approved ALS school, but a new ERC Manual must be used by each student.
6. The ERC will issue, by means of the National Resuscitation Council or national organisation approved by the ERC to give ALS courses, a certificate of attendance or completion of the course to the candidates who have successfully completed the ALS course.

3.3. Postresuscitation Care

3.3.1. INTRODUCTION

The goals of cardiopulmonary resuscitation (CPR) are to produce a patient with normal cerebral function, a stable cardiac output and rhythm, and adequate organ perfusion. The return of spontaneous circulation (ROSC) is just the first step in what may be a long period of recovery. All patients who regain spontaneous circulation after cardiac arrest should be admitted to an intensive care unit (ICU) or coronary care unit (CCU). Aspects of postresuscitation care have been reviewed previously [1,2], and in summary, the aims of postresuscitation care are to:
- Perform a rapid assessment of the patient's vital signs, and prevent another cardiac arrest.
- Transport to the intensive care unit or coronary care unit
- Limit organ damage
- Predict nonsurvivors

3.3.2. INITIAL ASSESSMENT

A patient who has survived a cardiac arrest must be stabilised as rapidly as possible in an attempt to reduce the risk of another cardiac arrest. The respiratory and cardiovascular systems must be optimised and electrolyte and metabolic abnormalities corrected.

AIRWAY AND BREATHING

The patient's airway must be protected. Those patients who have been rapidly defibrillated after a brief period of ventricular fibrillation (< 2 min) are likely to regain consciousness very quickly. These patients will not have been intubated and the rapid return of airway reflexes, will probably prevent the need for intubation in the postresuscitation period. However, these patients must be capable of adequate spontaneous ventilation and must be given supplementary oxygen. This should be delivered at the highest concentration available until an arterial blood gas sample has confirmed adequate oxygenation. Once the patient is peripherally well perfused, a pulse oximeter will provide a continuous indication of oxygenation. Prolonged hypoxia and inadequate ventilation increase the chances of further cardiac arrest and contribute to secondary cerebral injury. Therefore, comatose patients will require assisted ventilation via a tracheal tube. If not already intubated (during resuscitation) they will require intubation by a person skilled in advanced airway management. Having secured the airway, assess the patient's ventilation. Look for symmetrical chest movement, and listen to ensure that the breath sounds are equal on both sides. A tracheal tube which is too long will tend to go down the right main bronchus and fail to ventilate the left lung. If ribs have been fractured there is a significant chance of a pneumothorax (reduced or absent breath sounds). Listen for evidence of pulmonary oedema or aspiration of gastric contents. Obtain a chest X-ray immediately and check the position of the tracheal tube, central venous line, and nasogastric tube. An arterial blood gas will allow optimisation of the FiO_2 and minute ventilation. Oxygen saturation of haemoglobin should be maintained at > 95% (pulse oximeter). In head injured patients prolonged periods of extreme hyperventilation worsen neurological outcome [3]. Similar data from patients suffering cardiac arrest is not available but it would seem reasonable to ventilate these patients to normocapnoea or mild hypocapnoea (i.e., $PaCO_2$ of 4.5 kPa or 35 mmHg). After calibration against an arterial blood gas measurement, the end-tidal CO_2 will provide continuous monitoring of ventilation.

CIRCULATION

Immediately after ROSC the patient's heart rate, blood pressure and cardiac output are likely to be unstable. An arterial cannula will allow continuous blood pressure monitoring and repeated sampling for blood gas analysis. Continuous ECG monitoring is essential, and a 12-lead ECG should be obtained as soon as possible. If cardiac arrest has been precipitated by myocardial infarction (as is the case in about 20% of sudden deaths), conduction abnormalities may result in severe bradyarrhythmias, particularly after an inferior myocardial infarction. On the other hand, high levels of circulating catecholamines often precipitate dangerous tachyarrhythmias. These arrhythmias require immediate and appropriate treatment in order to prevent further cardiac arrest. Immediately after ROSC a number of factors may contribute to a very poor myocardial contractility:
- Myocardial infarction
- Myocardial stunning and reperfusion injury
- Severe metabolic acidosis

Adequate cerebral and coronary blood flow are essential if myocardial and neurological recovery are to be maximised. This may require the use of fluids and inotropic drugs. A pulmonary artery catheter (PAC) will guide inotrope and fluid therapy, but their use is controversial because of associated complications and, as yet, benefit has not been demonstrated by prospective randomised controlled trials. Noninvasive methods of measuring cardiac output, such as Doppler techniques, are not associated with the same complications but are not as accurate as the PAC.

NEUROLOGY

Although it is impossible to accurately predict neurological outcome immediately after ROSC, a rapid baseline neurological assessment of the patient should be documented. This should include pupillary response to light and Glasgow Coma Score (GCS). These responses may be modified by sedative/anaesthetic drugs (see below).

ELECTROLYTE AND METABOLIC ABNORMALITIES

Blood samples should be sent for urgent biochemical analysis. Electrolyte disturbances, in particular of the cations K^+, Mg^{2+}, and Ca^{2+} should be corrected. Immediately after cardiac arrest there is typically a short period of hyperkalaemia. This is followed by hypokalaemia as potassium is transported intracellularly by the action of catecholamines on β_2-adrenoreceptors. After cardiac arrest hypokalaemia is likely to provoke ventricular arrhythmias and the serum potassium should be maintained at 4.0–4.5 mmol l^{-1} with appropriate replacement therapy. The routine use of magnesium therapy is controversial but in the face of continued arrhythmias after ROSC, it is probably rational to administer 2 g of magnesium sulphate.

Acidaemia (high blood H^+ ion concentrations) should be corrected by addressing the underlying cause; poor peripheral perfusion is better managed by fluid and inotropes rather than by the administration of alkali such as bicarbonate. Bicarbonate may result in tissue acidosis as it is converted to carbon dioxide with the release of H^+ ions within the cell (paradoxical intracellular acidosis). Bicarbonate provides a significant plasma sodium load and any tendency to alkalosis will worsen tissue hypoxia by shifting the oxygen dissociation curve to the left and reducing cellular uptake of oxygen from haemoglobin. The resultant carbon dioxide will increase respiratory drive in an already acidaemic patient and, in the mechanically ventilated patient, will require an increase in minute ventilation. However, in the presence of profound acidaemia (pH < 7.1) when the excess H^+ ions may directly depress myocardial function, cardiac arrest associated with hyperkalaemia, or following tricyclic antidepressant overdose, small amounts of bicarbonate (0.5–1 mmol kg^{-1}) may be given. This should be guided by known acid-base status and its effect monitored by frequent arterial blood gas analysis.

Hyperglycaemia is believed to have detrimental effects on neurological outcome because high glucose levels provide substrate for continued anaerobic metabolism during ischaemia and low flow states [4]. Animal studies have demonstrated negative effects of hyperglycaemia after cardiac arrest [5,6]. Although this has never been proven after cardiac arrest in human studies, most clinicians would treat high blood glucose levels appropriately with insulin. The detrimental effects of prolonged hypoglycaemia are well documented and include disruption of cerebral blood flow autoregulation and reduced membrane stability [7]. After cardiac arrest, normoglycaemia (blood glucose 4–8 mmol dL^{-1}) is the aim and hypoglycaemia must be avoided.

3.3.3. TRANSPORT TO CCU/ICU

The most appropriate time to transfer the patient to the CCU or ICU will depend on the condition of the patient and where ROSC was achieved. Patients who have ROSC after only a short period of CPR, and have regained consciousness and have a stable rhythm, can be transferred rapidly to the CCU. After CPR, the indications for the transfer of a patient to the ICU include:
- Those who remain comatose with inability to protect the airway.
- The continued need for intubation, either for airway protection, or to provide mechanical ventilation. Mechanical ventilation will be required for comatose patients with inadequate ventilation or for patients who have sustained lung injury such as aspiration pneumonitis or contusion (from chest compressions).
- Haemodynamic instability that requires invasive monitoring and pharmacological or mechanical support which may not be available on the CCU.

The decision to transfer a patient to the ICU should be made only after discussion with senior members of the ICU team. Shortly after ROSC, it is impossible to predict the outcome of those patients remaining comatose (see below). Therefore, unless intensive care is otherwise inappropriate, liberal admission criteria are justified. Comatose and hypotensive patients will require interventions to achieve stability of the respiratory and cardiovascular systems. The resuscitation room of an emergency department may be well enough equipped to allow the clinician time to achieve full stabilisation before transfer to the ICU. This may include placement of invasive monitoring lines (arterial, central venous pressure) and commencement of infusions of inotropes. On the other hand, only immediately life-saving interventions should delay the transfer of a patient from a poorly equipped general ward.

Continuous monitoring (ECG with defibrillator, blood pressure, pulse oximetry and, if intubated, end-tidal CO_2) is essential during the transfer. The ICU team will usually have a transfer box containing all the relevant equipment and drugs for management of the airway and circulation. The transport trolley must be equipped with portable suction and an oxygen supply.

3.3.4. LIMIT ORGAN DAMAGE

The goal of critical care management after successful ROSC is to provide conditions that will maximise the potential for organ recovery. In the awake, spontaneously breathing patient this can be achieved on a CCU. Other postcardiac arrest patients will require the facilities and staffing levels provided by an ICU.

MYOCARDIUM

An adequate coronary perfusion pressure is essential to oxygenate the recovering myocardium. Consider the patient's normal blood pressure and avoid hypotension. Where cardiac arrest has been precipitated by myocardial infarction, urgent consideration should be given to the possibility of restoring coronary artery patency with thrombolytic drugs [8,9] or angioplasty. Coronary artery reperfusion using thrombolytic agents may provoke further arrhythmias.

Indications for Thrombolytic Therapy

— Chest pain suggestive of myocardial infarction lasting more than 30 min with ST-segment elevation > 0.2 mV in two or more adjacent chest leads, or > 0.1 mV in limb leads. Presumed new LBBB with typical history is also an indication.
— Time from onset of symptoms < 12 h.

Absolute Contraindications to Thrombolytic Therapy

— Major surgery, organ biopsy or trauma within 6 weeks.
— Gastro-Intestinal or Genito-Urinary bleeding within 6 months.
— History of bleeding disorder.
— Known or suspected aortic dissection.
— Known or suspected pericarditis.
— Stroke within 6 months.
— Known intracranial tumour or previous neurosurgery.
— Head trauma within one month.

Relative Contraindications to Thrombolytic Therapy

— Noncompressible vascular puncture.
— CPR greater than 10 min.
— Systolic blood pressure > 200 mmHg or diastolic blood pressure > 110 mmHg despite treatment.
— Recent Transient Ischaemic Attack or any previous stroke.
— Known or suspected active peptic ulceration.
— Pregnancy or < 10 days postpartum.
— Oral anticoagulation treatment.
— Source of clot such as abdominal aneurysm or large fibrillating atrium.
— Higher risk with small body size, > 75 years old.

BRAIN

Early after ROSC, there is a period of cerebral hyperaemia. However, this is maldistributed,

and there is likely to be some regional ischaemia. After 15–30 min of reperfusion, global cerebral blood flow decreases, resulting in generalised hypoperfusion. This situation may exist for 18–24 h after which regional cerebral blood flow may improve, correlating with functional recovery, or decline, resulting in progressive ischaemic damage and cell death. The available evidence indicates that intracranial pressure does not increase immediately after ROSC and therefore is not a major influence on early cerebral perfusion pressure. After a period of global ischaemia the normal cerebral autoregulation is lost, leaving cerebral perfusion dependent on mean arterial pressure [10,11]. At this stage, hypotension will severely compromise cerebral blood flow and will compound any neurological injury. Thus, after ROSC, mean arterial pressure should be maintained at that patient's normal level, using appropriate inotropes and fluids.

There is no good clinical evidence supporting any particular duration for elective mechanical ventilation after prolonged cardiac arrest. However, many clinicians elect to continue ventilation for 24 h in an effort to optimise the conditions for neurological recovery. The PaCO$_2$ should be maintained in the low to normal range (see above).

SEDATION

Intubated patients may require sedation and analgesia to prevent coughing or to counteract restlessness and anxiety. These stimuli will increase cerebral metabolism and cerebral oxygen consumption at a time when cerebral oxygen supply may be compromised. Adequate sedation will reduce cerebral oxygen consumption and optimise the conditions for neurological recovery. Agents with short elimination half-lives and lack of active metabolites (e.g., propofol) are the most suitable.

Temperature Control

Cerebral metabolic rate changes by about 8% per degree Celsius change in body temperature. An increase in regional cerebral metabolic rate may create imbalance between oxygen supply and demand and several animal studies have documented that even modest hyperthermia worsens outcome after an ischaemic insult [12,13]. In the postresuscitation period, hyperthermia must be treated aggressively.

Hypothermia reduces cerebral metabolic activity and controlled hypothermia is used successfully for cerebral protection during a variety of surgical procedures. In head injured patients with Glasgow coma scores of 5 to 7 on admission, treatment with moderate hypothermia (33°C) for 24 h improved outcome [14]. Animal studies have shown that after cardiac arrest, the beneficial effect of hypothermia reduces significantly when induced more than 15 min after resuscitation [2]. A recent human study has suggested an improved outcome following induction of moderate hypothermia in 22 patients initially surviving out of hospital cardiac arrest [15]. However, this study used historic controls and we must await the results of larger, prospective, randomised, controlled studies before routinely inducing hypothermia during postresuscitation care. Well recognised detrimental effects of hypothermia include increased blood viscosity, decreased cardiac output, and an increased susceptibility to infection.

Anticonvulsant Therapy

Seizures occur in about 5−15% of adult postarrest patients [16]. Seizures increase cerebral metabolism by up to 3−4 times and prolonged seizure activity can cause cerebral injury [17]. Seizures should be controlled with benzodiazepines, phenytoin, or a barbiturate.

Neuroprotective Drugs

A variety of drugs purported to have neuroprotective effects in animal studies have undergone clinical trials. Barbiturates [18] and calcium entry blocking drugs [19] have failed to improve outcome when given to humans after cardiac arrest.

RENAL FUNCTION

Urine output is a good monitor of renal perfusion. With the exception of those patients who had a very short period of CPR and rapid return to consciousness, all patients will require a urinary catheter and hourly measurements of urine. Prerenal oliguria should be treated with fluid and/or inotrope therapy, as appropriate. Patients who have had prolonged CPR and a long period of hypotension are at significant risk of acute tubular necrosis (ATN). This will require continuous renal replacement therapy (e.g., continuous veno-venous haemofiltration). In the absence of renal cortical necrosis, ATN will resolve spontaneously in 2−4 weeks.

3.3.5. PREDICTION OF NONSURVIVORS

Those working in critical care have a moral, ethical, and financial responsibility to treat only those patients who will benefit from it. About 80% of patients successfully resuscitated remain unconscious for variable lengths of time [20].The ability to accurately predict neurological outcome soon after ROSC remains an elusive goal [21]. One of the largest studies of prognostication following cardiac arrest followed up 262 patients who remained comatose 10 min after ROSC [22]. At this stage, the absence of pupil light response predicted poor outcome (death or persistent vegetative state) in 82% of cases. However, 16 of the 89 patients with absent pupil light response at this stage survived to regain consciousness. By day 3, absence of motor response to pain and absence of pupil light response both predicted permanent vegetative state or death with 100% accuracy. The authors concluded that after 3 days of observation in ICU, a sufficiently precise clinical prediction of poor neurological outcome can be made to allow limitation of further life support. Others have supported this conclusion [23]. In another study, a Glasgow coma score of < 5 on day 2 predicted severe cerebral disability or death in all 70 patients [24]. Among 63 patients resuscitated from cardiac arrest, no survivor had absence of corneal reflex, pupillary reflex, or reflex eye movement (oculocephalic, oculovestibular) by 6 h after cardiac arrest [25]. Using brain stem reflexes, Jorgensen was able to differentiate those patients who will regain consciousness from those who will remain unconscious within an hour of cardiac arrest [26]. However, this work has yet to be validated. Long-latency evoked potentials [27] and cerebrospinal fluid creatine kinase BB isoenzyme [28] also have the potential to predict outcome after CPR but neither are in routine clinical use.

3.3.6. CARE OF THE CARDIAC ARREST TEAM

All attempts at resuscitation should be formally audited. Audit data should be recorded using the standard Utstein template to allow comparison between different institutions. Regardless of outcome, the team should be debriefed at the earliest opportunity. This should take the form of positive critique and not develop a fault/blame culture. Whether the resuscitation attempt was successful or not, the patient's relatives will require considerable support. Equally, the pastoral needs of all those associated with the arrest, no matter how hard they may seem, should not be forgotten.

3.3.7. REFERENCES

1. Steen PA, Edgren E, Gustafson, Fuentes CG. Cerebral protection and postresuscitation care. A statement for the Advanced Life Support Working Party of the European Resuscitation Council. Resuscitation 1992;24: 233–237.

2. Abramson NS, Ebmeyer U, Wrad KR, Neumar RW. Bringing it all together; brain-orientated postresuscitation critical care. In, Paradis NA, Halperin HR, Nowak RM, editors, Cardiac Arrest. The Science and Practice of Resuscitation Medicine. Baltimore: Williams & Wilkins, 1996;923–934.

3. Muzilaar JP, Marmarou A, Ward JD et al. Adverse effects of prolonged hyperventilation in patients with severe head injury: a randomized clinical trial. J Neurosurg 1991;75:731–739.

4. Pulsineli W, Waldman S, Rawlinson D et al. Moderate hyperglycaemia augments ischemic brain damage: neuropathologic study in the rat. Neurology 1982;32: 1239–1246.

5. D'Alecy LG, Lundy EF, Barton KJ et al. Dextrose containing intravenous fluid impairs outcome and increases death after eight minutes of cardiac arrest and resuscitation in dogs. Surgery 1986;100:505–511.

6. Myers RE, Yamaguchi S. Nervous system effects of cardiac arrest in monkeys. Arch Neurol 1977;34: 65–74.

7. Ceber F, Koehler R, Derrer S et al. Hypoglycaemia and cerebral autoregulation in anesthetized dogs. Am J Physiol 1990;258:H1714–H1721.

8. Collins R, Peto R, Baigent C, Sleight P. Aspirin, heparin, and fibrinolytic therapy in suspected acute myocardial infarction. N Engl J Med 1997;336:847–860.

9. Gershlick AH, More RS. Treatment of myocardial infarction. Br Med J 1998;316:280–284.

10. Nemoto EM, Snyder JV, Carrol RG, Morita H. Global ischaemia in dogs: cerebrovascular CO_2 reactivity and autoregulation. Stroke 1975;6:425–431.

11. Kågström E, Smith ML, Siesjö BK. Cerebral circulatory responses to hypercapnia and hyperoxia in the recovery period following complete and incomplete ischemia in the rat. Acta Physiol Scand 1983;118:281–291.

12. Busto R, Dietrich WD, Globus MY-T et al. Small differences in intraischemic brain temperature critically determine the extent of ischemic neuronal injury. J Cereb Blood Flow Metab 1987;7:729–738.

13. Minamisawa H, Smith M, Siesjö BK. The effect of mild hyperthermia and hypothermia on brain damage following 5, 10, and 15 minutes of forebrain ischaemia. Ann Neurol 1990;28:26–33.

14. Marion DW, Penrod LE, Kelsey SF et al. Treatment of traumatic brain injury with moderate hypothermia. N Engl J Med 1997;336:540–546.

15. Bernard SA, Jones BMacC, Horne M. Clinical trial of induced hypothermia in comatose survivors of out-of-hospital cardiac arrest. Ann Emerg Med 1997; 30:146–153.

16. Roine RO, Kaste M, Kinnunen A et al. Nimodipine after resuscitation from out-of-hospital ventricular fibrillation. A placebo controlled double-blind randomized trial. J Am Med Ass 1990;264:3171–3177.

17. Nevander G, Ingvar M, Auer R, Siesjö BK. Status epilepticus in well-oxygenated rats causes neuronal necrosis. Ann Neurol 1985;18:281–290.

18. Brain Resuscitation Clinical Trial I Study Group. Randomized trial of thiopental loading in comatose survivors of cardiac arrest. N Engl J Med 1986;314: 397–403.

19. Brain Resuscitation Clinical Trial II Study Group. A randomized clinical study of a calcium-entry blocker (lidoflazine) in the treatment of comatose survivors of cardiac arrest. N Engl J Med 1991;324:1225–1231.

20. Longstreth WT, Diehr P, Inui TS. Prediction of awa-

kening after out of hospital cardiac arrest. N Engl J Med 1983;308:1378—1382.

21. Longstreth WT, Dikmen SS. Outcomes after cardiac arrest. Ann Emerg Med 1993;22:64—69.

22. Edgren E, Hedstand U, Kelsey S, Sutton-Tyrrell, Safar P. Assessment of neurological prognosis in comatose survivors of cardiac arrest. Lancet 1994;343:1055—1059.

23. Eleff SM, Hanley DF. Postresuscitation prognostication and declaration of brain death. In: Paradis NA, Halperin HR, Nowak RM (eds) Cardiac Arrest. The Science and Practice of Resuscitation Medicine. Baltimore: Williams & Wilkins, 1996;910—922.

24. Mullie A, Verstringe P, Buylaert W et al. Predictive value of glasgow coma score for awakening after out-of-hospital cardiac arrest. Lancet 1988;I:137—140.

25. Snyder BD, Gumnit RJ, Leppik IE, Hauser WA, Loewenson RB, Ramirez-Lassepas M. Neurologic prognosis after cardiopulmonary arrest. IV. Brainstem reflexes. Neurology 1981;31:1092—1097.

26. Jorgensen EO. Course of neurological recovery and cerebral prognostic signs during cardio-pulmonary resuscitation. Resuscitation 1997;35:9—16.

27. Madl C, Grimm G, Kramer L et al. Early prediction of individual outcome after cardiopulmonary resuscitation. Lancet 1993;341:855—858.

28. Tirschwell DL, Longstreth WT, Rauch-Mathews ME et al. Cerebrospinal fluid creatine kinase BB isoenzyme activity and neurologic prognosis after cardiac arrest. Neurology 1997;48:352—357.

4. Paediatric Life Support

CONTENTS:

4.1. Introduction

The Paediatric Working Group of the European Resuscitation Council published its recommendations for Paediatric Life Support in 1994 [1]. In 1997 the International Liaison Committee on Resuscitation (ILCOR) presented and published its deliberations [2] following examination of the recommendations of the American Heart Association [3], the Heart and Stroke Foundation of Canada, The European Resuscitation Council [1], the Australian Resuscitation Council [4] and the Resuscitation Council of Southern Africa [5]. The ILCOR document presented a framework of consensus for each national body to develop its own guidelines based on published data and peer-reviewed knowledge. It is interesting to note that the ILCOR working group found that few differences existed among the current national guidelines for paediatric life support.

The ERC paediatric working group has re-evaluated its 1994 recommendations in the light of the ILCOR statement. It discussed the points raised in the ILCOR statement and found no fundamental differences in the approach to or the procedures for paediatric life support. The following major changes in the basic life support protocol were agreed:

1. **Age definitions** – the ERC working group supported the ILCOR approach of trying to define an infant, child and adult based on considerations of anatomy, physiology and epidemiology. The definition of an infant as a child of less than 1 year of age remained unchanged. The working group agreed to adopt the definition of a young child as one up to approximately 8 years of age and an older child as greater than 8 years of age based mainly on anatomical and epidemiological considerations.

2. **Pulse check** – the ERC working group agreed to modify its recommendations for pulse check in line with the ILCOR statement following consideration of the recently published data on the reliability [6,7] and usefulness [8] of this procedure. The revised recommendations deal with the difficulty in making an accurate pulse check by recommending that if a pulse is not confidently detected within 10 s then further resuscitation interventions should not be delayed.

3. **Chest compressions (depth)** – the ERC working group agreed to modify its recommendations for the depth of chest compression from an absolute measurement to one of relative depth. It is now recommended to compress the chest to one-third of the resting chest diameter. The working group also endorsed the need for assessment of effectiveness of chest compression by the palpation of pulses, evaluation of carbon dioxide measurements and the analysis of arterial pressure waveforms.

In Paediatric Advanced Life Support the ERC working group agreed to adopt the concept of the ILCOR universal paediatric template thus simplifying the final treatment pathways in the algorithm to two:

1. *Nonventricular Fibrillation / Nonventricular Tachycardia* (including asystole and electromechanical dissociation).
2. *Ventricular Fibrillation / Ventricular Tachycardia*

This algorithm closely resembles that proposed for adult advanced life support. The ERC working group wished to emphasise the importance of the difference in epidemiology of paediatric from adult resuscitation by placing the Nonventricular Fibrillation/Nonventricular Tachycardia (the right hand pathway) first.

The following documentation is therefore a "sequence of actions" based on the original ERC paediatric life support recommendations [1] but reflecting the changes described above. A paediatric life support training programme has been appended to illustrate the minimum skill base required.

The document "Recommendations for Resuscitation of Babies at Birth" is a new document that was prepared by the European Resuscitation Council, which also reflects the recommendations of ILCOR [2], the American Heart Association [9] and the UK [10].

REFERENCES

1. European Resuscitation Council. Guidelines for paediatric life support. Resuscitation 1994;27:91–106.
2. Nadkarni V, Hazinski MF, Zideman DA, Kattwinkel J, Quan L, Bingham R, Zaritsky A, Bland J, Kramer E, Tiballs J. Paediatric life support: an advisory statement by the Paediatric Life Support Working Group of the International Liaison Committee on Resuscitation. Resuscitation 1997;34:115–127.
3. Emergency Cardiac Care Committee and Subcommittees of the American Heart Association. Guidelines for cardiopulmonary resuscitation and emergency cardiac care. J Am Med Assoc 1992;268:2171–2302.
4. Advanced Life Support Committee of the Australian Resuscitation Council. Paediatric advanced life support: the Australian Resuscitation Council guidelines. Med J Aust 1996;165:199–206.
5. Kloeck WGJ. Resuscitation Council of Southern Africa Guidelines: new recommendations for basic life support in adults, children and infants; obstructed airway in adults, children and infants; advanced life support for adults and children. Trauma Emerg Med 1993; 10(1):738–771.
6. Mather C, O'Kelly S. The palpation of pulses. Anaesthesia 1996;51:189–191.
7. Brearley S, Simms M, Shearman C. Peripheral pulse palpation: an unreliable sign. Yawn Roy Coll Surgeons 1992;74:169–172.
8. Connick M, Berg R. Femoral venous pulsations during open-heart cardiac massage. Yawn Emerg Med 1994; 24(6):1176–1179.
9. American Heart Association. Neonatal advanced life support. J Am Med Assoc 1996;255:2969–2973.
10. Royal College of Paediatrics and Child Health. Resuscitation of Babies at Birth. BMJ Publishing Group, 1997.

4.2. International Liaison Committee on Resuscitation: Paediatric Working Group Advisory Statement*

Writing group:
Vinay Nadkarni (Chairman, AHA), Mary Fran Hazinski (AHA), David Zideman (ERC), John Kattwinkel (AHA,AAP), Linda Quan (AHA), Robert Bingham (ERC), Arno Zaritsky (AHA), Jon Bland (ERC), Efraim Kramer (RCSA), James Tiballs (ARC).

Paediatric ILCOR participants:
Robert Bingham (ERC), David Burchfield (AHA/AAP), Brian Conolly (HSFC), Leon Chameides (AHA), Mary Fran Hazinski (AHA), John Kattwinkel (AHA,AAP), Efraim Kramer (RCSA), Vinay Nadkarni (AHA), Linda Quan (AHA), F.G. Stoddard (AHA), James Tiballs (ARC), Patrick Van Reempst (ERC), Arno Zaritsky (AHA), David Zideman (ERC), Jelka Zupan (WHO).

4.2.1. PURPOSE

This summary document reflects the deliberation of the Paediatric Working Group of the International Liaison Committee on Resuscitation (ILCOR). The ILCOR's goal is to improve consistency of guidelines issued by international resuscitation councils and associations. The purpose of this summary is to highlight areas of conflict or controversy in current paediatric basic and advanced life support guidelines [2–6], outline solutions considered, and recommendations reached by consensus of the Working Group. We also list unresolved issues and highlight a few areas of active guideline research interest and investigation. This document does not include a complete list of guidelines for which there is no perceived controversy. The algorithm/decision tree figures presented attempt to illustrate a common flow of assessments and interventions. Whenever possible, this has been coordinated to complement the BLS and ALS algorithms used for adult victims. Since arrest of the newly born infant presents unique resuscitation challenges in terms of etiology, physiology and required resources, we have developed a separate section addressing initial resuscitation of the newly born. Other areas of departure from the adult algorithms are noted and rationale explained in text.

In the absence of specific paediatric data (outcome validity), recommendations may be made or supported on the basis of common sense (face validity) or ease of teaching or skill retention (construct validity). Practicality of recommendations in the context of local resources (technology and personnel) and customs must always be considered. In compiling this document, it was surprising to the working group participants how few differences exist among current Paediatric guidelines advocated by the American Heart Association, Heart and Stroke Foundation of Canada, European Resuscitation Council, Australian Resuscitation Council, and Resuscitation Council of Southern Africa.

4.2.2. BACKGROUND

The epidemiology and outcome of paediatric cardiopulmonary arrest and the priorities, techniques and sequence of paediatric resuscitation assess-

*This statement was published in *Resuscitation* 1997 [1]

ments and interventions differ from those of adults. As a result, it is imperative that any guidelines developed for paediatric resuscitation address the unique needs of the newly born, infant, child and young adult. Unfortunately, specific data supporting these differences have been deficient in both quantity and quality for several reasons: a) paediatric cardiac arrest is uncommon, b) in most circumstances, survival from documented asystolic paediatric cardiac arrest is dismal, and c) most paediatric studies have failed to utilize consistent patient inclusion criteria and resuscitation outcome definitions and measures. Additional paediatric-specific data including data for the newly born are required to confirm or further refine paediatric resuscitation techniques.

In general, prehospital primary cardiac arrest is a less common etiology of arrest in children and young adults than in older adults [7–9], and primary respiratory arrest appears to be a more common etiology than primary cardiac arrest in children [10–14]. However, most reports of paediatric arrest contain insufficient patient numbers or utilize exclusion criteria that prohibit broad generalization of study results to general or international paediatric populations. In a 15-year retrospective study of prehospital cardiac arrest from the USA, only 7% of 10,992 victims of prehospital cardiac arrest were younger than 30 years, and only 3.7% were younger than 8 years [7]. Only 2% of victims of in-hospital cardiopulmonary resuscitation in the UK were 0–14 years of age [15].

Cardiac arrest in children is rarely sudden; it is typically the end result of deterioration in respiratory function or shock, and the terminal rhythm is typically bradycardia with progression to electrical mechanical dissociation or asystole [16,17]. Ventricular tachycardia and fibrillation have been reported in 15% or less of a subset of paediatric and adolescent victims of prehospital cardiac arrest [7,8], even when rhythm is assessed by first responders [18,19].

Survival following prehospital cardiopulmonary arrest averages only approximately 3–17% in most studies, and survivors are often neurologically devastated [8,10–12,16,18–24]. In addi-

tion, most paediatric resuscitation reports are retrospective in design and plagued with inconsistent resuscitation definitions and patient inclusion criteria. As a result, conclusions based upon statistical analysis of the efficacy of specific resuscitative efforts are unreliable. Some of these problems should be improved by application of uniform guidelines for reporting outcomes of advanced life support interventions outlined in the Paediatric Utstein-Style Guidelines [25]. Large, randomized, multicenter and multinational clinical trials are clearly needed.

AGE definitions: what defines an infant, child and adult?

The age of the victim is currently the primary characteristic which guides decisions for application of resuscitation sequences and techniques. Discrimination on the basis of age alone is inadequate. Further, any single age delineation of the "child" vs. the "adult" is arbitrary because there is no single parameter that separates the infant from the child from the adult. The following factors should be considered:

1. *Anatomy*: There is consensus that the age cutoff for infants should be at approximately 1 year. In general, cardiac compression can be accomplished using one hand for victims up to the age of approximately 8 years. However, variability in the size of the victim or the size and strength of the rescuer can require use of the two-handed "adult" compression technique for cardiac compression. For instance, the chronically ill infant may be sufficiently small to enable compression using circular hand technique, and a large 6- or 7-year-old may be too large for one-hand compression technique. A small rescuer may need to use two hands to effectively compress the chest of a child victim.

2. *Physiology*: The newly born infant provides an example of how physiologic considerations may affect resuscitative interventions. Perinatal circulatory changes during transition from fetus to newborn may result in profound extrapulmon-

ary shunting of blood. Fluid-filled alveoli may require higher initial ventilation pressures than subsequent rescue breathing. Lung inspiratory and expiratory time constants for filling and emptying and inflation volumes may need to be adjusted according to both anatomic and physiologic development.

3. *Epidemiology:* Ideally, the sequence of resuscitation should be determined by the most likely cause of the arrest. In the newly born infant, this will be most likely related to respiratory failure. In the older infant and child, it may be related to progression of respiratory failure, shock, or neurologic dysfunction. In general, paediatric prehospital arrest has been characterized as hypoxic, hypercarbic arrest, with respiratory arrest preceding asystolic cardiac arrest [11,26,27]. Therefore, a focus on early ventilation and early CPR (rather than early EMS activation and/or defibrillation) appears to be warranted. *Early effective oxygenation and ventilation must be established as quickly as possible.* Primary dysrhythmic cardiac arrest may occur, and should particularly be considered in patients with underlying cardiac diseaseor history consistent with myocarditis.

Resuscitation sequence/EMS activation

Local response intervals, dispatcher training and EMS protocols may dictate the sequence of early life support interventions. In addition, the sequence of resuscitation actions must consider the most likely causes of arrest in the victims. Respiratory failure and/or trauma may be primary etiologies of cardiopulmonary arrest in victims up to 40 years of age [7,9], with a relatively low incidence of primary ventricular fibrillation. One critical issue in determining the sequence of interventions is whether the primary cause of arrest is due to a cardiac or respiratory etiology. Probability of successful resuscitation based on that etiology is another important unresolved resuscitation question.

4.2.3. PAEDIATRIC BASIC LIFE SUPPORT

Determination of Responsiveness

Unresponsiveness mandates assessment and support of airway and breathing. Patients with suspected cervical spinal injury and infants should not be shaken to assess responsiveness.

Airway

Consensus continues to support use of the head tilt-chin lift or the jaw thrust (the jaw thrust especially when cervical spine instability or neck trauma is suspected) to open the airway. Other maneuvers, such as the tongue-jaw lift may be considered if initial ventilation is unsuccessful despite repositioning of the head. The most common cause of airway obstruction in the unconscious paediatric victim is the tongue [28]. Although the use of a tongue-jaw lift and visual mouth inspection prior to ventilation of any unconscious infant may be considered if foreign body airway obstruction is strongly suspected, there are no data to support the delay of attempted ventilation in all victims. Blind removal or attempted visualization of unsuspected foreign bodies is not likely to be effective for the following reasons: foreign bodies causing complete airway obstruction are unlikely to be visible with cursory inspection, the object may not be retrievable, and attempted intervention may result in displacement of the object further into the trachea. More data are needed regarding the optimal method of maintaining the airway in an open position to ensure effective ventilation during CPR.

Breathing

There is general consensus regarding the technique for rescue breathing for infants and children. The current recommendations for initial number of attempted breaths, however, vary from 2 to 5 [2−6]. There are no data to support any specific number of initial breaths. There was agreement that a minimum of two breaths be

MANOEUVRE	ADULT AND OLDER CHILD	YOUNG CHILD	INFANT	NEWBORN	CPR/RESCUE BREATHING
	Older child and adult	Approximately 1–8 years	Less than 1 year	Newly born	CHECK RESPONSIVENESS
AIRWAY	Head tilt-chin lift (If trauma, use jaw thrust)	Head tilt-chin lift (If trauma, use jaw thrust)	Head tilt-chin lift (If trauma, use jaw thrust)	Head tilt-chin lift (If trauma, use jaw thrust)	Open Airway Activate EMS
BREATHING Initial	2–5 breaths at approximately 1 1/2 s per breath	2–5 breaths at approximately 1 1/2 s per breath	2–5 breaths at approximately 1 1/2 s per breath	2–5 breaths at approximately 1 s per breath	CHECK BREATHING: If victim breathing: Place in recovery position
Subsequent	12 breaths/min (approximate)	20 breaths/min (approximate)	20 breaths/min (approximate)	30–60 breaths/min (approximate)	If no chest rise, Reposition airway and reattempt up to 5 times
Foreign body airway obstruction	Abdominal thrusts or back blows	Abdominal thrusts or back blows or chest thrusts	Back blows or chest thrusts (No abdominal thrusts)	Suction, (No abdominal thrusts or back blows)	
CIRCULATION					ASSESS FOR SIGNS OF LIFE:
Pulse check (Trained healthcare providers only*)	*Carotid	*Carotid	*Brachial	*Umbilical	If pulse present but breathing absent: provide rescue breaths
Compression landmarks	Lower half of sternum	Lower half of sternum	One finger width below intermammary line	*One finger width below intermammary line	If pulse not confidently felt > 60/min and poor perfusion: chest compressions
Compression method	Heel of one hand, other hand on top	Heel of one hand	Two or three fingers	*Two fingers or Encircling thumbs	
Compression depth	Approximately 1/3 the depth of the chest	Approximately 1/3 the depth of the chest	Approximately 1/3 the depth of the chest	*Approximately 1/3 the depth of the chest	Continue BLS: Integrate procedures appropriate for newborn, paediatric, or adult advanced life support at earliest opportunity
Compression rate	Approximately 100/min	Approximately 100/min	Approximately 100/min	*Approximately 120/min	
Compression/ ventilation ratio	15:2 (Single rescuer) 5:1 (Two rescuers)	5:1	5:1	3:1	

*Interventions recommended for suitably trained healthcare providers only.

FIG. 1. Paediatric Basic Life Support — a comparison of techniques at different ages.

attempted. The rationale for attempting to deliver more than two initial ventilations include: the need to provide effective ventilation for paediatric victims is based upon the likely hypoxic and hypercarbic etiology of arrest, suspected inability of the lay rescuer to establish effective ventilation with only two attempts, clinical impressions that more than two breaths may be required to improve oxygenation and restore effective heart rate in the apneic, bradycardic infant.

Initial breaths should be delivered slowly, over 1–1.5 s, with a force sufficient to make the chest clearly rise. Care and attention to abdominal distention caused by insufflation of gas into the stomach should be recognized and avoided [29–31].

Consideration of the optimal method for delivering breaths to infants supports the current recommendation of mouth to mouth-and-nose ventilation for infants up to 1 year of age. However, mouth-to-nose ventilation may be adequate in this population [32,33].

Consensus continues to support the emphasis on the provision of more ventilation (breaths per minute) for infants and children and more compressions per minute for adult victims. Current recommended ventilation rates are based on normal ventilatory rates for age, the need for coordination with chest compression and the perceived practical ability of the rescuer to provide them. Ideal ventilation frequency during CPR is unknown.

Circulation

Pulse Check

There is a lack of specific paediatric data on the accuracy and time course for determining pulselessness of victims who are apneic and unresponsive. Several reports have documented the inability of lay rescuers and health care providers to reliably locate or count the pulse of the victim [34,35]. The use of the pulse check during pae-

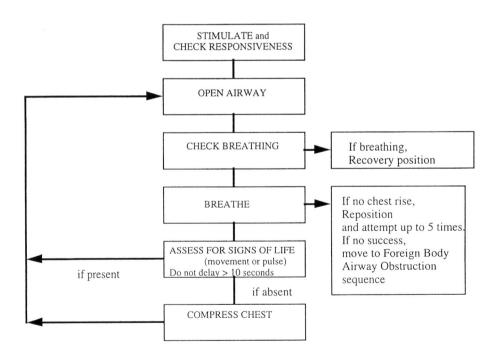

FIG. 2. ILCOR Universal Paediatric Basic Life Support Template

diatric CPR has been questioned [36]. Furthermore, the pulse check is difficult to teach to lay persons. It seems reasonable for health care providers to search for a pulse because it may be palpated by trained personnel, does not require sophisticated equipment, and there is no better alternative. However, resuscitative interventions should NOT be delayed beyond 10 s if a pulse is not confidently detected.

Chest Compression

WHEN TO START

There is consensus that all pulseless patients and patients determined to have heart rates too low to adequately perfuse vital organs warrant chest compressions. Because cardiac output in infancy and childhood is largely heart rate dependent, profound bradycardia is usually considered an indication for cardiac compressions.

LOCATION OF COMPRESSION

There is consensus for compression over the lower half of the sternum, taking care to avoid compression of the xiphoid.

DEPTH

Consensus supports recommendation of relative rather than absolute depth of compression (e.g., compress approximately one-third of the depth of the chest rather than compression of 4–5 cm depth).

Effectiveness of compression should be assessed by the health care provider. Methods of assessment include palpation of pulses, evaluation of end-tidal carbon dioxide, analysis of arterial pressure waveform (if inta-arterial monitoring is in place). Although it is recognized that pulses palpated during chest compression may reflect venous rather than arterial blood flow during CPR [37], pulse detection during CPR for health care providers remains the most universally practical "quick assessment" of chest compression efficacy.

RATE

Consensus supports a compression rate of approximately 100/min. With interposed ventilations, this will result in the actual delivery of less than 100 compressions to the patient in a 1-min period.

Compression – Ventilation Ratio

Ideal compression/ventilation ratios for infants and children are unknown. A single, universal compression ventilation ratio for all ages and both BLS and ALS interventions would be desirable from an educational standpoint. There is consensus among resuscitation councils currently for a compression to ventilation ratio of 3:1 for newborns and 5:1 for infants and children. The justification for this difference from adult guidelines includes: 1) respiratory problems are the most common etiology of paediatric arrest and therefore ventilation should be emphasized, and 2) physiologic respiratory rates of infants and children are faster than for adults, Although the actual number of delivered interventions is dependent on the amount of time the rescuer spends opening the airway and the effect of frequent airway repositioning on rescuer fatigue, there is insufficient evidence to justify changing the current recommendations for educational convenience at this time.

External chest compression must always be accompanied by rescue breathing in children. At the end of every compression cycle, a rescue breath should be given. Interposition of compressions and ventilations is recommended to avoid simultaneous compression/ventilation.

Activation of the EMS System

Ideally, the sequence of resuscitation is determined by the aetiology of the arrest. In paediatric arrest, dysrhythmias requiring defibrillation are relatively uncommon and some data suggest that early bystander CPR is associated with improved survival [10,37,38]. However, it is impractical to teach the lay public different resuscitation sequences based on arrest etiology. The consensus recommendation is ''phone fast'' rather than ''phone first'' for young victims of cardiac arrest, but the appropriate ''age cutoff'' for this recommendation remains to be determined. Local EMS response intervals and the availability of dispatcher-guided CPR may override these considerations.

Recovery Position

Although many recovery positions are used in the management of paediatric patients, particularly in those emerging from anaesthesia, no specific optimal recovery position can be universally endorsed on the basis of scientific study in children. There is consensus that an ideal recovery position considers the following: etiology of the arrest and stability of the C-spine, risk for aspiration, attention to pressure points, ability to monitor adequacy of ventilation and perfusion, maintenance of a patent airway, and access to the patient for interventions.

Relief of Foreign-Body Airway Obstruction

Consensus supports prompt recognition and treatment of complete airway obstruction. There are three suggested maneuvers to remove impacted foreign bodies: back blows, chest thrusts, and abdominal thrusts. The sequences differ slightly among resuscitation councils exist, but published data do not convincingly support one technique sequence over another. There is consensus that the lack of protection of the upper abdominal organs by the rib cage renders infants and newborns at risk of iatrogenic trauma from abdominal thrusts; therefore abdominal thrusts are not recommended in infants and newborns. An additional practical consideration is that back blows should be delivered with the victim positioned head down, which may be physically difficult in older children. Suctioning is recommended for newborns, rather than back blows which are potentially harmful to this age group.

Barrier Equipment

Health care professionals should utilize appropriate barrier devices and universal precautions whenever possible. However, issues related to efficacy of the devices in preventing bacterial or viral transmission, anatomical fit of masks, use of devices in paediatric patients with increased airway resistance and dead space ventilation, and the actual risk of paediatric disease transmissibility during paediatric resuscitative interventions are not resolved.

4.2.4. PAEDIATRIC ADVANCED LIFE SUPPORT

Automated External Defibrillators (AEDs) in Paediatrics

The true prevalence of ventricular fibrillation among paediatric victims of cardiopulmonary arrest is unknown. Early rhythm assessment for paediatric prehospital arrest is not frequently reported or reliable. In most studies, pulseless ventricular tachycardia or ventricular fibrillation have been documented in less than 10% of all paediatric arrest victims [7,16–18,39], even when the victim was evaluated by first responders within 6.2 min of emergency medical service call [8,19]. In some studies, ventricular fibrillation treated with early defibrillation, both at the scene and in the hospital, may result in better survival rates than those treated for asystole or electromechanical dissociation [21]. However, other studies contradict these data [18,19]. The development of AEDs have not yet addressed the energy levels required to treat ventricular tachycardia or fibrillation in children, or the reliability of these devices in the detection of ventricular tachycardia and fibrillation in children. The age-appropriate application of AEDs is assumed to be similar to current guidelines for initial defibrillator placement and energy delivery. Therefore, the conditions under which early detection and treatment of ventricular fibrillation should be emphasised requires further research.

Vascular Access

Vascular access for the arrested victim is needed for the delivery of resuscitative fluids and medications. However, establishment of adequate ventilation with BLS support of circulation is the first priority. The intravenous or intraosseous route for the delivery of medications is the preferred route [40–44], but the endotracheal route can be used for circumstances when vascular access is delayed. It is likely that drug delivery following endotracheal adrenaline epinephrine administration may be lower than that delivered by the intravascular approach. Drug doses may need to be increased accordingly, with attention to drug concentration, volume of vehicle, and delivery technique [45–48]. There is consensus that the tibial intraosseous route is useful for vascular access, particularly for victims up to the age of 6 years [49,50]. In the newly born, the umbilical vein is easy to find and frequently used for urgent vascular access.

Dose of adrenaline epinephrine

Consensus supports the initial dose of epinephrine (adrenaline) at 0.01 mg/kg (0.1 ml/kg of the 1:10,000 solution) by the intravascular/intraosseous route or 0.1 mg/kg (0.1 ml/kg of the 1:1,000 solution) by the endotracheal route. Because the outcome of asystolic and pulseless arrest in children is very poor and a beneficial effect of higher doses of adrenaline epinephrine has been suggested by some animal and a single retrospective paediatric study [51–55], second and subsequent intravenous doses and all endotracheal doses for unresponsive asystolic and pulseless arrest in infants and children should be 0.1 mg/kg (0.1 ml/kg of the 1:1,000 solution) as a class IIa recommendation. If no return of spontaneous circulation occurs beyond the second dose of adrenaline epinephrine despite adequate CPR, the outcome is likely to be dismal [12,18,22]. High-dose adrenaline epinephrine is of special concern for patients at high risk of intracranial hemorrhage, such as in the preterm newborn. Disappointing efficacy of "high-dose"

adrenaline epinephrine use when applied to adult study populations [56,57] and potential detrimental effects of high-dose adrenaline epinephrine therapy, including potential for systemic and intracranial hypertension (particularly in the newborn), myocardial hemorrhage or necrosis [58,59] suggest caution in advocating high-dose adrenaline epinephrine therapy unless further study is encouraging.

Sequence of Defibrillatory Shocks and Medications for Ventricular Fibrillation

Ventricular fibrillation and pulseless ventricular tachycardia are relatively uncommon in infants and children. Although there are minor differences between the names of the drugs, dose of second defibrillation, and number of defibrillations between medication doses based on local availability and custom. There is general consensus on medication/defibrillation dosage and sequence for ventricular fibrillation/pulseless ventricular tachycardia. The initial treatment is defibrillation with 2 J/kg increasing to a maximum of 4 J/kg in a series of three shocks. Subsequent series of up to three shocks following medication administration is based on local custom and training (i.e., first defibrillation up to three times (2 J/kg, 2–4 J/kg, 4 J/kg), then medication with adrenaline/epinephrine and circulation, then defibrillation up to three times (4 J/kg), then repeat adrenaline/epinephrine at higher dose, then defibrillation up to three times (4 J/kg) and consideration for other medications (lidocaine/lignocaine) and the treatment of reversible causes (see Fig. 4).

Complications from CPR

Reported complications from appropriately applied resuscitative techniques are rare in infants and children. The prevalence of significant adverse effects (rib fractures, pneumothorax, pneumoperitoneum, hemorrhage, retinal hemorrhages, etc.) from properly performed CPR appears to be much lower in children than in adults [60–67]. In the most recent study [60],

	ILCOR	AHA	HSFC	ERC	RCSA	ARC
Initial shock	2 J/kg	2 J/kg	2 J/kg	2 J/kg	2 J/kg	2 J/kg
Second shock	2–4 J/kg	4 J/kg	4 J/kg	2 J/kg	2 J/kg	2–4 J/kg
Third shock	2–4 J/kg	4 J/kg	4 J/kg	4 J/kg	4 J/kg	4 J/kg
First Medication	Epinephrine (Adrenaline) 0.01 mg/kg	Epinephrine 0.01 mg/kg	Epinephrine 0.01 mg/kg	Adrenaline 0.01 mg/kg	Adrenaline 0.01 mg/kg	Adrenaline 0.01 mg/kg
Shocks after 1st medication	4 J/kg *Up to 3* shocks	4 J/kg × 1 shock	4 J/kg × 1 shock	4 J/kg × 3 shocks	4 J/kg × 3 shocks	4 J/kg × 3 shocks
Second Medication	Epinephrine (Adrenaline) 0.1 mg/kg	Epinephrine and Lidocaine	Epinephrine and Lidocaine	Adrenaline	Adrenaline and Lignocaine	Adrenaline and Lignocaine
Shocks after 2nd medication	4 J/kg *Up to 3* shocks	4 J/kg × 1 shock	4 J/kg × 1 shock	4 J/kg × 3 shocks	4 J/kg × 3 shocks	4 J/kg × 3 shocks

FIG. 3. Examples of minor differences in recommendations for treatment of persistent ventricular fibrillation and pulseless ventricular tachycardia between the American Heart Association (AHA), Heart and Stroke Foundation of Canada (HSFC), European Resuscitation Council (ERC), Resuscitation Council of Southern Africa (RCSA), and Australian Resuscitation Council (ARC) and International Liaison Committee on Resuscitation (ILCOR).

despite prolonged CPR by rescuers with variable resuscitation training skill levels, medically significant complications were documented in only 3% of patients. Therefore, there is consensus that chest compressions should be provided for children if the pulse is absent or critically slow, or if the rescuer is uncertain if a pulse is present.

4.2.5. NEWBORN GUIDELINES

There is a need for International Newborn BLS guidelines. A review of information from the USA national database, World Health Organization, and Seattle/King County EMS Systems [67] demonstrates the importance of developing an early intervention sequence for the newly born. In the USA, approximately 1% of births occur out-of-hospital facilities, but neonatal mortality has more than doubled for these children born out of hospital. Worldwide, more than 5 million newborn deaths occur, with approximately 56%

of all births out-of-facility. Neonatal mortality is high, with birth asphyxia accounting for 19% of these deaths. These data only assess mortality, and morbidity from asphyxia and inadequate newborn resuscitation must be assumed to be much higher. The worldwide potential for saved lives from newborn asphyxia with simple airway interventions is estimated at greater than 900,000 infants per year. Therefore, the consensus supports Newborn/Newly born guidelines from ILCOR as a worthy goal.

Although the following are intended as preliminary BLS advisory guidelines, the difference between BLS and ALS interventions for the newly born may be subtle. The development of specific ILCOR advisory guidelines for new born ALS is beyond the scope of this document. It is hoped that ILCOR member organizations will address Newborn ALS in the near future. In the newborn, where birth can usually be anticipated, it is often possible to anticipate and have more personnel

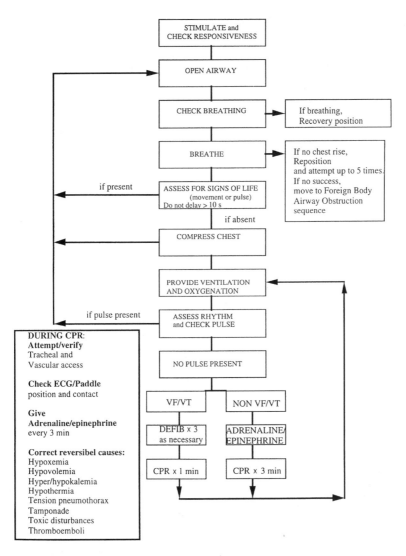

FIG. 4. ILCOR Universal Paediatric Advanced Support Template

and equipment on hand than may be available for unexpected BLS interventions in older children or adults. Ideally, the mother should give birth in a location where there is optimum equipment available and personnel are trained in newborn resuscitation. If this is not possible, then certain rudimentary equipment should be available at the birth site or should be brought to the birth attendant. Such equipment might include the following:

1. Bag/valve/mask ventilation device of appropriate size for the newborn
2. Suction device
3. Warm, dry towels and blanket
4. Clean (sterile, if possible) instrument for cutting the umbilical cord
5. Clean rubber gloves for the attendant

Most newly born infants will breathe spontaneously (usually manifested by a cry) within sec-

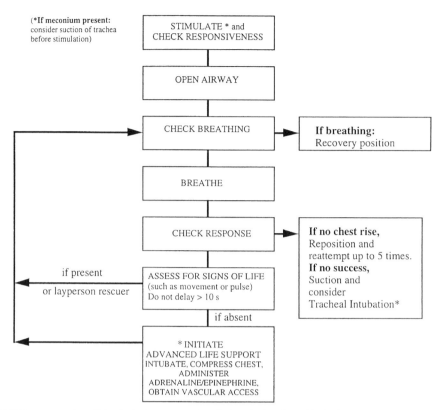

FIG. 5. ILCOR Universal Newborn Template.

onds after birth. During this time, an attendant should dry the newborn with a warm towel and remove wet linen to reduce heat loss. If the baby is limp and not crying, immediate resuscitation is required.

Basic Life Support for the Newborn

I. Stimulate and Check Responsiveness

a. Stimulation is best provided by drying the newborn with a towel and flicking the soles of the feet. Slapping, shaking, spanking, or holding the newborn upside down are contraindicated and potentially dangerous
b. Assess for a cry: a cry is the most common confirmation of adequate initial ventilation. If

present, further resuscitative efforts are probably not indicated.
c. Assess for regular respirations: Although the respiratory pattern may be irregular, respirations should be sufficient to result in adequate oxygenation (i.e., absence of persistent central cyanosis). Occasional "gasping", without normal breaths interspersed, is generally indicative of severe compromise and should be treated as inadequate respiration. If poor response, call or send for additional assistance.

II. Open Airway

a. Clear the airway of material, particularly if there is blood or meconium present. This has special importance in the newborn because of the narrow airway which creates high resistance to gas flow. Clearing the airway will also provide additional respiratory stimulation. Clearing of secretions should be accomplished with a suction device (bulb syringe, suction catheter); otherwise, removal of secretions may be accomplished with a cloth wrapped on the rescuer's finger.

b. Position the head to the "sniffing" position and particularly avoid excessive neck flexion or hyperextension which may result in airway obstruction.

c. If a suitably trained provider and equipment are available: if the newborn is stained with thick meconium the trachea should be suctioned as the initial resuscitative step. This is accomplished by intubating the trachea, applying suction directly to the tube using any of a variety of devices available for this purpose, and withdrawing the tube as suction is continued. If meconium is recovered, it may be necessary to repeat this procedure several times until the residual is sufficiently thin to permit suctioning through the tube, using a standard suction catheter.

III. Check Breathing

a. Assess for presence of a cry, If a strong cry is present, further resuscitation efforts are not indicated. If the cry is weak or absent: look, listen and feel for air entry and chest movement and feel for evidence of spontaneous respiration.

b. If respirations are absent or inadequate (gasping), assisted ventilation is necessary. Further attempts to stimulate the newborn, in this case, will waste valuable time.

IV. Breathe

a. Although it is recognized that a bag/valve/mask is the most effective piece of equipment for assisting ventilation, various other devices are available or are being developed. Use will be dictated by local availability, cost and custom.

b. If a resuscitation device is not available, consider using mouth-to-mouth-and-nose to assist ventilation. Although some controversy exists about whether mother's mouths can effectively seal their older infants' mouth-and-nose [32,33], consensus supports initial attempts at newborn ventilation via both the infant's mouth and nose. Because of the presence of maternal blood and other body fluids on the face of the newborn, there is a perceived risk of infection to the rescuer. Quickly wipe away as much of this material as possible before attempting mouth to mouth-and-nose ventilation.

c. Blow sufficient air into the newborn airway to cause the chest to rise visibly.

d. Watch for chest rise as an indication of ventilation efficacy. If inadequate, adjust head position, clear airway, achieve a seal over the mouth-and-nose on the face, and consider an increase in inflation pressure.

e. Ventilate at a rate of approximately 30–60 times per minute.

f. Note that INITIAL breaths may require a higher inflating pressure to overcome the resistance in small and fluid filled airways.

V. Assess Response

a. After assisting ventilation for 30 s to 1 min, check again for response. If still no response, deliver breaths watching closely for adequate chest rise with each delivered breath.

b. In addition to the presence of a cry and spontaneous respirations, the response may also be assessed by feeling for a pulse, although this may be difficult in the newborn and should not distract the rescuer from providing adequate ventilations. A pulse may be detectable by feeling the base of the umbilical cord and should be above 100 beats/min.

c. Continue to ventilate and assess (return to Step II) until there is either an adequate response (crying, breathing, and heart rate greater than 100/min), or additional medical assistance has arrived. If effective spontaneous respirations resume, consider positioning the newborn on its side in a recovery position.

VI. Compress Chest

A. *Laypersons:* Chest compressions in the newborn are not recommended for administration by persons untrained in neonatal resuscitation, particularly when rescue is being provided by a single individual. Ventilation is nearly always the primary need of the newly born and administration of chest compressions may decrease the efficacy of assisted ventilation [69].

B. *Trained health care providers:* If suitably trained health care providers are available, and adequate ventilations have not resulted in improvement, the following steps should be taken:

1. Feel for a pulse. In the newborn, a pulse is most easily palpated by lightly grasping the base of the umbilical cord between the thumb and index finger. If a stethoscope is available, a heartbeat may be detected by auscultating the chest.
2. Assess the heart rate for up to 10 s. If the heart rate is below 60 beats/min and not clearly rising, begin chest compressions. If the heart rate is above 60 and is rising, consider continuation of effective ventilations alone and reassess the heart rate in 60 s.
3. Chest compressions for the newborn are delivered in series of three, followed by a pause for delivery of a ventilation (ratio 3 compressions and 1 ventilation per cycle). The rate should be approximately 120 "events" (i.e., -c-c-c-v-c-c-c-v- 120) per minute.
4. Reassess the heart rate approximately every 60 s, until the heart rate improves to greater than 60–80/min or ALS resources are available for oxygen supplementation, endotracheal intubation, and administration of epinephrine.

VII. Other newborn issues

a. TEMPERATURE CONTROL

In addition to drying the newborn to decrease evaporative heat loss, drape the newborn in dry towels or a blanket during the resuscitation process. Remove the newborn from wet surfaces or pools of fluid. As soon as resuscitation has been successful, place the baby skin-to-skin on the mother's chest/breast and cover both with a blanket.

b. INFECTION CONTROL

Wash hands and wear gloves, using universal precautions for secretion contact, if available. Use clean towels, blankets and instruments and avoid rescuer exposure to blood and other fluids.

c. UMBILICAL CORD

It is not necessary to cut the umbilical cord before resuscitation of the newborn. This can be done after the baby is spontaneously breathing and the cord has stopped pulsating. The cutting instrument and cord ties should be sterilized, if possible. These may be sterilized by boiling in water for 20 min. A new, packaged razor blade does not require sterilization. If sterile equipment is not available, clean equipment should be used. Tie the cord in two places with a string. Cut the cord between the ties with a razor blade, scissors, or knife.

d. DO NOT FORGET THE MOTHER

Watch for and attend to potential complications of childbirth. Excessive vaginal bleeding, seizures and infection are the most common maternal complications of childbirth. Arrange for health care provider support to attend to mother and child, if possible.

4.2.6. RESEARCH

The paucity of paediatric and newborn clinical resuscitation outcome data makes scientific justification of recommendations difficult. Therefore, the development of prospective, paediatric-specific clinical studies and the development of laboratory and animal resuscitation models that specifically address paediatric and neonatal issues is of paramount importance. Collection of data should follow the paediatric Utstein-style guidelines [25,70]. Specific data on the aetiology of arrest, success of interventions, frequency and severity of complications, significant short- and long-term neurologic and overall performance outcomes, educational value, and costs associated with resuscitation techniques are urgently needed.

Areas of Controversy in Current Guidelines, Unresolved Issues and Need for Additional Research

The ILCOR Paediatric working group recognizes the difficulty in creating advisory statements for universal application. After careful review of the rationale for current guidelines that exist in North America, Europe, Australia and Southern Africa, the working group identified the areas of controversy where it was felt the greatest need for research exists before evolution to "universal" guidelines can occur.

Some of these areas are listed below:

1. Should initial resuscitation interventions and sequences be based on etiology of arrest or the likelihood of successfully resuscitating a presenting cardiac rhythm (e.g., etiology: hypoxia/asystole most likely for children but ventricular fibrillation treated with defibrillation most likely to have successful resuscitation)?

2. What is the prevalence of ventricular fibrillation during or following resuscitation?

3. What number of breaths should be initially attempted after opening the airway? (AHA/HSFC: 2 breaths, ERC: 5 breaths, ARC: 4 breaths, RCSA: 2 breaths: *ILCOR: 2–5 breaths*)

4. Is adult mouth to infant nose ventilation a better method than adult mouth to infant mouth-and-nose ventilation for newborn and/or infants?

5. What sequence of interventions for the conscious choking child is most appropriate: back blows vs. abdominal thrusts vs. chest thrusts and should visual inspection of the mouth for foreign body precede attempts at ventilation in infants?

6. What is an optimal recovery position for infants and children?

7. At what heart rate should chest compressions be initiated in ALS: When the pulse is absent or "too slow"? (Currently: AHA/HSFC: < 60 beats/min, ERC: < 60 beats/min, ARC: 40–60 beats/min, RCSA: < 60 beats/min: *ILCOR: < 60 beats/min*)

8. What is the optimal depth for chest compressions? (1/3–1/2 depth of chest or a specified number of inches or centimeters: *ILCOR approximately 1/3 the depth of the chest*)

9. What is an optimal compression/ventilation ratio for different age groups and can a universal compression/ventilation ratio be adopted that accommodates all victims from newborn to adulthood?

10. What is the appropriate dose of epinephrine? (*ILCOR: First dose of adrenaline/epinephrine 0.01 mg/kg, subsequent doses 0.1 mg/kg*)

11. What defibrillation dose and how many defibrillation shocks should be delivered after medication for ventricular fibrillation in children? (*ILCOR: 2 J/kg, 2–4 J/kg, 4 J/kg; one to three shocks at 4 J/kg after medications*).

12. Should alternative medications (e.g., Lidocaine/Lignocaine) be used for persistent ventricular fibrillation, if defibrillation and initial epinephrine doses are not successful?

13. Can automated external defibrillators accurately and reliably be applied to paediatric patients?

14. What sequence of interventions should be employed by advanced health care providers for the newborn?

15. What is the impact of implementing ILCOR guidelines on arrest prevention, successful resuscitation and neurologic performance outcome from potential or actual cardiopulmonary arrest in the newborn, infants and children?

4.2.7. SUMMARY

This document reflects on the deliberation of the Paediatric Working Group of the International Liaison Committee on Resuscitation (ILCOR). The epidemiology and outcome of paediatric cardiopulmonary arrest and the priorities, techniques and sequence of paediatric resuscitation assessments and interventions differ from those of adults. The working group identified areas of conflict and controversy in current paediatric basic and advanced life support guidelines, outlined solutions considered, and made recommendations by consensus. The working group was surprised by the degree of conformity which already exists in current guidelines advocated by the American Heart Association, Heart and Stroke Foundation of Canada, European Resuscitation Council, Australian Resuscitation Council, and Resuscitation Council of Southern Africa. Differences are currently based upon local and regional preferences, and training networks and customs, rather than scientific controversy. Unresolved issues with the potential for future universal application are highlighted. This document does not include a complete list of guidelines for which there are no perceived controversy and the algorithm/decision tree figures presented attempt to follow a common flow of assessments and interventions, in coordination with their adult counterparts.

Survival following paediatric prehospital cardiopulmonary arrest averages only approximately 3–17%, and survivors are often neurologically devastated. Most paediatric resuscitation reports have been retrospective in design and plagued with inconsistent resuscitation definitions and patient inclusion criteria. Careful and thoughtful application of uniform guidelines for reporting outcomes of advanced life support interventions using large, randomized, multicenter and multinational clinical trials are clearly needed. Paediatric advisory statements from ILCOR will, by necessity, be vibrant and involve guidelines fostered by national and international organizations intent on improving the outcome of resuscitation for infants and children worldwide.

4.2.8. ILCOR PAEDIATRIC ADVISORY STATEMENT REFERENCES

1. Nadkerni V, Hazinski M, Zideman D, Kattwinkel J, Quan L, Bingham R, Zaritsky A, Bland J, Kramer E, Tiballs J. Paediatric life support. An advisory statement by the Paediatric Life Support Working Group of the International Liaison Committee on Resuscitation. Resuscitation 1997;34:115–127.
2. Emergency Cardiac Care Committee and Subcommittees of the American Heart Association. Guidelines for cardiopulmonary resuscitation and emergency cardiac care. J Am Med Assoc 1992;268:2171–2302.
3. Paediatric Life Support Working Party of the European Resuscitation Council. Guidelines for paediatric life support. Br Med J 1994;308:1349–1355.
4. Advanced Life Support Committee of the Australian Resuscitation Council. Paediatric advanced life support: the Australian Resuscitation Council guidelines. Med J Aust 1996;165:199–206.
5. Roy RN, Bethera FR. The Melbourne chart – a logical guide to neonatal resuscitation. Anaesth Intens Care 1990;18:348–357.
6. Kloeck WGJ. Resuscitation Council of Southern Africa Guidelines: new recommendations for basic life support in adults, children and infants; obstructed airway in adults, children and infants; advanced life support for adults and children: Trauma Emerg Med 1993: 10(1):738–771.
7. Appleton GO, Cummins RO, Larson MP, Graves JR. CPR and the single rescuer: at what age should you "call first" rather than "call fast"? Yawn Emerg Med 1995;25:492–494.
8. Mogaysel C, Quan L, Graves JR, Tiedeman D, Fahrenbruch C, Herndon P. Out-of-Hospital Ventricular Fibrillation in children and Adolescents: causes and outcomes. Yawn Emerg Med 1995;25:484–491.
9. Hazinski MF. Is paediatric resuscitation unique? Relative merits of early CPR and ventilation versus early defibrillation for young victims of prehospital cardiac arrest. Yawn Emerg Med 1995;25:540–543.
10. Hickey RW, Cohen DM, Strausbaugh S, Dietrich AM. Paediatric patients requiring CPR in the prehospital setting. Yawn Emerg Med 1995;25:495–501.
11. Innes PA, Summers CA, Boyd IM, Molyneaux EM. Audit of paediatric cardiopulmonary resuscitation. Arch Dis Child 1993;68:487–491.
12. Zaritsky A, Nadkarni V, Getson P, Kuehl K. CPR in children. Yawn Emerg Med 1987;16;1107–1111.
13. Teach SJ, Moore Pe, Fleisher GR. Death and resuscitation in the paediatric emergency department. Yawn Emerg Med 1995;25:799–803.
14. Thompson JE, Bonner B, Lower GM. Paediatric cardiopulmonary arrests in rural populations. Paediatrics

1990;86:302–306.

15. Tunstall-Pedoe H, Bailey L, Chamberlain DA, Marsden AK, Ward ME, Zideman DA. Survey of 3765 cardiopulmonary resuscitations in British hospitals (the BRESUS study): methods and overall results. Br Med J 1992;304:1347–1351.

16. Eisenberg M, Bergner L, Hallstrom A. Epidemiology of cardiac arrest and resuscitation in children. Yawn Emerg Med 1983;12:672–674.

17. Walsh CK, Krongrad E. Terminal cardiac electrical activity in paediatric patients. Am J Cardiol 1983;51: 557–561.

18. Dieckmann RA, Vardis R. High-dose epinephrine in paediatric out-of-hospital cardiopulmonary arrest. Paediatrics 1995;95:901–913.

19. Losek JD, Hennes H, Glaeser PW, Smith DS, Hendley G. Prehospital countershock treatment of paediatric asystole. Am J Emerg Med 1989;7:571–575.

20. Ronco R, King W, Donley DK, Tilden SJ. Outcome and cost at a children's hospital following resuscitation for out-of-hospital cardiopulmonary arrest. Arch Pediatr Adolesc Med 1995;149:210–214.

21. Friesen RM, Duncan P, Tweed WA, Bristow G. Appraisal of paediatric cardiopulmonary resuscitation. Can Med Assoc J 1982;126:1055–1058.

22. Schindler MB, Bohn D, Cox P, McCrindle B, Jarvis A, Edmonds J, Barker G. Outcome of out-of-hospital cardiac or respiratory arrest in children. N Engl J Med 1996;335:1473–1479.

23. O'Rourke PP. Outcome of children who are apneic and pulseless in the emergency room. Crit Care Med 1986;14:466–468.

24. Torphy DE, Minter MG, Thompson BM. Cardiorespiratory arrest and resuscitation of children. Am J Dis Child 1984;138:1099–1102.

25. Zaritsky A, Nadkarni V, Hazinski MF, Foltin G, Quan L, Wright L, Fiser D, Zideman D, O'Malley P, Chameides L, Cummins RO, and the Paediatric Utstein Consensus Panel. Recommended guidelines for uniform reporting of paediatric advanced life support: the Paediatric Utstein Style. Circulation 1995;92(7): 2006–2020.

26. Nichols DG, Kettrick RG, Swedlow DB, Lee S, Passman R, Ludwig S. Factors influencing outcome of cardiopulmonary resuscitation in children. Pediatr Emerg Care 1986;2:1–5.

27. Barzilay Z, Somekh E, Sagy M, Boichis H. Paediatric cardiopulmonary resuscitation outcome. J Med 1988; 19:229–241.

28. Ruben HM, Elam JO, Ruben AM, Greene DG. Investigation of upper airway problems in resuscitation. I. Studies of pharyngeal X-rays and performance by laymen. Anesthesiology 1961;22:271–279.

29. Melker RJ. Asynchronous and other alternative methods of ventilation during CPR. Yawn Emerg Med

30. Melker RJ, Banner MJ. Ventilation during CPR: two-rescuer standards reappraised. Yawn Emerg Med 1985;14:397–402.

31. Bowman F, Menegazzi J, Check B, Duckett T. Lower oesophageal sphincter pressure during prolonged cardiac arrest and resuscitation. Yawn Emerg Med 1995; 26:216–219.

32. Tonkin SL, Davis SL, Gunn TR. Nasal route for infant resuscitation by mothers. Lancet 1995;345:1353–1354.

33. Segedin E, Torrie J, Anderson B. Nasal airway versus oral route for infant resuscitation. Lancet 1995; 346:382.

34. Mather C, O'Kelly S. The palpation of pulses. Anaesthesia 1996;51:189–191.

35. Brearley S, Simms MH, Shearman CP. Peripheral pulse palpation: An unreliable sign. Yawn Roy Coll Surg 1992;74:169–172.

36. Connick M, Berg RA. Femoral venous pulsations during open-heart cardiac massage. Yawn Emerg Med 1994;24:6:1176–1179.

37. Berg RA, Kern KB, Sanders AB, Otto CW, Hilwig RW, Ewy GA. Bystander cardiopulmonary resuscitation. Is ventilation necessary? Circulation 1993;88:4(1):1907–1915.

38. Kyriacou DN, Arcinue EL, Peek C, Kraus JF. Effect of immediate resuscitation on children with submersion injury. Paediatrics 1994;94:2(1):137–142.

39. Gillis J, Dickson D, Rieder M, Steward D, Edmonds J. Results of inpatient paediatric resuscitation. Crit Care Med 1986;14:469–471.

40. Kissoon N, Peterson R, Murphy S, Gayle M, Ceithaml E, Harwood-Nuss A. Comparison of pH and carbon dioxide tension values of central venous and intraosseous blood during changes in cardiac output. Crit Care Med 1994;22:1010–1015.

41. Kissoon N, Rosenberg H, Gloor J, Vidal R. Comparison of the acid-base status of blood obtained from intraosseous and central venous sites during steady- and low-flow states. Crit Care Med 1993;21(11): 1765–1769.

42. Warren D, Kissoon N, Sommerauer J, Rieder M. Comparison of fluid infusion rates among peripheral intravenous and humerus, femur, malleolus, and tibial intraosseous sites in normovolemic and hypovolemic piglets. Yawn Emerg Med 1993;22:2:183–186.

43. Andropoulos D, Soifer S, Schreiber M. Plasma epinephrine concentrations after intraosseous and central venous injection during cardiopulmonary resuscitation in the lamb. J Pediatr 1990;116:2:312–315.

44. Emerman C, Pinchak A, Hancock D, Hagen J. Effect of injection site on circulation times during cardiac arrest. Crit Care Med 1988;16:11:1138–1141.

45. Mazkereth R, Paret G, Ezra D, Aviner S, Peleg E,

Rosenthal T, Barzilay Z. Epinephrine blood concentrations after peripheral bronchial versus endotracheal administration of epinephrine in dogs. Crit Care Med 1992;20:1582–1587.

46. Jasani M, Nadkarni V, Finkelstein M, Mandell G, Salzman S, Norman M. Crit Care Med 1994;22:1174–1180.

47. Quinton D, O'Byrne G, Aitkenhead A. Comparison of endotracheal and peripheral venous intravenous adrenaline in cardiac arrest: is the endotracheal route reliable. Lancet 1987;1:828–829.

48. Roberts J, Greenberg M, Knaub, Kendrick Z, Baskin S. Comparison of the pharmacological effects of epinephrine administered by the intravenous and endotracheal routes. J Am Coll Emerg Phys 1978;7:260–264.

49. Fiser D. Intraosseous infusion. N Engl J Med 1990;322:1579–1581.

50. Rosetti VA, Thompson BM, Miller J, Mateer JR, Aprahamian C. Intraosseous infusion: an alternative route of paediatric intravascular access. Yawn Emerg Med 1985;14:885–888.

51. Brown C, Werman H. Adrenergic agonist during cardiopulmonary resuscitation. Resuscitation 1990;19:1–16.

52. Goetting M, Paradis N. High-dose epinephrine improves outcome from paediatric cardiac arrest. Yawn Emerg Med 1991;20:22–26.

53. Berkowitz ID, Gervais H, Schleien C, Koehler R, Dean J, Traystman R. Epinephrine dosage effects on cerebral and myocardial blood flow in an infant swine model of cardiopulmonary resuscitation. Anesthesiology 1991;75:6:1041–1050.

54. Callaham M, Madsen C, Barton C, Saunders C, Pointer J. A randomized clinical trial of high-dose epinephrine and norepinephrine vs. standard-dose epinephrine in prehospital cardiac arrest. J Am Med Assoc 1992;268:2667–2672.

55. Patterson M, Boenning D, Klein B. High dose epinephrine in paediatric cardiopulmonary arrest. Paediatr Emerg Care 1994;10:310.

56. Stiell I, Hebert P, Weitzman B, Wells G, Raman S, Stark R, Higginson K, Ahuja J, Dickinson G. High-dose epinephrine in adult cardiac arrest. N Engl J Med 1992;327:1045–1050.

57. Brown CG, Martin D, Pepe P, Stueven H, Cummins R, Gonzalez E, Jastremski M and the Multicenter High-dose epinephrine study group. A comparison of standard-dose and high-dose epinephrine in cardiac arrest outside the hospital. N Engl J Med 1992;327:1051–1055.

58. Berg R, Otto C, Kern K, Hilwig R, Sanders A, Henry C, Ewy G. A randomized, blinded trial of high-dose epinephrine versus standard-dose epinephrine in a swine model of paediatric asphyxial arrest. Crit Care Med 1996;24:1695–1700.

59. Callaham M. High-dose epinephrine in cardiac arrest. West J Med 1991;155:289–290.

60. Bush CM, Jones JS, Cohle S, Johnson H. Paediatric injuries from cardiopulmonary resuscitation. Yawn Emerg Med 1996;28:1:40–44.

61. Spevak M, Kleinman P, Belanger P, Primack C. Cardiopulmonary resuscitation and rib fractures in infants: a postmortem radiologic-pathologic study. J Am Med Assoc 1994;272:8:617–618.

62. Kaplan J, Fossum R. Patterns of facial resuscitation injury in infancy. Am J Forensic Med Pathol 1994;15:3:187–191.

63. Feldman K, Brewer D. Child abuse, cardiopulmonary resuscitation and rib fractures. Paediatrics 1984;73:3:339–342.

64. Nagel E, Fine E, Krischer J, Davis J. Complications of CPR. Crit Care Med 1981;9:5:424.

65. Powner D, Holcombe P, Mello L. Cardiopulmonary resuscitation-related injuries. Crit Care Med 1984;12:1:54–55.

66. Parke T. Unexplained pneumoperitoneum in association with basic cardiopulmonary resuscitation efforts. Resuscitation 1993;26:2:177–181.

67. Kramer K, Goldstein B. Retinal hemorrhages following cardiopulmonary resuscitation. Clin Paediatrics 1993;32(6):366–368.

68. Kattwinkel J (AAP/AHA Neonatal Resuscitation Programme), Zupan J (World Health Organisation), Quan L (Seattle/King County Emergency Medical Systems). Personal communications 1996.

69. Dean JM, Koehler R, Schleien C, Michael J, Chantatrojanasiri T, Rogers M, Traystman R. Age related changes in chest geometry during cardiopulmonary resuscitation. J Appl Physiol 1987;62:2212–2219.

70. Becker BL, Idris AH. Proceedings of the second Chicago symposium on advances in CPR Research and guidelines for laboratory research. Yawn Emerg Med 1996;27:5:539–541.

4.3. The 1998 European Resuscitation Council Guidelines for Paediatric Life Support. Sequence of Actions

4.3.1. PAEDIATRIC BASIC LIFE SUPPORT

To be read in conjunction with the International Liaison Committee on Resuscitation Paediatric Working Group Advisory Statement (April 1997).

Definitions

An **infant** is a child under the age of 1 year.
A **child** is aged between 1 and 8 years of age. Children over the age of 8 years will still be treated as younger children but may require different techniques to attain adequate chest compressions.

Sequence of Actions

Text Note: In the following descriptions
– the masculine includes the feminine.
– unless specified a "child" includes an "infant".

1. Ensure safety of rescuer and child

2. Check the child's responsiveness

* Gently stimulate the child and ask loudly: "Are you all right?"

– Infants, and children with suspected cervical spinal injuries, should *not* be shaken.

3A. If the child responds by answering or moving:

* Leave the child in the position in which you find him (provided he is not in further danger).

* Check his condition and get help if needed.

* Reassess him regularly

3B. If the child does not respond:

* Shout for help

* Open the child's airway by tilting his head and lifting his chin (Figs. 1,2).

– If possible with the child in the position in which you find him, place your hand on the child's forehead and gently tilt his head back.
– At the same time, with your fingertip(s) under the point of the child's chin, lift the chin to open the airway. Do not push on the soft tissues under the chin as this may block the airway.
– If you have any difficulty, carefully turn the child on to his back and then open the airway as described.

Avoid head tilt if trauma (injury) to the neck is suspected.

If neck injury is suspected use only the jaw thrust method of opening the airway.

4. Keeping the airway open, look, listen and feel for breathing (Figs. 1 and 3):

– Look for chest movements
– Listen at the child's nose and mouth for breath sounds
– Feel for air movement on your cheek.

* Look, listen and feel for up to 10 s before deciding that breathing is absent.

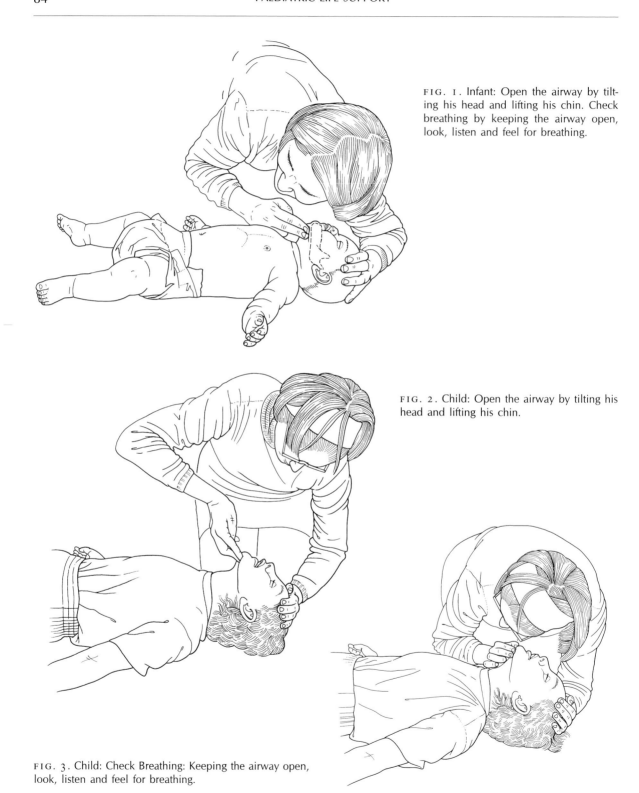

FIG. 1. Infant: Open the airway by tilting his head and lifting his chin. Check breathing by keeping the airway open, look, listen and feel for breathing.

FIG. 2. Child: Open the airway by tilting his head and lifting his chin.

FIG. 3. Child: Check Breathing: Keeping the airway open, look, listen and feel for breathing.

5A. If the child *is* breathing:

* Turn the child on his side.

* Check for continued breathing.

5B. If the child is *not* breathing:

* Carefully remove any obvious airway obstruction.

* Give up to five rescue breaths, each of which makes the chest rise and fall.

For a child (Fig. 4)

— Ensure head tilt and chin lift.
— Pinch the soft part of his nose closed with the index finger and thumb of your hand on his forehead.
— Open his mouth a little, but maintain the chin in an up position.
— Take a breath and place your lips around his mouth, making sure that you have a good seal.
— Blow steadily into his mouth over about 1—12 s watching for his chest to rise.
— Maintain head tilt and chin lift, take your mouth away from the victim and watch for his chest to fall as air comes out.
— Take another breath and repeat this sequence up to 5 times (a minimum of two effective rescue breaths must be given).

For an infant (Fig. 5)

— Ensure head tilt and chin lift.

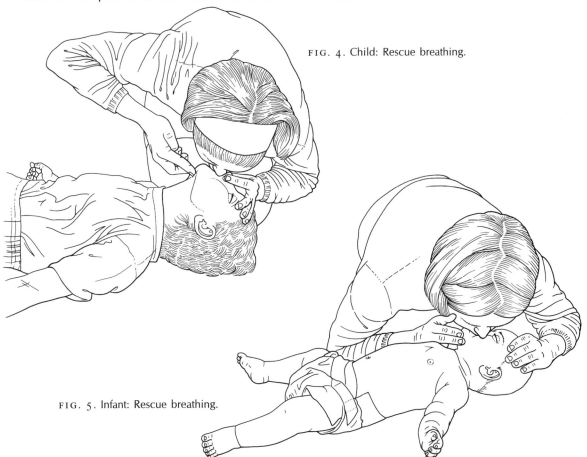

FIG. 4. Child: Rescue breathing.

FIG. 5. Infant: Rescue breathing.

– Take a breath and cover the mouth and nasal apertures of the infant with your mouth, making sure you have a good seal.
– Blow steadily into the infants mouth and nose over 1–12 s sufficient to make the chest visibly rise.
– Maintain head tilt and chin lift, take your mouth away from the victim and watch for his chest to fall as air comes out.
– Take another breath and repeat this sequence up to 5 times (a minimum of two effective rescue breaths must be given).

* If you have difficulty achieving an effective breath, the airway may be *obstructed*

– Open the child's mouth and remove any obstruction
– Ensure that there is adequate head tilt and chin lift but also that the neck is not over extended.
– Make up to five attempts in all to achieve at least 2 effective breaths
– If still unsuccessful, move on to foreign body airway obstruction sequence.

6. Assess the child

* Take *no more than 10 s* to:
– Check the pulse

Child – feel for the carotid pulse in the neck (Fig. 6)

Infant – feel for the brachial pulse on the inner aspect of the upper arm (Fig. 7)
– Look for any movement, including swallowing or breathing (more than an occasional gasp)

7A. If you are *confident* that you can detect signs of a circulation within 10 s

* Continue rescue breathing, if necessary, until the child starts breathing effectively on his own.

* Turn the child on to his side (into the recovery position) if he remains unconscious.

7B. If there are *no* signs of a circulation, or you are at all unsure (or, in infants, the pulse rate is very slow – less than one per second):

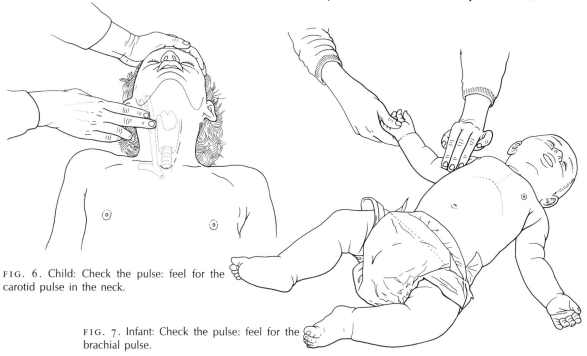

FIG. 6. Child: Check the pulse: feel for the carotid pulse in the neck.

FIG. 7. Infant: Check the pulse: feel for the brachial pulse.

* Start chest compression

* Combine rescue breathing and compression

For a child

– Locate and place the heel of one hand over the lower half of the sternum ensuring that you do not compress on or below the xiphisternum.
– Lift the fingers to ensure that pressure is not applied over the child's ribs.
– Position yourself vertically above the victim's chest and, with your arms straight, press down on the sternum to depress it approximately 1/3 of the depth of the child's chest.
– Release the pressure, then repeat at a rate of about 100 times a minute (a little less than two compressions a second).

– After five compressions tilt the head, lift the chin and give one effective breath.
– Return your hands immediately to the correct position on the sternum and give five further compressions
– Continue compressions and breaths in a ratio of 5:1

For a child over the age of 8 years (Fig. 8)

In children over the age of approximately 8 years, it may be necessary to use the "adult" two-handed method of chest compression to achieve an adequate depth of compression.

– Locate the lower half of the sternum and place the heel of one hand there, with the other hand placed on top.

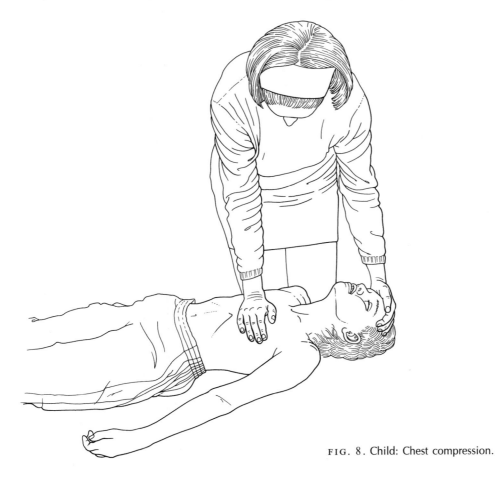

FIG. 8. Child: Chest compression.

— Interlock the fingers of both hands and lift them to ensure that pressure is not applied over the child's ribs.

— Position yourself vertically above the victim's chest and, with your arms straight, press down on the sternum to depress it approximately 1/3 of the depth of the child's chest.

— Release the pressure, then repeat at a rate of about 100 times a minute (a little less than two compressions a second).

— After 15 compressions tilt the head, lift the chin and give two effective breaths.

— Return your hands immediately to the correct position on the sternum and give 15 further compressions.

— Continue compressions and breaths in a ratio of 15:2

For an infant (Fig. 9)

— Locate the sternum and place the tips of two fingers, one fingers breadth below an imaginary line joining the infants nipples.

— With the tips of two fingers, press down on the sternum to depress it approximately 1/3 of the depth of the infant's chest.

— Release the pressure, then repeat at a rate of about 100 times a minute (about two compressions a second).

— After five compressions tilt the head, lift the chin and give 1 effective breath.

— Return your fingers immediately to the correct position on the sternum and give five further compressions.

— Continue compressions and breaths in a ratio of 5:1

8. Continue resuscitation until:

— The child shows signs of life (spontaneous respiration, pulse).

— Qualified help arrives.

— You become exhausted.

When to call for assistance

It is vital for rescuers to get help as quickly as possible when a child collapses.

* When more than one rescuer is available, one should start resuscitation while another rescuer goes for assistance.

* If only one rescuer is present, they should perform resuscitation for about **1 min** before going for assistance. It may be possible to take the infant or small child with you whilst summoning help.

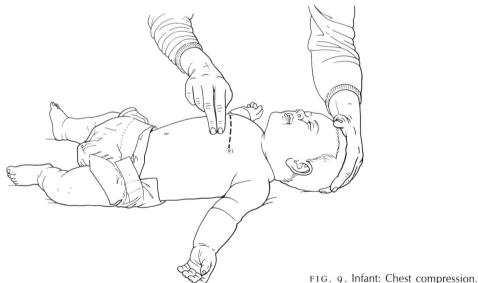

FIG. 9. Infant: Chest compression.

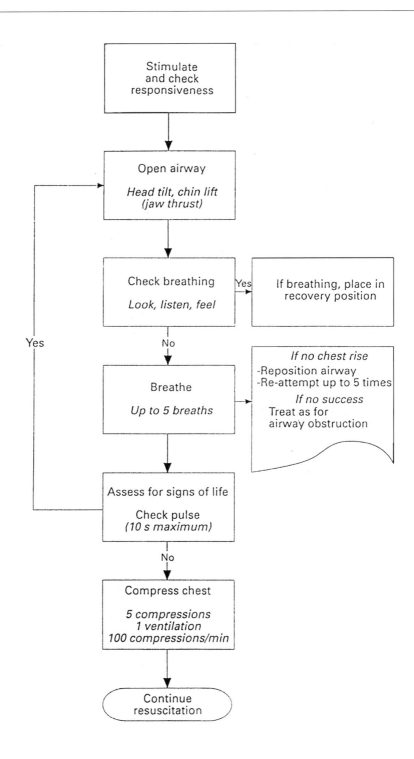

TABLE I. Algorithm for paediatric basic life support.

Recovery position

An unconscious child whose airway is clear, and who is breathing spontaneously, should be turned on his side into the recovery position. This prevents the tongue falling back to obstruct the airway, and reduces the risk of inhalation of stomach contents. There are a number of different recovery positions, each of which has its advocates. The important principles to be followed are:

– the child should be in as near to the true lateral position as possible with his mouth dependant to allow free drainage of fluid.
– the position should be stable. In an infant this may require the support of a small pillow or rolled up blanket placed behind the infants back to maintain the position.
– any pressure on the chest that impairs breathing should be avoided.
– it should be possible to turn the child onto his side and to return him back easily and safely, paying particular attention to the possibility of cervical spine injury.
– good observation and access to the airway should be possible.

Obstructed Airway

* If you have difficulty achieving an effective breath

– Recheck the child's mouth and remove any obvious obstruction
– Recheck that there is adequate head tilt and chin lift but also that the neck is not overextended.
– Make up to five attempts in all to achieve at least two effective breaths
– If still unsuccessful, move on to foreign body airway obstruction sequence.

Foreign Body Obstruction Sequence

There are a number of different foreign body obstruction sequences, each of which has its advocates.

If the child is breathing spontaneously his efforts to clear the obstruction should be encouraged. Intervention is necessary only if these attempts are clearly ineffective and breathing is inadequate.

– Do not perform blind finger sweeps of the mouth or upper airway as these may further impact a foreign body or cause soft tissue damage.

– Use measures intended to create a sharp increase in pressure within the chest cavity, such as an artificial cough.

1. Perform up to FIVE Back blows

* Hold the child in a prone position and try to position the head lower than the chest.

* Deliver five smart blows to the middle of the back between the shoulder blades.

* If this fails to dislodge the foreign body proceed to chest thrusts.

2. Perform up to FIVE Chest thrusts

* Turn the child into a supine position.

* Give five chest thrusts to the sternum.

– The position of chest thrusts is similar to that for chest compressions.

– Chest thrusts should be sharper and more vigorous than compressions and carried out at a rate of about 20 per minute.

3. Check mouth (Fig. 10)

* After five back blows and five chest thrusts check the mouth.

* Carefully remove any visible foreign bodies.

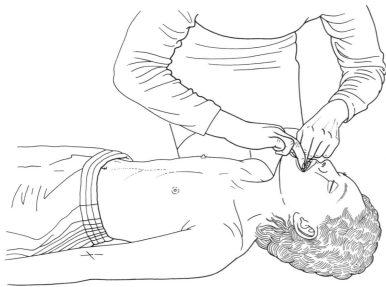

FIG. 10. Obstructed Airway: Check the child's mouth and remove obvious obstruction.

4. Open airway

* Reposition the airway by the head tilt and chin lift (jaw thrust) manoeuvre.

* Reassess breathing.

5A. If the child is breathing

* Turn the child on his side

* Check for continued breathing.

5B. If the child is not breathing:

* Attempt up to five rescue breaths, each of which makes the chest rise and fall.

— the child may be apnoeic or the airway partially cleared, in either case the rescuer may be able to achieve effective ventilation at this stage.

* If the airway is still obstructed repeat the sequence:

For a child (Fig. 11a, 11b)

* Repeat the cycle (1–5 above) but substitute five abdominal thrusts for five chest thrusts

— Abdominal thrusts are delivered as five sharp thrusts directed upwards towards the diaphragm.

— Use the upright position if the child is conscious (Fig. 11a).

— Unconscious children should be laid supine and the heel of one hand placed in the middle of the upper abdomen (Fig. 11b).

* Repeat the cycles of alternate chest thrusts and abdominal thrusts.

* Repeat the cycles until the airway is cleared or the child breathes spontaneously.

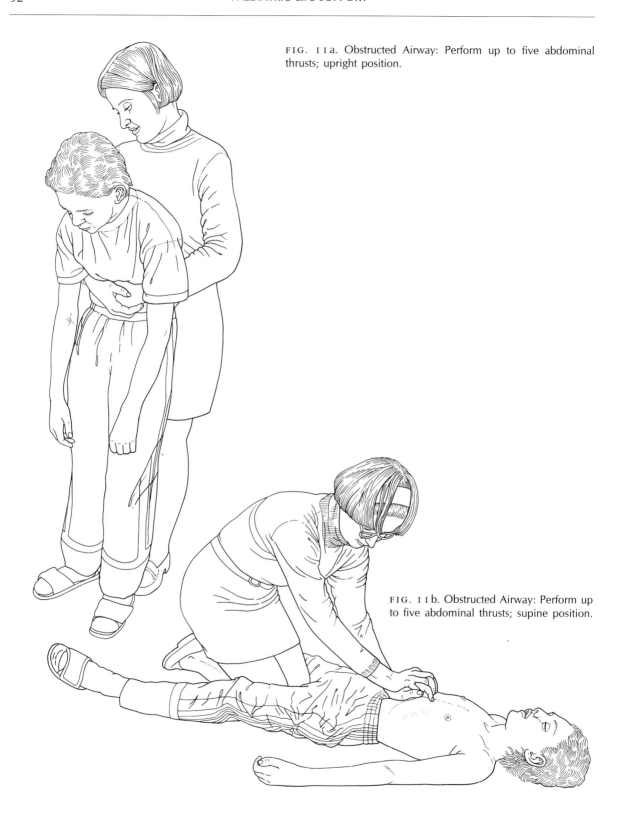

FIG. 11a. Obstructed Airway: Perform up to five abdominal thrusts; upright position.

FIG. 11b. Obstructed Airway: Perform up to five abdominal thrusts; supine position.

For an infant (Fig. 12a, 12b)

* Abdominal thrusts are not recommended in infants because they may rupture the abdominal viscera.

* Perform cycles of five back blows and five chest thrusts only.

* Repeat the cycles until the airway is cleared or the infant breathes spontaneously.

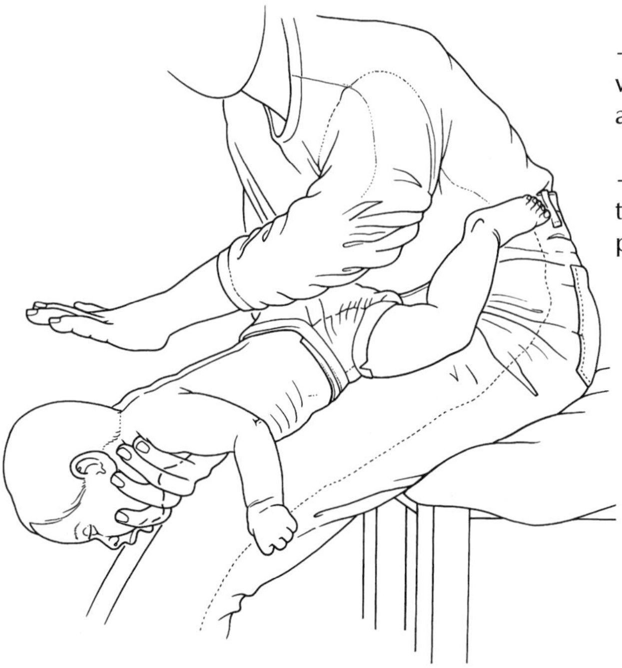

FIG. 12a. Infant: Obstructed Airway: Perform up to five back blows.

4.3.2. PAEDIATRIC ADVANCED LIFE SUPPORT

To be read in conjunction with the International Liaison Committee on Resuscitation Paediatric Working Group Advisory Statement (April 1997).

1. Establish basic life support

2. Oxygenate, Ventilate (Fig. 13)

* Provide positive pressure ventilation with a high inspired oxygen concentration

3. Attach a Defibrillator or Monitor

* Monitor the cardiac rhythm:

— Place the defibrillator paddles on the chest wall; one just below the right clavicle, the other at the left anterior axillary line.

— For infants, when using this method of monitoring, it may be more appropriate to apply the paddles to the front and back of the infants chest.

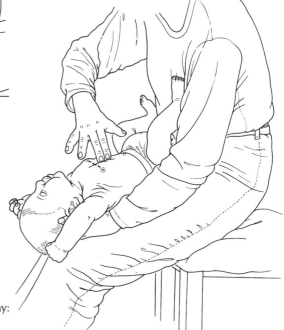

FIG. 12b. Infant: Obstructed Airway: Perform up to five Chest thrusts.

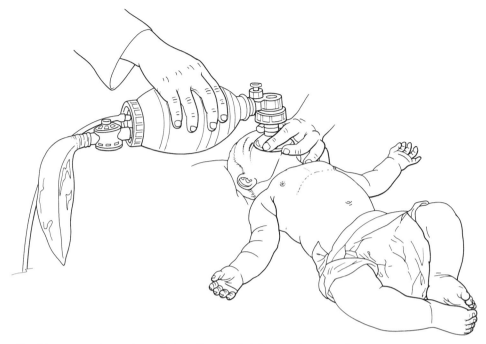

FIG. 13. Provide oxygenation and ventilation: One-handed face mask application.

— Place monitoring electrodes in the conventional chest positions and monitor with a cardiac monitor.

4. Assess Rhythm (± check for pulse)

* Check the pulse

Child — feel for the carotid pulse in the neck.

Infant — feel for the brachial pulse on the inner aspect of the upper arm.

* Take **no more than 10 s**

* Assess the rhythm on the monitor as being:
— Non-Ventricular fibrillation (Non-VF) or non-pulseless ventricular tachycardia (Non-VT) (Asystole or Electromechanical Dissociation)
— Ventricular fibrillation (VF) or pulseless ventricular tachycardia (VT)

5A. Non-VF/VT — Asystole, Electromechanical Dissociation

* This is more common in children

* Administer adrenaline/epinephrine

— If direct venous or intraosseous access has been established, give 10 **mcg**/kg adrenaline/epinephrine (0.1 ml/kg of 1 in 10,000 solution) (Fig. 14).
— If venous access has not been established consider giving 100 mcg/kg adrenaline/epinephrine via the tracheal tube (1 ml/kg of 1 in 10,000 or 0.1 ml/kg of 1 in 1000 solution).

* Perform 3 min of basic life support.

* Repeat the administration of adrenaline/epinephrine.

— If direct venous or intraosseous access has been established, give 100 mcg/kg adrenaline/

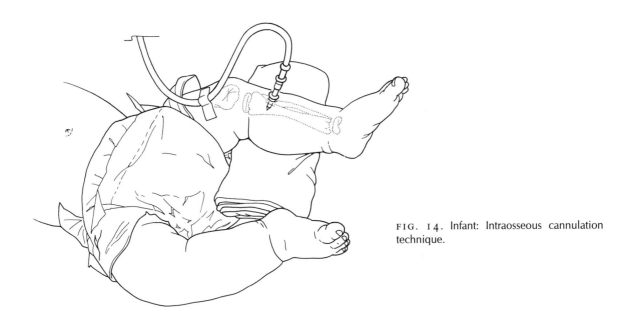

FIG. 14. Infant: Intraosseous cannulation technique.

epinephrine (1 ml/kg of 1 in 10,000 or 0.1 ml/kg of 1 in 1000 solution).

* Repeat the cycle of 100 mcg/kg adrenaline/epinephrine followed by 3 min of basic life support.

* Consider the use of other medications and treat reversible causes

5B. VF/VT

* This is less common in paediatric life support but the rescuer must always be aware of the possibility of treating this arrhythmia rapidly and effectively.

* Defibrillate the heart with three defibrillation shocks:
2 J/kg
2 J/kg
4 J/kg

(Accuracy of dosage may be difficult using defibrillators with stepped energy levels.)

– Place the defibrillator paddles on the chest wall; one just below the right clavicle, the other at the left anterior axillary line.
– For infants, when using this method of monitoring, it may be more appropriate to apply the paddles to the front and back of the infants chest.

* If VF/VT persists perform 1 min of basic life support.

* Defibrillate the heart with three defibrillation shocks:
4 J/kg
4 J/kg
4 J/kg
Repeat the cycle of defibrillation and 1-min basic life support until defibrillation is achieved. Consider the use of other medications and treat reversible causes.

6. Advanced life support procedures during CPR

* Establish a definitive airway.

− Attempt tracheal intubation
− Verify the position of the tracheal tube at regular intervals.
* Establish ventilation

− Ventilate with 100% oxygen using a self-inflating resuscitation bag.

* Establish vascular access
− Gain access to the circulation by:
  · Direct venous access
  · Intraosseous access

* Give adrenaline/epinephrine every 3 min

* Consider giving Bicarbonate to correct severe acidosis

* Correct reversible causes:
  Hypoxia
  Hypovolaemia
  Hyper/hypokalaemia
  Hypothermia
  Tension pneumothorax
  Tamponade
  Toxic/therapeutic disturbances
  Thromboemboli

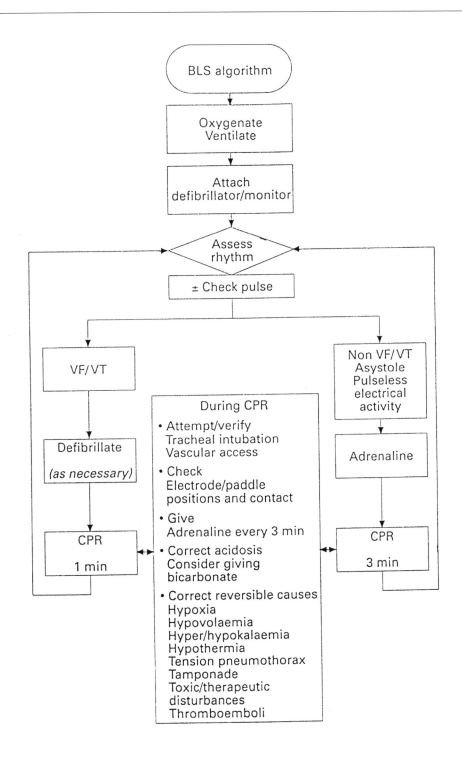

TABLE 2. Algorithm for paediatric advanced life support.

4.4. Paediatric Life Support Training Programme

Training in paediatric life support should be developed along flexible guidelines that will allow students to develop adequate and accurate skills in:

- Basic Life Support (BLS)
- Advanced Life Support (ALS)

Notes:

- BLS should form part of the fundamental training in resuscitation.
- All students must be competent in BLS before progressing to ALS.
- Both BLS and ALS are skill-based courses and should contain both theoretical and practical course elements.
- Completion of both BLS and ALS courses must be by a short written and practical examination.
- Certification must be for "successful completion" of a course and not be issued on a pass/fail or competency basis.

Paediatric Life Support

Course Content

The Course must contain adequate instruction, both theoretical and practical, for each student to be able to demonstrate an adequate knowledge of:

(A) Fundamental Principles

The difference in the *aetiology and epidemiology* between paediatric and adult resuscitation.

An understanding of the *age definitions* for:

> A newborn
> An infant
> A child (age < 8 years)
> An older child (age > 8 years)

An understanding of the importance of *prevention* especially in relation to the epidemiology of paediatric life support.

(B) Basic Life Support

Determination of responsiveness

Airway:
  Head Tilt – Chin Lift
  Jaw Thrust

Breathing:
  Determination of effective spontaneous respiration
  Expired air resuscitation
      Mouth-to-Mouth
      Mouth-to-Mouth and -Nose

Circulation
  Determination of the need for chest compressions:
      "Signs of life"
      Pulse Check
  External Chest Compressions:
      Compression landmarks
      Compression method
      Compression depth
      Compression rate
      Compression/ventilation ratio

Activation of Emergency Medical Services

Recovery position

Relief of foreign-body airway obstruction:
    Back slaps
    Chest thrusts
    Abdominal thrusts

The use of simple airway adjuncts and barrier equipment

(C) Advanced Life Support

Airway:
    Simple airway adjuncts:
        Oral airway
        Nasal airway
    Tracheal intubation:
        Oral
        Nasal
    Surgical airway techniques

Breathing:
    Bag, valve, mask ventilation
    Bag, valve, tracheal tube ventilation

Circulation:
    Rhythm assessment (confined to relevant resuscitation rhythms only)
    Vascular access:
        Direct venous
            Peripheral
            Central
        Intraosseous
        Tracheal

Drug and Fluid administration:
    Pharmacology of the commonly used resuscitation drugs and fluids.
    Drug dosages
    Fluid volumes
    Side effects

Defibrillation:
    Technique
    Energy levels
    Sequence

Treatment algorithm for advanced life support.

Complications of resuscitation

Audit:
    Collection of data
    Analysis of data
    Knowledge of current results of paediatric life support.

Note: It may be considered appropriate to consider instructing candidates on:

The arrested child
The seriously ill child
The seriously injured child

MANOEUVRE	OLDER CHILD	CHILD	INFANT	NEWBORN AT BIRTH	CPR/RESCUE BREATHING
	Older child	Approximately 1–8 years	Less than 1 year	Newborn at birth	**CHECK RESPONSIVENESS**
AIRWAY	Head tilt-chin lift (If trauma, use jaw thrust)	Head tilt-chin lift (If trauma, use jaw thrust)	Head tilt-chin lift (If trauma, use jaw thrust)	Head tilt-chin lift (If trauma, use jaw thrust)	Open Airway Activate EMS
BREATHING **Initial**	2–5 breaths at approximately 1 1/2 s per breath	2–5 breaths at approximately 1 1/2 s per breath	2–5 breaths at approximately 1 1/2 s per breath	2–5 breaths at approximately 1 s per breath	**CHECK BREATHING:** If victim breathing: Place in recovery position If no chest rise, Reposition airway and reattempt breaths up to 5 times
Subsequent	12 breaths/min (approximate)	20 breaths/min (approximate)	20 breaths/min (approximate)	30–60 breaths/min (approximate)	
Foreign body airway obstruction	Back blows and/or abdominal thrusts	Back blows and/or chest thrusts and/or abdominal thrusts	Back blows and/or chest thrusts (No abdominal thrusts)	Suction, (No abdominal thrusts or back blows)	
CIRCULATION					**ASSESS FOR SIGNS OF LIFE:**
Pulse check (Trained healthcare providers only*)	*Carotid	*Carotid	*Brachial	*Umbilical	If pulse present but breathing absent: provide rescue breaths
Compression landmarks	Lower half of sternum	Lower half of sternum	One finger width below intermammary line	*One finger width below intermammary line	If pulse not confidently felt > 60/min and poor perfusion: chest compressions
Compression method	Heel of one hand, other hand on top	Heel of one hand	Two or three fingers	*Two fingers or Encircling thumbs	
Compression depth	Approximately 1/3 the depth of the chest	Approximately 1/3 the depth of the chest	Approximately 1/3 the depth of the chest	*Approximately 1/3 the depth of the chest	**Continue BLS:** Integrate procedures appropriate for newborn, paediatric, or adult advanced life support at earliest opportunity
Compression rate	Approximately 100/min	Approximately 100/min	Approximately 100/min	*Approximately 120/min	
Compression/ ventilation ratio	15:2 (Single rescuer) 5:1 (Two rescuers)	5:1	5:1	*3:1	

*Interventions recommended for suitably trained healthcare providers only.

4.5. The 1998 European Resuscitation Council Guidelines for Resuscitation of Babies at Birth

4.5.1. INTRODUCTION

The International Liaison Committee on Resuscitation, ILCOR, in its 1997 advisory statement on paediatric life support [1] recognised the need to develop consistent international guidelines, to be promulgated by national resuscitation councils and associations. These guidelines, known as advisory statements, are based on specific data (outcome validity), but in the absence of specific data were developed and supported on the basis of common sense (face validity) or ease of teaching or skill retention (construct validity). The ILCOR advisory statement [1] makes specific recommendations for basic resuscitation of the newborn infant. These guidelines have developed and enhanced these concepts and extended them into advanced life support. They are an extension of the guidelines already published by the ERC [2–4] and take into account recommendations made by other national [5,6] and international [7] organisations.

ILCOR estimated that worldwide there was the potential to save 800,000 babies per year from morbidity or mortality from newborn asphyxia by using simple airway interventions. A relatively small number of newborn babies need any resuscitative intervention beyond gentle stimulation to breathe. Of the few that do need supplemental help the majority will require only assisted ventilation for a short period of time, the remaining minority will need advanced interventions including circulatory support and drug administration. Palme-Kilander analysing the results from 100,000 babies born in Sweden in 1 year found, that for babies over 2.5 kg in weight, 10 per 1,000 (1%) needed ventilation by mask or tracheal intubation. Of those babies requiring ventilation, eight responded to mask ventilation and

two required intubation [8]. The same study tried to assess the unexpected need for resuscitation at birth and found that for low-risk babies, born at > 32 weeks after an apparently normal labour, 0.2% required resuscitation unexpectedly; 90% responded to mask ventilation alone while the remaining 10% required intubation at birth. Another study, carried out in the UK, compared the frequency of tracheal intubation in two large but similar maternity units [9] and found a 5-fold difference in frequency of intubation, 10% vs. 2%. From the accumulated data it is therefore difficult to estimate the need for basic or advanced resuscitation skills.

It is therefore essential that personnel trained in the fundamental skills of newborn life support should be in attendance at every delivery. The care of the baby should be their sole responsibility. One person trained in the advanced life support techniques for the newborn should also be available for normal low risk deliveries and in attendance for all deliveries considered associated with a high risk for neonatal resuscitation. Appendix 1 lists types of deliveries where the baby may be considered to be at risk. The list has been included to act as a starting point for those who wish to develop local guidelines. The decision for a skilled resuscitator to be alerted or requested to attend a delivery will depend on local circumstances. It is recommended that local guidelines be developed based on current practice and clinical audit.

An organised educational programme in the standards and skills required for resuscitation of the newborn is therefore essential for any institution in which deliveries occur. Teamwork is essential for good results especially where advanced resuscitation techniques are required. Each hospital should develop a protocol delineating lines of responsibility for the implementation of such a programme.

4.5.1.1. Home deliveries

The recommendations for those who should attend a home delivery vary widely from country to country but it is universally accepted that the decision to undergo a home delivery, once agreed by the medical and midwifery staff, should not result in a compromise of the standard of newborn resuscitation at the time of delivery [6]. In an ideal situation at least two trained professionals (doctors or midwives) should be present at all home deliveries. At least one of the two professionals must be fully trained and experienced in neonatal basic life support including bag and mask ventilation. It must be agreed prior to delivery which professional will have responsibility for resuscitation of the baby.

4.5.1.2. The equipment and environment

Resuscitation at birth should be and often is a predictable event. It is therefore somewhat simpler to prepare the environment and the equipment prior to delivery of the baby than is the case in adult resuscitation that is often unpredictable. Where there is a need for resuscitation a warm, well-lit, draught-free area with a padded resuscitation surface should be prepared, and the resuscitation equipment made ready. A suggested list of equipment and drugs is presented in Appendix 2. All equipment must be checked daily and there should be a signed acknowledgement that this has been carried out. Furthermore, prior to each delivery, the attendant responsible for care of the new born baby should personally check the resuscitation equipment, making sure that no item is missing and that all are in working order.

When a birth takes place in a nondesignated delivery area, the recommended minimum set of equipment should include a bag/valve/mask ventilation device of appropriate size for the newborn, a suction device with a selection of suitably sized suction catheters, warm dry towels and a blanket, a clean (sterile) instrument for cutting the umbilical cord and clean rubber gloves for the attendant [1].

All newborn babies have difficulty in tolerating a cold environment. A wet newborn baby can cool rapidly at birth, and compromised babies have a particularly unstable thermo-regulatory system [10]. Exposure of the newborn to cold stress will result in a lower arterial oxygen tension [11] and an increased metabolic acidosis [12]. Heat loss is prevented by:

1. Maintaining a warm (25°C) delivery room. Keep all doors and windows closed.
2. Placing the baby under a preheated radiant warmer.
3. Quickly drying the baby immediately after delivery and thereafter covering the body, including the scalp with a warm towel to prevent further heat loss.

These steps which only take a few seconds, are appropriate for all babies following delivery but are especially important for small and/or asphyxiated babies.

4.5.1.3. Initial assessment

The Apgar scoring system [13] has been widely used as an indicator for the need for resuscitation at birth. The need for resuscitation can, however, be more accurately assessed by evaluating the heart rate, respiratory activity and colour than by the total Apgar score [14]. Since even a short delay in initiating resuscitation may result in a long delay in establishing spontaneous and regular respiration, resuscitation should be started immediately when indicated and not delayed for the assessment of the 1-min score.

A. Respiratory activity. This is initially assessed by the cry of the baby. A cry is the most common confirmation of adequate ventilation. The effectiveness of respiration should then be evaluated by observing the rate, depth and symmetry of respiration, together with any abnormal breathing pattern such as gasping, grunting etc.

B. Heart rate. This can be evaluated either by listening to the apex beat with a stethoscope, feeling the pulse in the base of the umbilical cord or palpating the brachial or femoral artery.

C. Colour. Observe whether the baby is centrally pink, cyanosed or pale. Peripheral cyanosis is common and does not, by itself, indicate hypoxemia.

Note: It is essential for good clinical care and for medicolegal reasons that the findings at each assessment and the actions taken are fully documented.

D. Tactile stimulation. Drying the baby usually produces enough stimulation to induce effective respiration in most who are not breathing adequately immediately after birth. If this fails additional safe methods can be used including slapping or flicking the soles of the feet, and gently rubbing the baby's back. More vigorous methods of stimulation should be avoided. If the baby fails to establish spontaneous and effective respirations following a brief period of stimulation, basic and/or advanced life support will be required.

E. Classification according to initial assessment. On the basis of the initial assessment, the babies can be divided into four groups.

1. Fit and healthy baby,
Vigorous effective respiratory efforts
Centrally pink
Heart rate > 100/min.
This baby requires no intervention other than drying, wrapping in a warm towel and, where appropriate, handing to the mother. The baby will usually remain warm by skin-to-skin contact with mother and may be put to the breast at this stage.

2. Breathing inadequately or apnoeic
Central cyanosis
Heart rate > 100/min
This group of babies may respond to tactile stimulation and/or facial oxygen but often need basic life support.

3. Breathing inadequately or apnoeic
Pale or white due to poor cardiac output and peripheral vasoconstriction
Heart rate < 100/min.
These babies sometimes improve with initial basic life support but normally require immediate intubation and positive pressure ventilation.

4. Breathing inadequately or apnoeic
Pale or white due to poor cardiac output and peripheral vasoconstriction
No detectable heart rate although this was documented up to 15–20 min before delivery.
These babies will require immediate ventilation, chest compressions, and full advanced life support including resuscitation drugs.

4.5.2. BASIC LIFE SUPPORT

Basic life support should be commenced if the baby has failed to cry by 30 s, to establish regular respiration by 1 min, or has a heart rate of below 100 beats/min before that. It can usually be achieved by means of a simple positive pressure ventilation device.

4.5.2.1. Airway (Fig. 1)

Look, listen and feel for respiratory efforts. The neonate should be on his or her back with the neck in a neutral or slightly extended position. A 2-cm thickness of the blanket or towel placed under the baby's shoulder is helpful in maintaining proper head position. If respiratory efforts are present but not producing tidal gas exchange, the airway is obstructed and immediate efforts must be made to clear the airway.

Clear the airway by gentle suction of the mouth and nares to remove any residual debris or fluid. Aggressive pharyngeal suction can delay the onset of spontaneous breathing and cause laryngeal spasm and vagal bradycardia [15]. It is not indicated unless the amniotic fluid is stained with thick meconium or blood. If suction is required, a 10 FG (or if preterm, an 8 FG) suction catheter should be connected to a suction source not exceeding −100 mmHg. This should

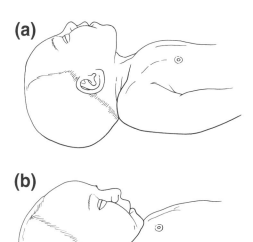

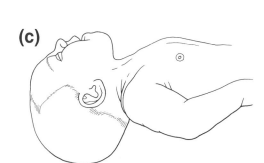

FIG. 1. Positioning the airway in newborn; (a) Correct position (slightly extended); (b) incorrect position; (c) incorrect position (too much extended).

not continue for longer than 5 s in the absence of meconium. The catheter should normally not be inserted further than about 5 cm from the lips.

4.5.2.2. Breathing

The main role of oxygen flowing over the face via a loose fitting face mask or funnel is to provide a cold stimulus to breathing. It has been traditional to use 100% oxygen as the resuscitation gas but there are increasing data indicating that in term babies 100% oxygen has little advantage and may increase oxygen-free radical

damage. Although there is no experimental animal or infant data to show that the use of lower oxygen concentrations leads to improved neurological survival, there are now data to show that resuscitation is as effective if air is used rather than 100% oxygen [16–20]. If gas-mixing facilities are available, 40% oxygen is sometimes used.

A. Face masks [21] (Figs. 2–3)

A well-fitting face mask, which covers the mouth and nose but does not cover the eyes or overhang the chin, though forms an effective air seal, is essential for effective inflation of the lungs. This is best provided by a round mask with a soft seal cuff. A range of sizes should be available.

Face mask ventilation systems

1. *Self-inflating bags.* These bags refill independently of gas flow and should incorporate a pressure-limited pop-off valve preset at 20–30 cmH_2O. In a minority, this pressure may be inadequate to achieve lung expansion at birth and the facility to override this is useful for a few babies. The volume of the bag should be at least 500 ml, so that the inflation pressure can be maintained for at least 0.5 s.

2. *Face mask T-piece resuscitation* [22]. In this system, compressed air/oxygen is fed to one arm of a T-piece attached to the face mask. The baby's lungs are inflated by occluding the open arm of the T-piece. It is obviously essential to have a safety pressure release system (set at 20–30 cmH_2O) incorporated in the gas supply tubing. A method for monitoring the peak pressures will also be required. This system has the advantage that it requires only one hand for normal operation and the inflation pressures can be maintained for longer than with the self-inflating bags.

3. *Paediatric anaesthetic circuit.* The anaesthetic rebreathing bag depends on a continuous flow of

air or oxygen. The anaesthetic circuit requires more training than the self-inflating bag, or the face mask T-piece system, but provides a greater range of peak inspiratory pressures which can be important in newborn resuscitation.

The technique of ventilation is different for the first few breaths. Maintain the inspiration for 1−2 s for the first five or six breaths. Prolonging the first inspiration for 2−3 s will more than double the first inspiratory volume and is more likely to lead to the immediate formation of a functional residual capacity [23]. The chest wall should be seen to be moving by the fifth breath. After the initial breaths ventilate the lungs at a rate of 30−40 breaths per minute. If the heart rate is >100 beats per minute continue ventilation until spontaneous respiration is established.

If the baby does not respond to face mask resuscitation some authorities recommend that the attendant should proceed to tracheal intubation immediately. Tracheal intubation requires training and experience to be performed effectively and if this is not available and the heart rate is falling, the attendant should proceed to chest compressions whilst calling a colleague who has advanced newborn resuscitation skills including the ability to intubate the trachea.

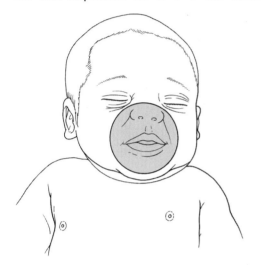

FIG. 2. Positioning the face mask.

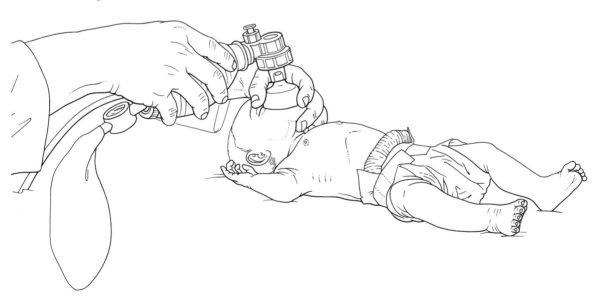

FIG. 3. Positive pressure ventilation using a bag, valve and mask.

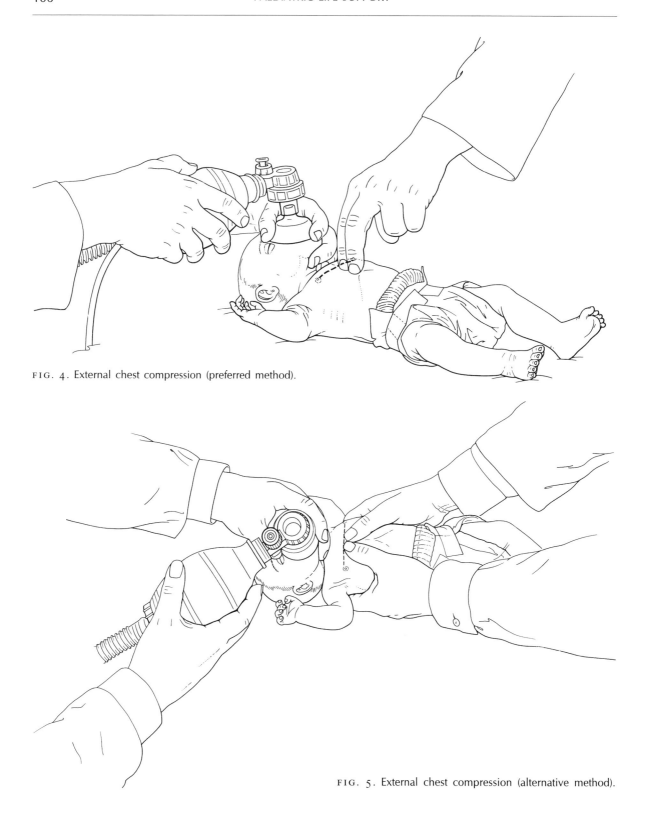

FIG. 4. External chest compression (preferred method).

FIG. 5. External chest compression (alternative method).

4.5.2.3. Circulation (Figs. 4–5)

Asphyxia causes peripheral vasoconstriction, tissue hypoxia, acidosis, poor myocardial contractility, bradycardia and eventually cardiac arrest. Prompt and effective ventilation and oxygenation can often avoid this critical state. Chest compression should be performed, however, if:

1. The heart rate is less than 60 beats/min.
2. The heart rate is less than 100 beats/min and falls despite adequate ventilation.

The optimal technique is to place the two thumbs side by side over the lower one-third of the sternum with the fingers encircling the torso and supporting the back [24–26]. The lower third of the sternum [27] is compressed 2–3 cm in a term baby at a rate of 120 compressions per minute. The compressions should be smooth and not jerky and each compression should last 50% of the compression/relaxation cycle. The thumbs should not be lifted off the sternum during the relaxation phase, but the chest wall should be allowed to return to its relaxed position between each compression. Alternatively, the index and middle finger of one hand can compress the lower sternum. Although this is less effective, it does free the other hand that may be needed for other resuscitation or assessment tasks.

A ratio of three compressions to one ventilation is recommended, as the respiratory rate will otherwise be too slow. Pulse rate should be checked after 1 min and periodically thereafter. Chest compressions should only be discontinued when the spontaneous heart rate reaches 100 beats/min and is rising.

4.5.3. ADVANCED LIFE SUPPORT

4.5.3.1. Airway

Advanced life support requires intubation of the trachea. Position the baby's head by gently extending the neck into the "sniffing" position, if necessary, with an assistant. Holding the laryngoscope handle in the left hand, pass the laryngoscope blade down into the mouth making sure that it is in the midline, with the tongue pushed to the left, until the epiglottis comes into view. Most clinicians find a straight bladed laryngoscope preferable. The tip of the blade can then be positioned either proximal to or immediately over the epiglottis so that the cords are brought into view. A gentle backward pressure may need to be applied over the larynx at this stage. This can be done with the 5th finger of the left hand during laryngoscopy or by an assistant. As the airway tends to be filled with fluid, the upper airway may have to be cleared with a suction catheter held in the right hand.

Once the cords are visible, pass the tracheal tube using the right hand and remove the laryngoscope blade taking care that this does not displace the tube out of the larynx. Then attach the tracheal tube to a ventilation system. Confirm that air is entering both lungs equally by listening for breath sounds in each axilla and over the upper abdomen. If there are no breath sounds over the lungs, the most likely cause is that the tracheal tube is lying in the oesophagus.

WHEN THERE IS ANY DOUBT ABOUT THE POSITION OR PATENCY OF THE TUBE REMOVE THE TRACHEAL TUBE IMMEDIATELY AND REINTUBATE AFTER A BRIEF PERIOD OF OXYGENATION USING FACE MASK VENTILATION.

Straight tubes can be used but may need introducers to make them more rigid. Particular care

Guidelines for tracheal tube size

Tracheal Tube Size (mm. Internal Diameter)	Weight (g)	Gestation (weeks)
2.5	<1000	<28
3	1000–2500	28–36
3.5	>2500	>36

These are only guidelines and tubes 0.5 mm larger and smaller should always be available.
The initial breath may need a higher pressure to inflate the alveolae and establish a functional residual capacity (see above).

is then required to ensure that the end of the introducer does not protrude beyond the tip of the tracheal tube to avoid laryngeal or tracheal trauma. An alternative approach is to pass a naso-tracheal tube through the nares, and then advance the tip into the larynx with Magill forceps, using the laryngoscope to ensure clear visualisation of the glottis. Advance the tube, until the black marking just disappears into the larynx. If a shouldered (Cole Tube) is used the shoulder must be positioned just above the cords. Do not force the shoulder through the cords as this will damage the cords.

4.5.3.2. Breathing

If a T-piece connector is used, maintain the initial inflation pressure for 2–3 s. This will help lung expansion (Fig. 6). The baby can subsequently be ventilated at a rate of 30/min allowing approximately 1 s for each inflation. If a self-inflating bag system or an anaesthetic rebreathing bag is used, squeeze the bag sufficiently to achieve visible chest wall movement.

If auscultation indicates that oxygen is entering one lung only, usually the right, the tube may have been passed too far down the trachea. Correct this by withdrawing the tracheal tube by 1 cm while listening over the left lung. Again

ensure bilateral and equal air entry to both lungs before securing the tube. If there is no improvement, carefully check the equipment for disconnection or lack of oxygen flow, then consider other possible causes including pneumothorax, pleural effusion or diaphragmatic hernia.

Ventilatory support should be continued until the baby is pink, well-perfused and making active respiratory efforts.

4.5.3.3. Circulation

Chest compressions should be carried out as described in Basic Life Support above, i.e., if the heart rate is 60 beats/min or less than 100 beats/min and falls despite adequate ventilation. If there is no prompt improvement, and direct venous access has yet to be established, inject 10–30 mcg/kg (0.1–0.3 ml/kg of 1/10,000) adrenaline/epinephrine via the tracheal tube during a brief period of disconnection from the positive pressure ventilation system. Although data on adults indicate that higher doses of adrenaline/epinephrine should be given when the tracheal route is used, there is currently no information to show that this is safe or more effective in neonates. Despite the tracheal administration of adrenaline/epinephrine being widely practised there is little evidence that it is effective but further

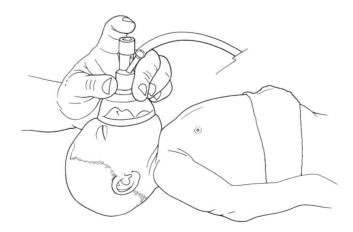

FIG. 6. Using a T-piece, valve and mask.

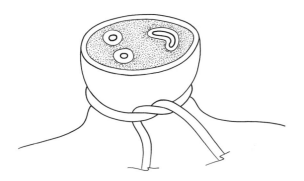

FIG. 7. The umbilical cord prepared for venous cannulation.

research is required to determine its true efficacy [20,28,29]. It may be least effective if given before the lungs have been fully inflated.

Lack of improvement of the heart rate is usually due to inadequate ventilation: check the seal of the face mask or the position of the tracheal tube first. When satisfied that there is optimal airway control and in the absence of continued improvement, the umbilical vein should be catheterised using a 4.5–5 FG umbilical catheter. This is achieved by transecting the cord 1–2 cm away from the abdominal skin and inserting a catheter until there is a free flow of blood up the catheter. A further dose of adrenaline/epinephrine 10–30 mcg/kg (0.1–0.3 ml/kg of 1:10,000 solution) should then be given via the umbilical venous catheter, flushing the adrenaline/epinephrine through the catheter with 2 ml of saline. If venous access fails, an intraosseous needle can be inserted into the tibia and this route used instead of the venous umbilical catheter (Fig. 7).

If there is still no response the baby should be given 1–2 mmol/kg body weight of sodium bicarbonate slowly over 2–3 min. Use a 4.2% bicarbonate solution or mix a volume of 8.4% sodium bicarbonate solution with an equal volume of 5 or 10% dextrose or sterile water. This results in a concentration of 0.5 mmol/ml solution. Basic life support must be continued. Sodium bicarbonate is a hyperosmolar solution and should be administered by slow infusion in

preterm babies below 32 weeks because of the risk of inducing intracerebral bleeding.

Repeat doses of adrenaline/epinephrine (10–30 mcg/kg) may be given intravenously through the umbilical catheter if there is still no response. Subsequent larger doses, up to 100 mcg/kg of adrenaline/epinephrine may be considered in resistant cases but there is evidence that the need for adrenaline/epinephrine during resuscitation is associated with a poor prognosis [30]. Repeat doses of sodium bicarbonate (1–2 mmol/kg may also be considered although fully correcting the metabolic component of the acidosis is not intended. Sodium bicarbonate is best administered using the results of blood gas analysis data.

Volume expanders

Volume expanders are indicated in the presence of hypovolaemia that should be considered in any baby who requires resuscitation.
Indications include:

1. Evidence of acute fetal blood loss.
2. Pallor which persists after oxygenation.
3. Faint pulses with a good heart rate and poor response to resuscitation including adequate ventilation.

The volume expander can be given as plasma or 4.5% albumin in normal saline or other plasma substitutes. Uncrossmatched Group O Rhesus negative blood can be given. 10–20 ml/kg of the selected fluid should be infused. Volume replacement should be infused as quickly as possible when severe hypovolaemia is evident, for example, after a large fetal or placental bleed or if there is continuing haemorrhage, although these are rare events.

4.5.3.4. Naloxone

Naloxone hydrochloride is a narcotic antagonist. Naloxone should be given to all babies who become pink and who have obviously satisfactory circulation on resuscitation, though fail to start adequate respiratory efforts and in whom

there is a history of recent therapeutic administration of opiates to the mother. Naloxone, 100
mcg/kg, should then be given intramuscularly.
Following a satisfactory response the baby should
be observed carefully for further signs of respiratory depression and an additional 100 mcg/kg
may be given intramuscularly to prevent relapse.
Naloxone can, if required, be administered via
the tracheal route.

*Do not give Naloxone to the baby of an opi-
ate-dependent mother as this will precipitate a
severe withdrawal crisis.*

4.5.3.5. Special situations

(a) *Meconium aspiration*

Where the liquor is contaminated by thick meconium, the oropharynx should be sucked out
while the baby's head is on the perineum. Direct
laryngoscopy should then be carried out immediately after birth. If this shows meconium in the
pharynx and trachea, intubate the baby immediately and apply suction. One approach is to
attach the tracheal tube to the suction source,
then suck up the free fluid while removing the
tracheal tube. Providing the baby's heart rate
remains above 100 beats/min, the trachea can
be reintubated and this procedure can be
repeated until meconium is no longer recovered.
It is rarely necessary to repeat this procedure
more than 3–4 times. Finally the trachea is reintubated and the baby oxygenated and ventilated
if necessary. There is currently a debate on the
efficacy of upper airway suction after the delivery
of the head and also whether there is a need for
tracheal intubation and suction for meconium
aspiration in the absence of fetal asphyxia.
Some centres advocate performing broncho-
alveolar lavage with saline. However, the balance
of opinion remains in favour of an active
approach to the problem.

(b) *Preterm babies*

Babies born with a gestation of > 35 weeks do
not differ from full-term babies in their requirements for resuscitation. At lower gestations morbidity and mortality are likely to be reduced by
adopting a more active intervention policy.

However, there is no evidence that outcome is
improved by routinely intubating all babies
whose gestation is less than 28 or 30 weeks.
Although there are no data to recommend elective intubation for all babies, even at the borders
of viability, other factors, for example, the need
to transfer the baby considerable distances to the
neonatal unit, or the prophylactic use of surfac-
tants may mean that intubation is advisable.
Nasal CPAP may also be beneficial in helping
to achieve and maintain an adequate respiratory
pattern. However, if the preterm baby fails to cry
by 15 s or to establish regular respiration by 30
s, face mask resuscitation should be commenced
and intubation carried out if the baby has not
achieved satisfactory respiratory exchange within
a further 30 s.

4.5.4. INDICATIONS FOR DISCONTINUING RESUSCITATION

Local and National Committees will determine
the indications for discontinuing resuscitation.
However, the Working Group felt that it was
important to include a simple guide as a baseline
within this text.

Resuscitatory efforts should be discontinued if
the baby does not have a cardiac output by 15
min or if the baby is failing to make any respiratory efforts despite Naloxone therapy by 30 min.
Those who make independent respiratory efforts
but are unable to maintain adequate tidal exchange should be transferred to a neonatal unit
for further respiratory support and reassessed after
24–48 h.

Communication with the parents

It is vitally important that the team caring for the
newborn baby informs the parents of the baby's
progress. At delivery the routine local plan
should be adhered to and, if possible the baby
handed to the mother at the earliest opportunity.
If resuscitation is required the parents should be

informed of the procedures being undertaken and why they are required. It is important to be as frank and honest as possible, especially if the baby unexpectedly requires resuscitation.

Decisions to discontinue resuscitation or to resuscitate an extremely preterm baby should closely involve the parents and senior paediatric staff. Where a difficulty has been foreseen, for example, in the case of severe congenital malformation, the options and prognosis should be discussed with the parents, midwives, obstetricians and birth attendants before delivery. Some special situations require further clarification or discussion with the parents about further advanced therapeutic manoeuvres that may be required (e.g., spinal shock, transverse spinal lesion or syndrome, hematomyelia, neonatal myasthenia, maternal intoxication) and the long-term prognosis in terms of the quality of the baby's life.

All discussions and decisions should be carefully recorded in the mother's notes prior to delivery and also in the baby's records after birth.

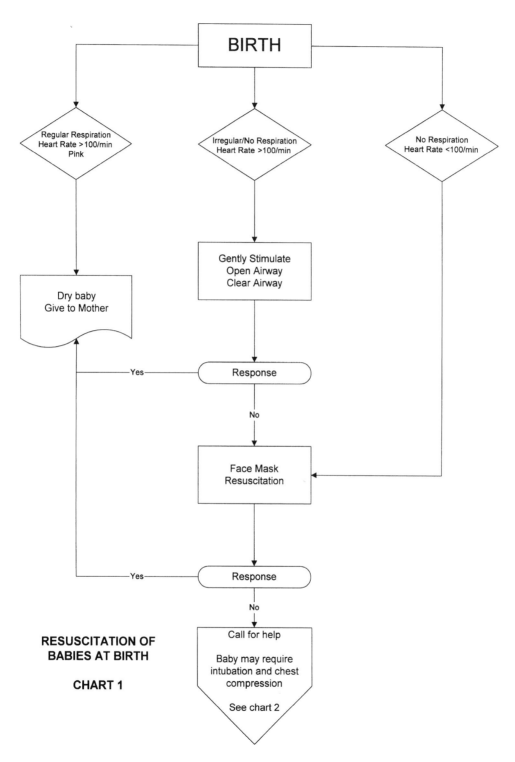

**RESUSCITATION OF
BABIES AT BIRTH**

CHART 1

Note: If there is thick meconium and the baby is unresponsive, proceed immediately to chart 2

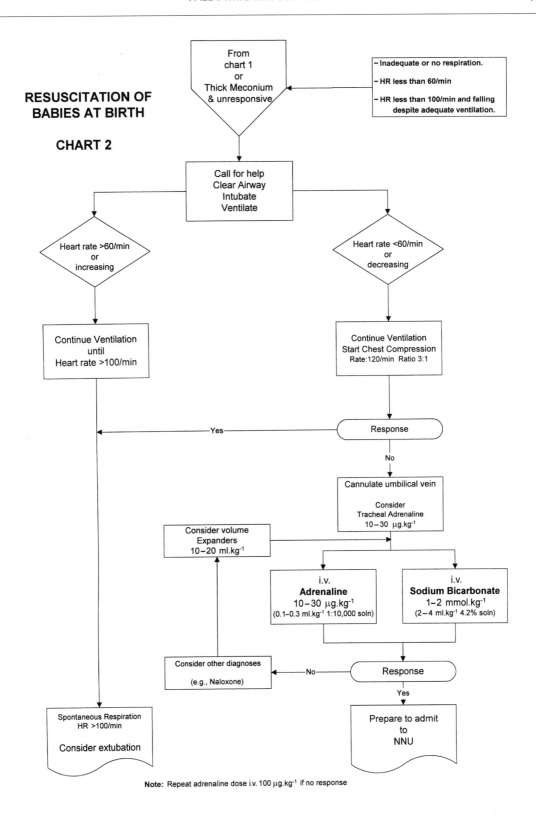

RESUSCITATION OF BABIES AT BIRTH

CHART 2

From chart 1 or Thick Meconium & unresponsive

- Inadequate or no respiration.
- HR less than 60/min
- HR less than 100/min and falling despite adequate ventilation.

Call for help
Clear Airway
Intubate
Ventilate

Heart rate >60/min or increasing

Heart rate <60/min or decreasing

Continue Ventilation until Heart rate >100/min

Continue Ventilation
Start Chest Compression
Rate:120/min Ratio 3:1

Response — Yes

No

Cannulate umbilical vein

Consider
Tracheal Adrenaline
10 – 30 µg.kg⁻¹

Consider volume Expanders
10 – 20 ml.kg⁻¹

i.v.
Adrenaline
10 – 30 µg.kg⁻¹
(0.1–0.3 ml.kg⁻¹ 1:10,000 soln)

i.v.
Sodium Bicarbonate
1 – 2 mmol.kg⁻¹
(2 – 4 ml.kg⁻¹ 4.2% soln)

Consider other diagnoses
(e.g., Naloxone) — No — Response — Yes

Spontaneous Respiration
HR >100/min

Consider extubation

Prepare to admit to NNU

Note: Repeat adrenaline dose i.v. 100 µg.kg⁻¹ if no response

APPENDIX 1: Deliveries where the baby may be considered to be at risk.

This list has been included to act as a starting point for those who wish to develop local guidelines.

Delivery
  Fetal distress
  Reduced fetal movement before onset of labour
  Abnormal presentation
  Prolapsed cord
  Prolonged rupture of the membranes
  Antepartum haemorrhage
  Thick meconium staining of liquor
  Forceps delivery
  Ventouse-assisted delivery
  Caesarean section

Maternal
  Severe pregnancy-induced hypertension
  Heavy sedation
  Drug addiction
  Diabetes mellitus
  Chronic illness
  Concern of attending staff

Fetal
  Multiple pregnancy
  Preterm ($<35/52$)
  Postterm ($>42/52$)
  Growth restriction
  Rhesus isoimmunisation/Hydrops
  Hydramnios and oligohydramnios
  Congenital abnormalities
  Intrauterine infection

The decision as to the need for attendance of an advanced skilled person will depend on local circumstances. It is recommended that local committees establish formal protocols based on current clinical practice and clinical audit.

APPENDIX 2: Recommended equipment and drugs for resuscitation of the newborn

Padded shelf/resuscitation trolley
Overhead heater
Overhead light
Clock
Stethoscope
Oxygen supply (variable up to 10 l/min flow rate)
Reserve oxygen cylinders
Face masks (different sizes)
Oro-pharyngeal airways (sizes 0, 00)
Resuscitation system (face mask, T-piece, valve, mask and reservoir)
Airway pressure manometer and pressure relief valve
Mechanical and/or manual suction device (manual with double trap); maximum level = 100 mmHg (13.3 kPa)
Suction catheters (sizes 6, 8, 10 FG)
Two laryngoscopes with spare blades
Tracheal tubes (sizes 2, 2.5, 3, 3.5 and 4 mm ID)
Tracheal tube introducer
Umbilical vein catheter set
2, 5, 10 and 20 ml syringes with needles
Method of securing the tracheal tube and intravenous lines

Drugs:

Recommended drug doses and volumes are contained in the text of the document

Volume expanders 4.5% Albumin
                 Plasma
                 Uncrossmatched Group O
                 Rhesus negative blood
Adrenaline/epinephrine (100 mcg/ml or 1/10,000 concentration)
Naloxone hydrochloride (400 mcg/ml),
Alkalising agent   Sodium bicarbonate (0.5 mmol/ml or 4.2% concentration)
                    (1.0 mmol/ml or 8.4% concentration)
                    (Trishydroxymethyl amino methane (TRIS) 3.6% concentration)
Sodium chloride (0.9%)
Dextrose (5—10% solutions)

Additional monitoring equipment may include: ECG monitor, Pulse Oximeter, Carbon Dioxide monitor.

REFERENCES

1. International Liaison Committee on Resuscitation (ILCOR) – Advisory statement on Paediatric Life Support. Resuscitation 1997;34:115–128.
2. European Resuscitation Council. Guidelines for basic life support. Resuscitation 1992;24:103–110. Br Med J 1993;306:1587–1589.
3. European Resuscitation Council. Guidelines for advanced life support. Resuscitation 1992;24:111–121. Br Med J 1993;306:1589–1593.
4. European Resuscitation Council. Guidelines for paediatric life support. Resuscitation 1994;27:91–106. Br Med J 1994;308:1349–1355.
5. Royal College of Paediatrics and Child Health. Resuscitation of Babies at Birth. BMJ Publishing Group, 1997.
6. British Paediatric Association. Neonatal Resuscitation – The report of a BPA Working Group 1993. British Paediatric Association, London.
7. American Heart Association. Neonatal advanced life support. J Am Med Assoc 1996;255:2969–2973.
8. Palme-Kilander C. Methods of resuscitation in low Apgar score newborn infants – a national survey. Acta Paediatr 1992;81:739–744.
9. Hospital and Health Board Comparisons in Obstetrics 1988–90. Information & Statistics Division, Scottish Health Service Common Services Agency, 1992, p. 57.
10. Dahn LS, James LS. Newborn temperature and calculated heat loss in the delivery room. Pediatrics 1972;49:504–513.
11. Stephenson JM, Du JN, Oliver TK. The effect of cooling on blood gas tensions in newborn infants. J Pediatr 1970;76:848–852.
12. Gandy GM, Adamson K, Cunningham N et al. Thermal environment and acid-base homeostasis in human infants during the first few hours of life. J Clin Invest 1964;43:751–758.
13. Apgar V, James LS. Further observations of the newborn scoring system. Am J Dis Child 1962;104:419–428.
14. Chamberlain G, Banks J. Assessment of the Apgar Score. Lancet 1974;ii:1225–1228.
15. Codero L, How EH. Neonatal bradycardia following nasopharyngeal suction. J Pediatr 1971;78:441.
16. Lundstrom KE, Pryds O, Greisen G. Oxygen at birth and prolonged cerebral vasoconstriction in preterm infants. Arch Dis Childh 1995;73:F81–F86.
17. Svenningsen NW, Stjernquist K, Stavenow S, Hellstrom-Vestas L. Neonatal outcome of extremely low birth weight liveborn infants below 901 g in a Swedish population. Acta Paed Scand 1989;78:180–188.
18. Ramji S, Ahuja S, Thirupuram S, Rootwelt T, Rooth G, Saugstad OD. Resuscitation of asphyxic newborn infants with room air or 100% oxygen. Pediatr Res 1993;34(Suppl 6):809–812.
19. Ballot DE, Rothberg AD, Davies VA, Smith J, Kirsten G. Does hypoxemia prevent brain damage in birth asphyxia? Med Hypotheses 1993;41(Suppl 4):344–347.
20. Lucas VW, Preziosi MP, Burchfield DJ. Epinephrine absorption following endotracheal administration: effects of hypoxia-induced low pulmonary blood flow. Resuscitation 1997;27:31–34.
21. Palme C, Nystrom B, Tunell R. An evaluation of the efficiency of face masks in the resuscitation of the newborn infants. Lancet 1985;i:207–210.
22. Hoskyns EW, Miner AD, Hopkin IE. A simple method of face mask resuscitation at birth. Arch Dis Child 1987;62:376–379.
23. Vyas H, Milner AD, Hopkin IE, Boon AW. Physiologic responses to prolonged slow rise inflation in the resuscitation of the asphyxiated newborn infant. J Pediatr 1981;99:635–639.
24. Thaler MM, Stobie GHC. An improved technique of external cardiac compression in infants and young children. N Engl J Med 1963;269:606–610.
25. Todres ID, Rogers MC. Methods of external cardiac massage in the newborn infant. J Pediatr 1975;86:781–782.
26. David R. Closed chest cardiac massage in the newborn infant. Pediatrics 1988;81:552–554.
27. Phillips G, Zideman DA. Relation of infant heart to sternum: its significance in cardiopulmonary resuscitation. Lancet 1986;i:1024–1025.
28. Lindemann R. Tracheal administration of epinephrine during cardiopulmonary resuscitation. Am J Dis Child 1982;136:753.
29. Mullett CJ, Kong JQ, Romano JT, Polak MJ. Age related changes in pulmonary venous epinephrine concentration and pulmonary vascular response after intratracheal epinephrine. Paediatr Res 1992;31:458–461.
30. Sims DG, Heal CA, Bartle SM. The use of adrenaline and atropine in neonatal resuscitation. Arch Dis Child 1994;70:F3–F10.

5. Automated External Defibrillation

CONTENTS:

5.1. Advisory Statement on Early Defibrillation

An advisory statement by the Advanced Life Support working group of the International Liaison Committee on Resuscitation [1]

5.1.1. THE CONCEPT OF EARLY DEFIBRILLATION

Most adults who can be saved from cardiac arrest are individuals in ventricular fibrillation or pulse-less ventricular tachycardia. Electrical defibrillation provides the single most important therapy for the treatment of these patients. Resuscitation science, therefore, places great emphasis upon early defibrillation. The greatest chances of survival result when the interval between the start of VF and the delivery of defibrillation is as brief as possible. To achieve the earliest possible defibrillation, ILCOR strongly endorses the concept that, in many settings, nonmedical individuals must be allowed and encouraged to use defibrillators [2].

ILCOR recommends that resuscitation personnel be authorized, trained, equipped and directed to operate a defibrillator, if their professional responsibilities require them to respond to persons in cardiac arrest.

This recommendation includes all first responding emergency personnel, in both the hospital and out-of-hospital setting, whether physicians, nurses, or nonmedical ambulance personnel.

The widespread availability of automated external defibrillators (AEDs) provides the technological capacity for early defibrillation both by ambulance crews and by lay responders.

5.1.2. EARLY DEFIBRILLATION BY AMBULANCE PERSONNEL

ILCOR urges the medical profession to increase the awareness of the public, and of those responsible for emergency medical services, of the importance of early defibrillation by ambulance personnel.

Every ambulance service which responds to emergencies should carry a defibrillator and staff trained in its use.

In some locations the medical profession will need to encourage medical and regulatory authorities to initiate changes in regulations and legislation.

Leaders of Emergency Medical Service (EMS) systems may need to overcome obstacles that include: nonenabling legislation, economic priorities, unsuitable EMS structure, lack of awareness, inadequate motivation and tradition.

ILCOR recommends that early defibrillation programmes by nonmedical ambulance personnel operate with control systems that:

- Set written policies and guidelines similar to those already developed by major resuscitation organisations.
- Establish a training and quality maintenance programme that ensures a high level of supervision.
- Place the programme under the direction and responsibility of a physician, or the direct representative of a physician acting on his/her behalf.

Writing group: L. Bossaert, V. Callanan and R. Cummins.
Members of the ALS working group: W. Kloeck, R. Cummins, D. Chamberlain, L. Bossaert, V. Callanan, P. Carli, J. Christenson, B. Connolly, J. Ornato, A. Sanders and P. Steen.

- Use only AEDs (except for fully trained paramedics who may use manual defibrillators by local agreement).
- Require that all defibrillators contain internal recording facilities that permit documentation and review of all clinical uses of the AED.

5.1.3. EARLY DEFIBRILLATION BY IN-HOSPITAL RESPONDERS

The concept of early defibrillation applies not only to the out-of-hospital setting, but also to in-hospital resuscitation efforts.

ILCOR strongly encourages the development of early defibrillation programmes for nonphysician in-hospital responders. ILCOR recommends that these programmes comply with these guidelines:

- Regularly train all hospital staff, who may need to respond to a sudden cardiopulmonary emergency, in basic life support.
- Establish and encourage AED training as a basic skill for health care providers working in settings where advanced life support professionals are not immediately available.
- Extend training and authorization to use conventional or AEDs to all appropriate nonphysician staff, including nurses, respiratory therapists, and physician assistants.
- Reduce the time from collapse to defibrillation by making conventional defibrillators or AEDs readily available in strategic areas throughout a facility.
- Document all resuscitation efforts accurately by recording specific treatment interventions, event variables, and outcome variables. The In-Hospital Utstein guidelines [3,4] provide a recommended Standard Reporting Form for in-hospital cardiopulmonary resuscitation.
- Collect and review the patient variables, event variables and outcome variables that are contained in the set of uniform data elements in the In-hospital Utstein guidelines.
- Establish an interdisciplinary committee, with expertise in cardiopulmonary resuscitation, to assess the quality and efficacy of the facilities resuscitation efforts.

5.1.4. EARLY DEFIBRILLATION BY FIRST RESPONDERS IN THE COMMUNITY

A first responder is defined as a trained individual, acting independently within a medically controlled system. In the community these may include police, security officers, lifeguards, airline cabin attendants, railway station personnel, voluntary aiders and those assigned to provide first aid at their own place of work or in the community, and are trained in how to use an AED.

ILCOR advises that physicians should be involved with any first responder defibrillation programme in the community and makes the following recommendations:

- Establish acceptance, support and coordination by responsible community medical and EMS authorities.
- In some specific situations, consider combining training programmes for bystander defibrillation with training in basic life support with careful monitoring of results.
- Arrange for review of all clinical application of an AED by a medically qualified programme coordinator or a designated representative.
- Plan for critical programme evaluation at two levels: individual clinical uses and overall EMS system effects.
- Ensure the availability of debriefing and counselling for every first responder following the clinical use of an AED, especially when the victim did not survive.
- Use only AEDs; for practical considerations manual defibrillators should not be used by laypersons.
- Continue innovations to produce simple, lightweight, economically priced and highly reliable AEDs.

5.1.5. EARLY DEFIBRILLATION AND THE CHAIN OF SURVIVAL CONCEPT

Early defibrillation addresses only part of the problem of sudden cardiac death. Early defibrillation initiatives will succeed only when implemented as part of the chain of survival concept. The links of the chain of survival include early recognition of cardiopulmonary arrest, early activation of trained responders, early cardiopulmonary resuscitation (CPR), early defibrillation when indicated, and early advanced life support. The chain of survival concept, while originally described in the context of out-of-hospital cardiac arrest, is equally valid for in-hospital resuscitation. Establishment of early defibrillation within a strong chain of survival will ensure the highest possible survival rate for both out-of-hospital and in-hospital events.

5.1.6. REFERENCES

1.　Bossaert L, Callanan V, Cummins R. Advisory statement on early defibrillation. An advisory statement by the Advanced Life Support working group of the International Liaison Committee on Resuscitation. Resuscitation 1997;34:113–114.

2.　Weisfeldt ML, Kerber RE, Mc Goldrick P, et al. Public access defibrillation: A statement for healthcare professionals from the American Heart Associaton Task Force on automatic external defibrillation. Circulation 1995;92:2763.

3.　Cummins R, Chamberlain D, Abramson N, Allen M, Baskett P, Becker L, Bossaert L et al. Special report: Recommended guidelines for uniform reporting of data from out-of-hospital cardiac arrest. Resuscitation 1991;22:91–26.

4.　Cummins R, Chamberlain D, Hazinski MF, Nadkarni V, Kloeck W, Kramer E, Becker L, Robertson C, Koster R, Zaritsky A, Bossaert L, Ornato J, Callanan V, Allen M, Steen P, Conolly B, Sanders A, Idris A, Cobbe S. Recommended guidelines for reviewing, reporting and conducting research on in-hospital resuscitation, the "in-hospital Utstein style". Resuscitation 1997; 34:151–185.

5.2. The 1998 European Resuscitation Guidelines for the Use of Automated External Defibrillators by EMS Providers and First Responders

Statement by the Early Defibrillation Task Force of the European Resuscitation Council

5.2.1. INTRODUCTION

1. Electrical defibrillation is the single most important therapy for the treatment of ventricular fibrillation. The time interval between the onset of ventricular fibrillation and the delivery of the first shock is clearly the main determinant of survival. Studies have shown that survival falls by approximately 7–10% for every minute after collapse for patients found in ventricular fibrillation [1]. The ERC strongly endorses the concept of early defibrillation within the Chain of Survival. To achieve the goal of early defibrillation it is mandatory to allow individuals other than physicians to defibrillate. The scientific and clinical evidence overwhelmingly reinforces this as the only acceptable strategy [2–7].

2. Having accepted this principle, the medical profession is urged to place pressure on the public, those responsible for directing emergency services within the hospital and prehospital, and those with regulatory powers, to permit changes in practice and legislation where necessary.

3. The remit of the ERC is to produce guidelines for automated defibrillation performed by first responders other than physicians, defined as a trained individual acting independently within a medically controlled system.

These include:
- first responding professional or volunteer Emergency Medical Service (EMS) personnel; and
- first responders other than EMS personnel prior to the arrival of the emergency medical services.

4. The ERC recommends:

- That every ambulance in Europe which might respond to a cardiac arrest must carry a defibrillator with personnel trained and permitted to use it.
- That defibrillation should be one of the core competencies of doctors, nurses and other health care professionals.
- That defibrillators should be widely placed on general hospital wards.
- To investigate the feasibility and efficacy of allowing all those assigned to the management of cardiac arrest in the community to be trained and permitted to defibrillate. These first responders could include police, security officers, lifeguards and volunteer first aiders.

5. All first responder defibrillation programmes must operate under strict medical control by physicians qualified and experienced in emergency programme management, who will have responsibility for ensuring that each link of the Chain of

Survival is in place and who have appropriate access to patient outcome information permitting systems audit using the Utstein template.

5.2.2. SYSTEMS DESIGN AND SPECIFICATION FOR DEFIBRILLATION BY EMERGENCY MEDICAL SERVICE PERSONNEL

1. There is clear evidence that EMS personnel such as ambulance staff can be trained to be reliable in defibrillation.
2. Professional Basic Life Support (BLS) providers should be trained to use an AED and each front-line ambulance must have the capability of providing defibrillation.

EMS Advanced Life Support (ALS) providers (such as ambulance personnel) may be trained in the use of either the manual defibrillator or the automated external defibrillator (AED).

Advanced Life Support EMS providers have the additional capability of providing advanced airway care, achieving access to the circulation and administering drugs, interpreting the ECG, and manually overriding the automated external defibrillator controls.

This will enable more EMS providers to treat ventricular fibrillation and pulseless ventricular tachycardia (VF and VT).

3. ERC emphasises that:
- Defibrillation by EMS providers is recognised as only one of the components of the Chain of Survival. The programme organisers and medical directors must ensure that the other links in the Chain of Survival are in place. EMS defibrillation will be of limited value unless it is supported by early access, early bystander CPR and early advanced life support.
- It is essential that reliable mobile communications are available to EMS providers to ensure contact with the other links in the Chain.
- A continuous training programme for EMS providers must be in place to ensure a high standard of care.

5.2.3. SYSTEMS DESIGN AND EQUIPMENT SPECIFICATION FOR DEFIBRILLATION BY FIRST RESPONDERS

1. As many vital minutes may elapse between the onset of ventricular fibrillation and the arrival of the EMS, immediate defibrillation by first responders is the next logical step after implementation of defibrillation by ambulance personnel.

2. Programmes designed to implement first responder defibrillation should be medically supervised, clinically audited, and critically evaluated in order to confirm that first responder defibrillation is of clinical benefit.

3. Areas for investigation could be defibrillation by fire fighters, security personnel and police officers, lifeguards, transport attendants (aeroplanes, railways, and ships), staff appointed to mass-gathering events, and persons appointed to provide first aid at their place of work. Defibrillators for first responder defibrillation could be placed in transport terminals, shopping malls, sports stadia and entertainment complexes, office buildings, and other public places, and their effectiveness evaluated.

4. Although, in the future, we could foresee the ready availability of defibrillators for bystanders with minimal training, this approach is neither recommended nor within our scope at the present time.

5. There is no place for manual defibrillators in first responder defibrillation programmes.

6. ERC emphasises that:
- Early defibrillation by a member of the EMS or by a first responder is recognised as only one of the components of the Chain of Survival and the programme organisers must ensure that appropriate attention is paid to the other links in the Chain.
- Thus it is essential that equipment for effective radio or telephone communications is available. At present, however, no reliable data

are available about interference between the AED and mobile radio or telephone equipment.

- Specific training programmes should be developed for first responders aimed at the successful combined application of automated external defibrillation with Basic Life Support techniques.
- The medical programme coordinator should review each case when a first responder defibrillator has been used.
- Arrangements should be made to provide critical incident debriefing to first responders who have used their defibrillator for a cardiac arrest.

5.2.4. EQUIPMENT SPECIFICATION

1. It is essential that AEDs are:
  - utterly reliable,
  - highly specific for shockable rhythms,
  - easy to use,
  - low weight,
  - low cost, and
  - require minimal maintenance

All AEDs should have recording facilities.

2. ERC urges defibrillator manufacturers to consider approaches aimed at standardising, wherever possible of:
  - the controls
  - the voice and screen prompts
  - the cable connections and defibrillation pad electrodes system
  - the data output interface
  - the testing procedures upon standardised ECG data banks

3. It is not possible at present to specify a standard for battery capacity.

4. Automated external defibrillators should be configurable to accommodate future changes in guidelines.

5. The energy levels recommended for monophasic defibrillators are currently those embodied within the ALS algorithm for defibrillation of the ERC (200, 200 and 360 J). Alternative waveforms, e.g., biphasic waveforms, and energy levels are acceptable if demonstrated to be of equal or greater net clinical benefit in terms of safety and efficacy.

6. ERC emphasises that:
- Defibrillators designed for use in ambulance services must have recording facilities (solid-state electronic ECG/voice memory modules, PC cards or tape-based ECG/voice recorders or similar), to facilitate medical control within the emergency medical system.
- Defibrillators available for Advanced Life Support personnel should, in addition, have an ECG display and the facility for manual override of the defibrillator controls.

5.2.5. GUIDELINES FOR THE USE OF AUTOMATED EXTERNAL DEFIBRILLATORS

1. The algorithm for the management of cardiac arrest employing an AED is shown in Table 1.

2. This algorithm has been made flexible to accommodate the practice of either first responder or EMS provider either single or working as a pair and, where appropriate, with the ability to provide Advanced Life Support.

3. Explanation of the guidelines is provided by margin notes and reference points.

ad 1. Arrival of rescuers

● **If two rescuers assign tasks, defibrillation has priority.**
The guidelines can be adapted to one or two rescuers. If two EMS providers are available, one should rapidly approach the patient and start defibrillation sequence whilst the other requests for backup help if appropriate, brings additional equipment to the arrest and assists with CPR.

● **Fetch AED and activate EMS:** A single first responder should activate the EMS and collect

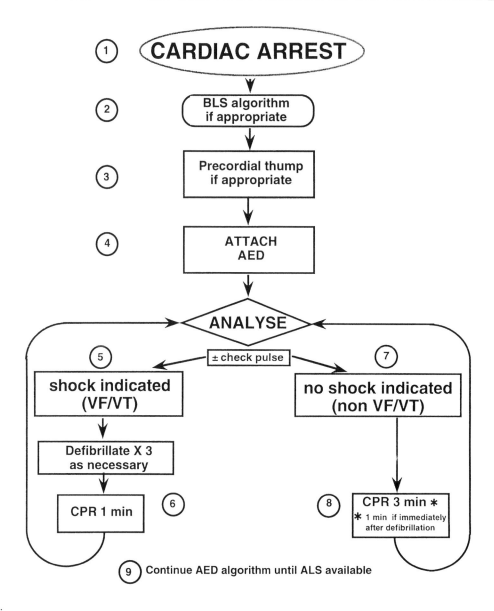

TABLE I.

the defibrillator as rapidly as possible. In practice, it would be unusual for him to have to leave the patient without anyone else being available to give CPR.

• **Use mobile communications:** It is essential that, when defibrillators are used, communications are available simultaneously to activate the other components of the Chain of Survival. When defibrillation is provided by Basic Life Support EMS providers within a 2-tiered system, it is essential that they have access to mobile communications in order to contact the ALS providers. In the future, this may be achieved automatically when a first responder defibrillator is removed from its base.

ad 2. BLS if appropriate

Check response, open airway and check for breathing, check circulation.

Where an automated external defibrillator is immediately to hand, time should not be wasted performing the two ventilations after checking for breathing. Those trained in defibrillation should be taught to perform a pulse check, which is an important part of checking for signs of a circulation. Where no defibrillator is available, the approved Basic Life Support algorithm should be followed.

ad 3. Precordial thump if appropriate

If the rescuer is trained in ALS, and cardiac arrest is witnessed or monitored, a precordial thump may be given before the defibrillator is attached. Those trained only in BLS should not delay to give a precordial thump.

ad 4. Attach the defibrillator

The carrying pouch with the automated external defibrillator must provide some strong scissors for cutting through clothing and a disposable razor for shaving chest hairs in order to obtain good electrode contact.

ad 5. Shock indicated

No pulse checks during first three shocks
When a shock is indicated, the priority is rapid defibrillation. Checking the pulse between the first three shocks is counterproductive because it interferes with proper rhythm analysis.

ad 6. After the first three shocks uninterrupted CPR should be given for 1 min. There should be no "check pulse" or "analyse" prompts and the CPR interval (usually four cycles of one-rescuer CPR) will be timed by the AED timer.

ad 7. No shock indicated

No pulse or analyse prompts during his period. Follow the AED timer

When no shock is indicated, the rhythm is likely to be either asystole or an organised but nonperfusing rhythm (electromechanical dissociation or pulseless electrical activity). In these circumstances, at the first analysis, uninterrupted CPR should be given for 3 min in line with the guidelines for Advanced Life Support. During these 3 min there should be no "check pulse" or "press analyse" prompts as these will interrupt the performance of CPR. CPR itself may produce an artefact which may be recognised as a shockable rhythm.

After 3 min a voice prompt should indicate that CPR should be stopped and the "press analyse" button pressed. If this confirms no shock indicated then the pulse should be checked.

ad 8. When no shock is indicated for the first time after an episode of ventricular fibrillation, the period of CPR before the next analysis is only 1 min.

ad 9. Continue the AED algorithm until ALS available.

When no shock is indicated and no pulse is present, CPR should be uninterrupted and sustained either during transport to an ALS facility, until an Advanced Life Support unit arrives or until life is pronounced extinct according to local procedures.

If the automated external defibrillator is being used by ALS-trained EMS providers, they should then continue with the ALS algorithm (intubation, ventilation, i.v. access, drug delivery, etc.).

In persisting VF/VT, the course of action of the rescuers would be dictated by local policy. In some systems, it is unacceptable to move the patient until the arrival of Advanced Life Support rescuers. In others, it is thought that, after a number of shocks (e.g., 12) when transport is available, it is permissible to move the patient to an Advanced Life Support facility whilst continuing CPR.

5.2.6. TRAINING IN THE USE OF AUTOMATED EXTERNAL DEFIBRILLATORS

1. Initial training in resuscitation involving AEDs should take about 8 h. This is usually the amount of time which is required to achieve the competencies in:
- knowledge of the Chain of Survival and defibrillation algorithms,
- BLS, and
- defibrillation,

and to allow practice and testing in simulated scenarios.

Depending on previous training and experience in life support, the time taken to achieve competence with an AED might be considerably shorter.

2. Refresher training should be carried out at least every 6 months. Reinforcement of the skills and knowledge learned is most important in the early stages of the programme. Refreshment in the use of the equipment controls and the checking of the apparatus should be at least every 6 months. The amount of time which is usually required for a refresher training is 2 h, depending on previous training and experience.

3. Training should be given by specifically certified instructors working within a medically controlled system.

4. Registration. The satisfactory completion of a course in the use of the AED (and the associated certification in competency) does not in itself imply any licence to use the equipment or skills. Licensing should be provided by the medical controller of the system who should be required to maintain a register of first responder providers.

5. Contents for courses in automated external defibrillator use for first responders and EMS providers are annexed.

5.2.7. REFERENCES

1. Larsen M, Eisenberg M, Cummins R, Hallstrom A. Predicting survival from out-of-hospital cardiac arrest: a graphic model. Ann Emerg Med 1993;22:1652–1658.
2. The 1998 European Resuscitation Council Guidelines for Adult Basic Life Support. Resuscitation 1998;37(2): (in press) (see also this volume Chapter 2.2, pp. 6–29).
3. The 1998 European Resuscitation Council Guidelines for Adult Advanced Life Support. Resuscitation 1998; 37(2):(in press) (see also this volume Chapter 3.1, pp. 36–47).
4. Report of a task force of the European Society of Cardiology and the European Resuscitation Council. The Pre-hospital Management of Acute Heart Attacks. Resuscitation 1998;37(2): (in press) (see also this volume Chapter 8, pp. 169–204).
5. Bossaert L. Fibrillation and defibrillation of the heart. BJA 1997;79:203–225.
6. Weisfeldt ML, Kerber RE, McGoldrick P et al. Public access defibrillation: A statement for healthcare professionals from the American Heart Associaton Task Force on automatic external defibrillation. Circulation 1995;92:2763.
7. Advanced Life Support Working Group of the International Liaison Committee on Resuscitation. Early defibrillation. An advisory statement by the Advanced Life Support Working Group of the International Liaison Committee on Resuscitation. Resuscitation 1997;34: 113–115.

5.3. Course Content

5.3.1. PROGRAMME FOR TRAINING IN AUTOMATED EXTERNAL DEFIBRILLATION BY EMERGENCY MEDICAL CARE PROVIDERS

Objectives

To teach EMS providers skills and competency associated with the safe use of an automated external defibrillator within the Chain of Survival.

Prerequisites

Candidates must fulfil local course requirements for EMS personnel certification.

Course content

1. Introduction
- defining the cardiac arrest problem in the community;
- emphasising the role of the ambulance team within the Chain of Survival; and
- emphasising why early defibrillation should be performed by ambulance personnel.

2. Refreshing the basic anatomy and physiology of the heart, applied to cardiac arrest and its symptoms and signs.

3. If not done previously within a separate training session, refreshing the techniques of:
- one and two-rescuer Basic Life Support (according to the ERC guidelines); and
- artificial ventilation and supplementary oxygen usage.

4. Training in the understanding, control and safe operation of the automated external defibrillator.

5. Intensive training of the combined application of Basic Life Support and automated external defibrillation techniques according to the ERC protocol for automated external defibrillators by EMS providers. A training manikin allowing rhythm simulation and defibrillation should be used. Training will be done in teams of two rescuers.

6. Advanced Life Support EMS providers will be expected to operate the automated external defibrillator within the training provided by comprehensive Advanced Life Support instruction.

7. Maintenance of the AED equipment.

8. The completion of a suitable record form according to the Utstein style.

Instructor/trainee ratio

For practical sessions a total of no more than six trainees per instructor is recommended.

Assessment

Trainees will demonstrate their full competence on the AED protocol during simulated cardiac arrests on a manikin. Testing will be done in pairs giving each trainee the opportunity to demonstrate all the required skills. Theoretical questions may be asked but the emphasis lies on the evaluation of practical skills.

Refresher training

This should include a demonstration of the competency in two-rescuer CPR and the safe and effective application of the automated external defibrillator in a variety of situations.

5.3.2. PROGRAMME FOR TRAINING IN AUTOMATED EXTERNAL DEFIBRILLATION BY FIRST RESPONDERS

Objective

To teach a first responder to recognise a cardiac arrest. To activate the emergency medical services, to be able to safely and effectively use an automated external defibrillator and to provide cardiopulmonary resuscitation.

Prerequisites

Previous first aid knowledge or experience is desirable.

Course content

1. Introduction:
   - defining the cardiac arrest problem in the community;
   - emphasising the role of bystanders within the Chain of Survival; and
   - emphasising why cardiac arrest victims with ventricular fibrillation should be immediately defibrillated by first responders.

2. Describing cardiac arrest and the meaning of ventricular fibrillation.

3. Providing training and demonstrating competency in Basic Life Support including Basic Airway Management and Ventilation.

4. Intensive training on the combined application of Basic Life Support and automated external defibrillation techniques according to the ERC algorithm.

A training manikin allowing rhythm simulation and defibrillation should be used. Only the one-rescuer protocol should be used unless specific circumstances (e.g., hospital wards) dictate otherwise.

5. Maintenance of AED equipment.

6. The completion of a suitable clinical record form according to the Utstein style.

Trainee/instructor ratio

For practical sessions, a total of no more than six trainees per instructor is recommended.

Assessment

Trainees will demonstrate their competency in using the algorithm during simulated cardiac arrests on a manikin. Only the one rescue protocol would normally be tested. Though theoretical questions may be asked, the emphasis lies on the evaluation of practical skills.

Refresher training

Refresher training should include the demonstration of competency in one-rescuer Basic Life Support and the safe and effective application of the automated external defibrillator in a manikin scenario.

6. The 1998 ERC Guidelines for the Management of the Airway and Ventilation During Resuscitation

CONTENTS:

6.1. INTRODUCTION

Guidelines for the management of the airway and ventilation during resuscitation have been published previously by the Airway and Ventilation Management Working Group of the European Resuscitation Council [1,2]. This subject has been reviewed recently [3]. Prompt assessment, control of the airway and establishment of ventilation are essential in order to prevent hypoxic injury to vital organs, particularly the brain.

Basic life support is undertaken without the use of specific equipment. Advanced life support implies the use of a variety of techniques, devices, and drugs. With the guidelines below we have extended basic airway and ventilation management to include simple airway adjuncts such as suction, oropharyngeal airways, and ventilation devices such as the pocket mask and bag-valve-mask. Often, health care personnel, particularly ward nurses, will be taught to use this equipment during their basic life support training. Tracheal intubation clearly falls into the category of advanced airway management and is generally taught to medical staff as well as paramedics and possibly a few specialist nurses. The laryngeal mask and Combitube provide alternatives for those without intubation skills or where intubation is otherwise not possible.

6.2. CAUSES OF AIRWAY OBSTRUCTION

Obstruction of the airway may be partial or complete and can occur at any level (Table 1: Guideline 1). In the unconscious patient the tongue and other soft tissues commonly occlude the airway at the pharynx. Obstruction may also be caused by vomit, blood or foreign material following trauma. Laryngeal obstruction may occur as a result of oedema, "spasm" or an inhaled foreign body. Obstruction of the airway below the larynx is less common but may occur due to bronchospasm, pulmonary oedema, mucosal oedema, excessive bronchial secretions, aspiration of gastric contents, or pulmonary haemorrhage. Unless the airway is cleared to allow ventilation within a very short period (generally

Causes of airway obstruction
Guideline 1

Cardiac arrest, Coma, Trauma	→	Tongue displacement
Anaphylaxis, Foreign body, Irritants	→	Tongue oedema / Oropharynx obstruction / Laryngeal spasm
Foreign body	→	Laryngeal, tracheal or bronchial obstruction
Trauma	→	Laryngeal damage
Infection, Anaphylaxis	→	Laryngeal oedema
Asthma, Foreign body, Irritants, Anaphylaxis	→	Bronchospasm
Irritants, Anaphylaxis, Infection, Near drowning, Neurogenic shock, Cardiac failure	→	Pulmonary oedema

TABLE I. Guideline 1. Causes of airway obstruction.

accepted as 2–5 min, except in unusual circumstances, e.g., hypothermia or intoxication with sedative or narcotic drugs), cerebral, neurological or other vital system damage will occur which may be irreversible or fatal.

6.3. BASIC AIRWAY MANAGEMENT

6.3.1. Basic Airway and Ventilation Assessment

The airway can be assessed simply by checking

for responsiveness, looking for chest movement, listening for breath sounds and feeling air flow on the cheek of the rescuer ("look, listen, and feel") (Table 2: Guideline 2). Unusual voice quality, abnormal breath sounds and wheeze or stri-dor indicate a partially obstructed airway. Inspira-tory "stridor" is caused by upper airway obstruction whereas expiratory "wheeze" indi-cates obstruction of the lower airways (e.g., asth-ma). Complete airway obstruction in a patient

Assessment of the airway and ventilation
Guideline 2

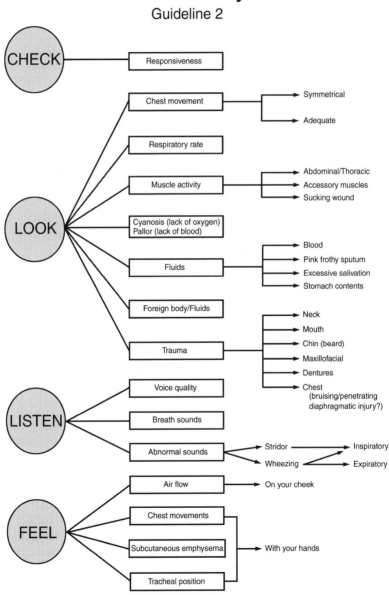

TABLE 2. Guideline 2. Basic airway and ventilation assessment.

who is making respiratory efforts results in paradoxical chest and abdominal ("seesaw") movement, often exaggerated by the use of accessory
muscles. During the assessment other signs
should be sought such as cyanosis, pallor, excessive salivation, gastric contents or foreign body in
the mouth or pharynx and maxillofacial or neck
trauma. The assessment in unresponsive patients

should be made in the position in which they are
found especially if traumatic injury is suspected.
If there is no obvious breathing, turn the patient
into the supine position and apply head tilt, chin
lift and, if necessary, jaw thrust. Head tilt is
omitted if there is a contraindication to moving
the patient's head and neck, e.g., suspected cervical spine injury.

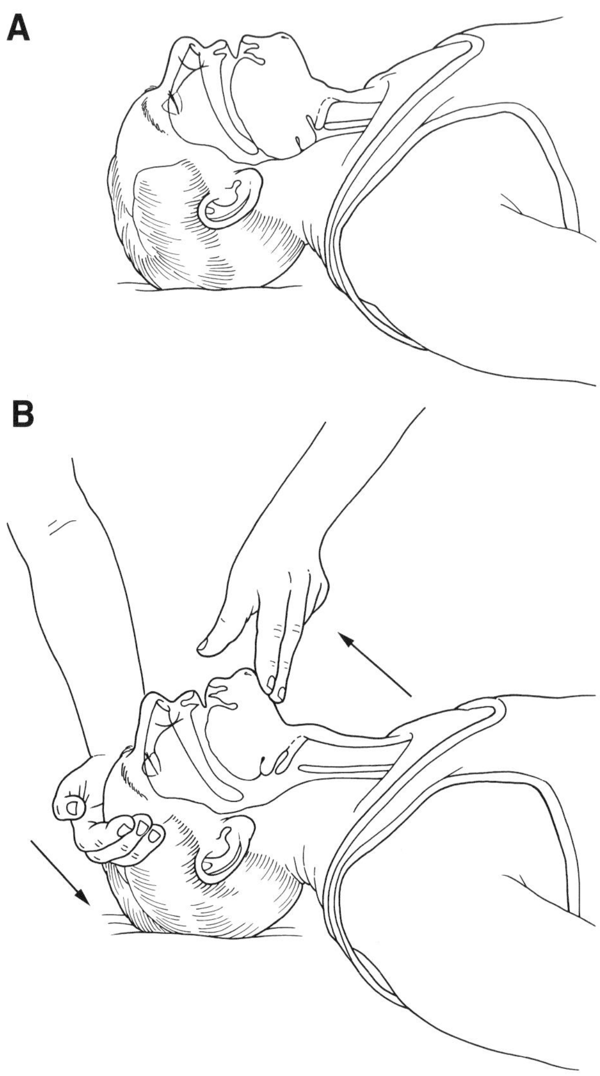

6.3.2. Management of the Airway by basic methods

Head tilt

This manoeuvre lifts the relaxed tongue from the
posterior pharyngeal wall and lifts the epiglottis
from the laryngeal opening by stretching the
anterior tissues of the neck (Fig. 1) [4−9]. Anaesthetic practical experience confirms that the
"sniffing the morning air" position of the head
and neck provides optimal head and neck alignment. A small pillow placed beneath the occiput
will flex the neck and extend the head at the
atlanto-occipital joint.

Chin lift

In some patients upper airway patency can be
improved by placing two fingers under the chin
and lifting it up (Fig. 2). This method further
encourages anterior displacement of the tongue
and complements head tilt.

Jaw thrust

Jaw thrust displaces the mandible (and with it the
tongue) forwards using the index fingers placed
just proximal to the angle. The thumbs reach
forward to depress the point of the chin slightly
to open the mouth (Fig. 3). This technique can be
used in combination with head tilt to maximise
displacement of the tongue from the posterior
pharyngeal wall. However, it is tiring and techni-
cally more difficult to perform and is recommended for health care providers only.

FIG. 1. Head tilt. This manoeuvre lifts the relaxed tongue
from the posterior pharyngeal wall and lifts the epiglottis
from the laryngeal opening by stretching the anterior tissues of the neck.

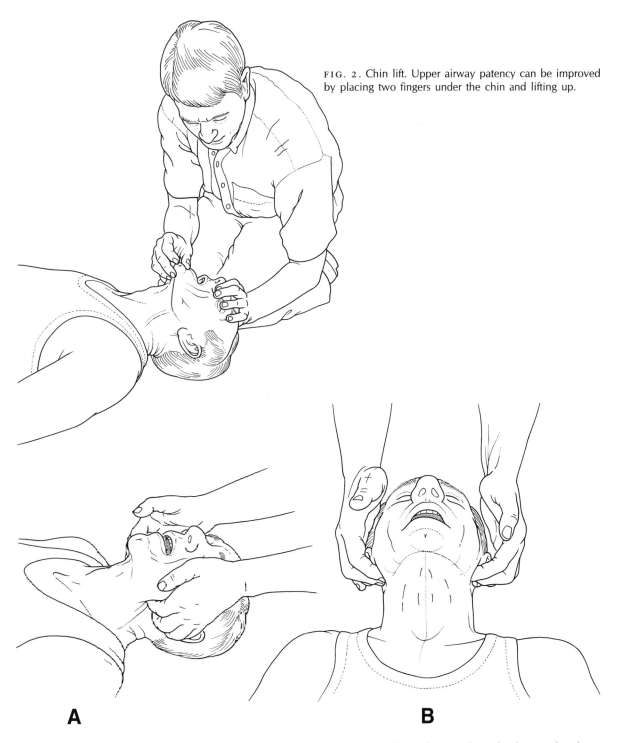

FIG. 2. Chin lift. Upper airway patency can be improved by placing two fingers under the chin and lifting up.

A

B

FIG. 3. Jaw thrust. Jaw thrust displaces the mandible (and with it the tongue) forwards using the index fingers placed just proximal to the angle. The thumbs reach forward to depress the point of the chin slightly to open the mouth.

6.3.3. Airway Management in Patients With Suspected Cervical Spine Injury

If spinal injury is suspected (e.g., if the victim has sustained a fall, been struck on the head or neck, or has been rescued after diving into shallow water) particular care must be taken during handling and resuscitation to maintain alignment of the head, neck, chest, and lumbar region in the neutral position. In these patients head tilt may aggravate the injury and cause damage to the cervical spinal cord. The recommended method [10] for establishing a clear upper airway in these circumstances is jaw thrust in combination with manual in-line stabilisation (MILS) of the head and neck by an assistant (Fig. 4) [11]. If life-threatening airway obstruction persists despite effective application of jaw thrust, it is then reasonable to apply chin lift and limited head tilt until the airway opens.

6.3.4. Adjuncts to Basic Airway Management

6.3.4.1. The oropharyngeal airway

The oropharyngeal airway limits airway ob-struction due to backward displacement of the tongue. It provides relief for the rescuer from having to apply prolonged jaw thrust, although chin lift is frequently necessary. The airway does not protect against aspiration of foreign material. A variety of sizes (000–4) are available. Sizes 2 or 3 are suitable for the average adult (Fig. 5).

Indications

- Upper airway obstruction due to backward displacement of the tongue and absent glosso-pharyngeal reflexes.
- To act as a protective bite block when other airways such as a tracheal tube or laryngeal mask airway are in place.

Contraindications

- Clenched jaws,
- Vulnerable dentition,
- Active glossopharyngeal reflexes,
- Active bleeding within the hypopharynx, and
- Imminent danger of regurgitation or vomiting of stomach contents.

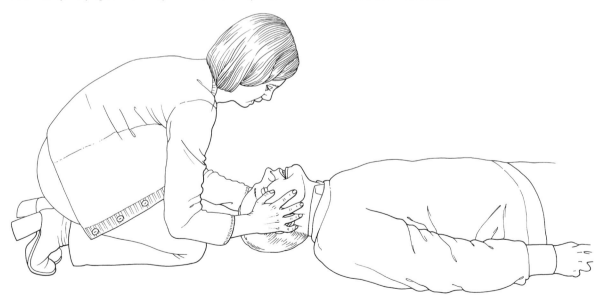

FIG. 4. Airway management in patients with suspected cervical spine injury. Jaw thrust in combination with manual in-line stabilisation (MILS) of the head and neck by an assistant.

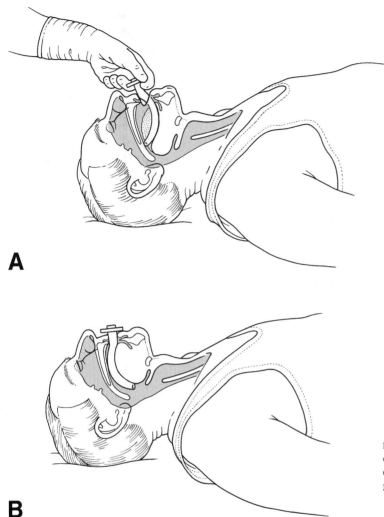

A

B

FIG. 5. The oropharyngeal airway. The oropharyngeal airway limits airway obstruction due to backward displacement of the tongue.

Equipment

- Suitable sized airway(s). The length of the airway should equal the distance from the incisors to the angle of the mandible.
- Lubrication jelly.

Procedure

- Place the patient in the supine or lateral position.
- Introduce the lubricated airway into the mouth in the inverted position and rotate it through 180° as it passes over the palate.

- Check for unimpeded air entry (additional chin lift and jaw thrust may be required).

Hazards

- Trauma to lips, teeth or palate.
- Provocation of retching, vomiting or laryngeal spasm if active reflexes are present. Remove the airway immediately at the first sign of these events.

Limitations

The airway does not protect against aspiration of

foreign material. Ventilation must be applied with a face mask.

Modifications

The cuffed oropharyngeal airway (COPA) may be more effective than the traditional oropharyngeal device. The relevant data is awaited.

6.3.4.2. Suction apparatus

An effective suction apparatus is essential to enable the oropharynx to be cleared of secretions, blood, regurgitated gastric contents and vomit. In hospitals wall-mounted or anaesthetic machine suction apparatus is connected to a central vacuum unit. These units are typically supported by portable battery-powered suction units. The battery-powered units are also ideal for out of hospital use. Manual (hand or foot-operated) suction units are inexpensive and can be distributed widely to first-aiders and provide back-up to the battery-powered units (Fig. 6).

6.3.5. Basic Management of Ventilation

Expired air ventilation has been accepted as the technique of choice since the late 1950s

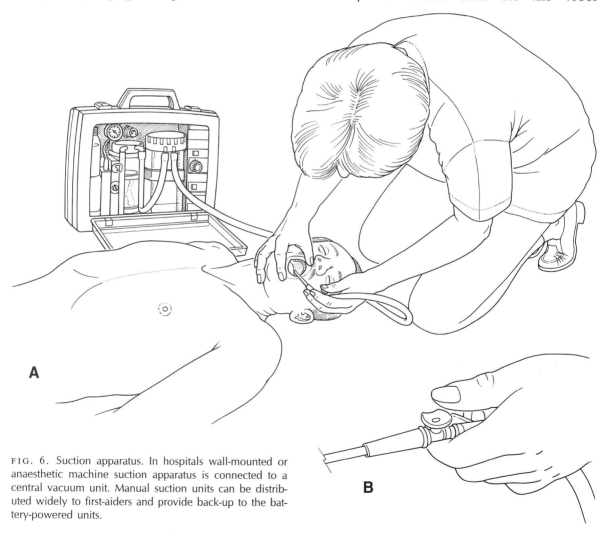

FIG. 6. Suction apparatus. In hospitals wall-mounted or anaesthetic machine suction apparatus is connected to a central vacuum unit. Manual suction units can be distributed widely to first-aiders and provide back-up to the battery-powered units.

[4,12−15]. It has been shown to be effective practice for both professionals and lay persons including young children over 5 years of age. Ventilation using the expired air of the rescuer can be applied to the mouth or nose of the adult victim and to the mouth and nose of the infant.

6.3.5.1. Mouth to mask ventilation

A moulded face mask similar to that used in anaesthesia may be used to provide mouth to mask ventilation. A unidirectional valve diverts the patient's expired air away from the rescuer and traps any macroscopic particles emerging from the patient. This valve improves the aesthetics and reduces risk of cross-infection. The mouth to mask method is a two-handed technique which produces a better seal than that obtained during single-person bag-valve-mask ventilation. As with mouth-to-mouth ventilation it is possible to generate high tidal volumes, high airway pressures and increase the risk of gastric inflation [16,17]. The addition of a port for the administration of supplemental oxygen increases the inspired oxygen concentration [18,19] (Fig. 7).

6.3.5.2. Face shield ventilation

Inexpensive protection devices made from a piece of plastic film with a valvular orifice to cover the mouth and nose will provide protection and reduce aesthetic worries of direct contact with the patient's vomitus, saliva, sputum or blood. The main disadvantage is that the film device requires repositioning for each sequence of breaths. In the community the bystander is likely to be a relative, friend or colleague of the victim and resuscitative efforts should not be deterred by the unavailability of a protective device as the risk is very small.

6.3.5.3. Bag-valve-mask ventilation

The self-inflating bag can be connected to either a facemask, a tracheal tube, a laryngeal mask, or a Combitube. When used on its own the bag-valve-mask will allow ventilation of the patient with ambient air (21% oxygen). This can be increased to around 50% by attaching an oxygen supply at 5−6 l/min directly to the bag next to the air inlet valve. Normally, however, a reservoir bag should be attached, which with oxygen flows of 8−10 l/min, will provide inspired oxygen concentrations of 90% (Fig. 8).

Certain ideal criteria have been laid down for bag-valve-mask devices used in resuscitation [20−25]. The requirements recommended include:

- The bag material should be transparent and convey a satisfactory "feel". It should not absorb anaesthetic or noxious gases and should possess sufficient recoil to draw in gases from a reservoir or a draw over anaesthesia circuit.
- Both inlet and outlet valves should be of robust construction, competent in preventing rebreathing or leaks, incapable of malfunction or jamming with a fresh gas flow (of oxygen) up to 15 l/min.
- The valves should be easy to take apart, clean and reassemble (except in disposable models); incorrect reassembly should be impossible.
- The inlet valve should be capable of being fitted with a filter (to exclude noxious gases) and an oxygen reservoir bag.
- The patient valve should have standard ISO 15/22 mm fittings.
- The patient valve should incorporate, or be capable of being fitted with, a PEEP valve.
- The bag should be capable of delivering a tidal volume of up to 1,500 ml in the adult version and ventilation rates of up to 45/min in the paediatric version.
- Infant, paediatric and adult versions of the device should be available.
- The device should function adequately during all common environmental conditions and temperature extremes.

There have been several reports of the performance of bag valve devices under varying conditions:

- Some bags deliver ventilation volumes of 1,500 ml, others produce volumes ranging from 1,500 to 1,000 ml. In circumstances of reduced compliance (20 ml/mbar) most bags only deliver 80% of their normal volumes and when compliance is further reduced to 10 ml/mbar, the output falls to approximately 60% of the normal volume. At increased resistance, delivered volumes fall to about 90% of the initial values [26−28].

- Few bags do not have forward and backward leaks; the leaks observed range from 40 to 50 ml (forwards) and 10 ml (backwards).
- Valve obstruction occurs in some cases at low

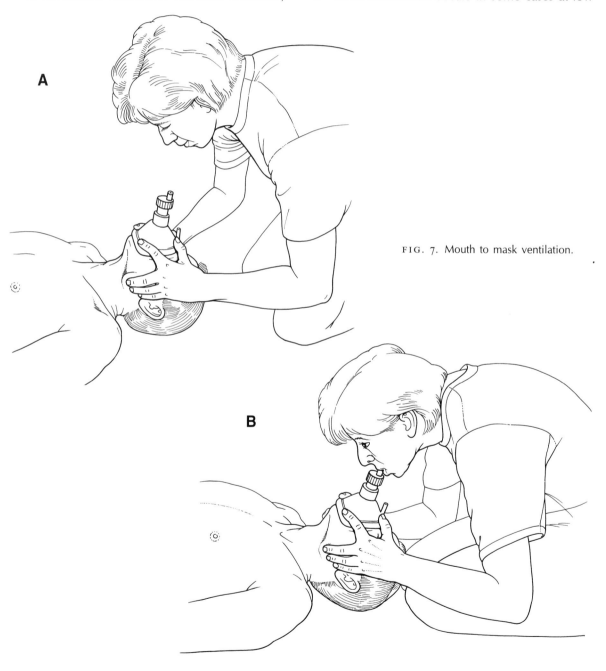

FIG. 7. Mouth to mask ventilation.

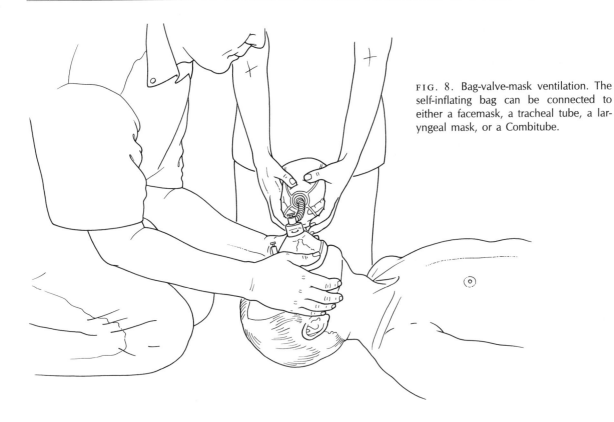

FIG. 8. Bag-valve-mask ventilation. The self-inflating bag can be connected to either a facemask, a tracheal tube, a laryngeal mask, or a Combitube.

flows, whereas in others 30 l/min are required to impair valve function. Most bag valve devices are rated as easy to operate with a few as more complex [23].

- Nearly all disposable devices meet national and international minimum standards under laboratory conditions [22,23].

When used by one person, a considerable degree of skill is required to maintain a patent airway and gas-tight seal with one hand, while squeezing the bag with the other [29]. This is only likely to be achieved by someone who regularly uses a bag-valve-mask device. Too much air leak will result in hypoventilation, while excessive tidal volumes may result in gastric insufflation and increased risk of regurgitation. If ventilation has to continue with a bag-valve-mask, the two-person technique is preferable; one person holds the facemask in place using both hands and an assistant squeezes the bag. In this way a better seal is achieved, the jaw thrust manoeuvre is more easily maintained and the patient's lungs can be ventilated more effectively.

Recommendations

Taking these considerations into account, the European Resuscitation Council recommends that:

- Bag valve devices should meet the criteria set out above.
- To minimise the possibility of gastric inflation, two rescuer operations are recommended when the bag valve device is used with a face mask.
- Emphasis should be placed on the achievement of an FiO_2 of 1.0 using a reservoir or demand valve.
- Particular care should be taken to avoid hyperinflation and barotrauma when the bag valve is connected to a tracheal tube.

6.3.5.4. Ventilation volumes

During external chest compressions, in comparison to a spontaneous circulation, pulmonary blood flow and thus the delivery of carbon dioxide to the lungs is considerably reduced [30–32]. The risk of gastric insufflation is increased with large tidal volumes and high inspiratory flow rates. For these reasons the tidal volumes of 400–500 ml are adequate during CPR. These volumes will be produce visible lifting of the chest [33]. Each inflation should take 1.5–2 s. The rescuer should wait for the chest to fall fully during expiration before giving another breath. This should normally take about 2–4 s; each sequence of 10 breaths will therefore take about 40–60 s to complete. The exact timing of expiration is not critical; the chest should be allowed to fall before another breath is given.

6.3.5.5. Oxygen

Expired air contains approximately 17% oxygen. Aim to deliver the highest concentrations available. Concerns about adverse effects of high concentration of oxygen on hypoxic drive in some patients with COPD are not applicable during cardiopulmonary resuscitation.

6.4. ADVANCED AIRWAY MANAGEMENT
(Table 3: Guideline 3)

6.4.1. Adjuncts to Advanced Airway Management

6.4.1.1. The nasopharyngeal airway

The nasopharyngeal airway is passed through the nose so that the tip lies behind the tongue in the hypopharynx just above the glottis. The modern nasopharyngeal airway is made of soft plastic material and has a flange collar at its proximal end to prevent it disappearing into the nasal cavity. If a purpose-made device is not available, one can be made from an uncuffed nasal endotracheal tube of the appropriate size shortened to 14–16 cm long with a large safety pin placed through the proximal end. Nasopharyngeal airways do not protect against aspiration of foreign material. Several sizes are available: 6.0–8.0 mm diameter is suitable for the average adult (Fig. 9).

Indications

Upper airway obstruction particularly in patients with clenched jaws, seizures or dentition at risk. The nasopharyngeal airway, once in situ, is often better tolerated than the oropharyngeal airway.

Contraindications

- Bilaterally obstructed or deformed nasal passages.
- Imminent danger of regurgitation or vomiting of stomach contents.

Relative contraindications

- Suspicion of fracture of base of skull.

Procedure

- Introduce the well-lubricated tube of appropriate size into the right nostril directing the tip backwards, not upwards. If obstruction to advance occurs, withdraw and try the left nostril.
- Insert the airway with rotation until the flange impinges on the nostril.
- Check for unimpeded air entry.

Hazards

- Severe nasal haemorrhage.
- Damage to nasal mucous membrane, bone or cartilages.
- Inadvertent passage into the cranial cavity through a fractured cribriform plate (ensure that the airway is directed backwards not upwards).
- Nasopharyngeal airways with relatively small flanges may disappear into the nose. The attachment of a safety pin to the flange should prevent this complication.

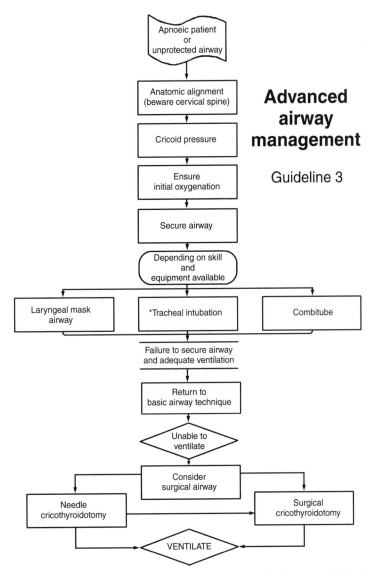

Advanced airway management

Guideline 3

Apnoeic patient or unprotected airway

Anatomic alignment (beware cervical spine)

Cricoid pressure

Ensure initial oxygenation

Secure airway

Depending on skill and equipment available

Laryngeal mask airway | *Tracheal intubation | Combitube

Failure to secure airway and adequate ventilation

Return to basic airway technique

Unable to ventilate

Consider surgical airway

Needle cricothyroidotomy | Surgical cricothyroidotomy

VENTILATE

*Tracheal intubation is best. The Laryngeal Mask Airway or Combitube are initial alternatives.

TABLE 3. Guideline 3. Advanced airway management.

- Provocation of retching, vomiting or laryngeal spasm (less likely than with the oropharyngeal airway).

Limitations

Difficulty in placement or nasal haemorrhage. The nasopharyngeal airway does not protect against aspiration of foreign material. Ventilation must be applied via a face mask.

6.4.1.2. Tracheal intubation

Introduction

Tracheal intubation provides the definitive clear

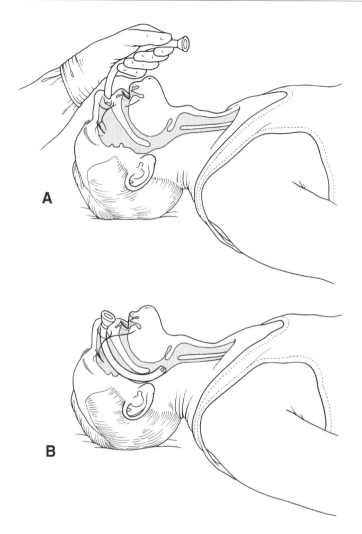

FIG. 9. The nasopharyngeal airway. The naso-pharyngeal airway is passed through the nose so that the tip lies behind the tongue in the hypo-pharynx just above the glottis.

and secure airway through which ventilation and oxygenation can be provided during a cardio-respiratory arrest. The distal cuff prevents gas leakage during use of the high inspiratory pressures often required during a resuscitation attempt, and protects the tracheobronchial tree from aspiration of gastric contents (Fig. 10).

Tracheal intubation can be performed on a patient of any age. A range of tube sizes is available to accommodate neonates (3–4 mm ID) to large adults (8–9 mm ID). In emergency kits of limited dimensions sizes 3, 5 and 7 mm ID will be suitable for short-term use in the majority of patients. In comparison with the oral route, naso-tracheal intubation is unreliable, particularly when the patient is apnoeic (the patient's breath sounds normally guide the intubator). Thus, oro-tracheal intubation is the recommended technique and nasotracheal will not be discussed.

Indications

- To provide a clear and secure airway in any case of cardiorespiratory arrest lasting more than 2–3 min.
- To provide a clear airway for cerebral resuscitation after cardiorespiratory arrest.
- To gain access to the lower respiratory tract for aspiration of inhaled foreign material.

Contraindications

- Absence of trained personnel and appropriate equipment.

Equipment

- Appropriate laryngoscopes in working order (Macintosh-curved blade, Magill-straight blade, etc.).
- Appropriate range of tracheal tubes (6.0–9.0 mm internal diameter for adults) cut to the correct length with connections (usually 15/22 mm) to fit the ventilating apparatus.
- Suction apparatus.
- Intubating forceps (Magill or Kelly), lubricant jelly and swabs.
- 10-ml syringe for cuff inflation.

- Clamp or one-way valve to secure inflated cuff.
- Gum elastic bougie/stylet.
- Scissors.
- Tape or tie to secure tube in place.
- Catheter mount.
- Facility to ventilate the lungs, e.g., self-inflating bag-valve device.
- Facility to confirm correct location of tracheal tube, e.g., stethoscope, oesophageal detector device.

Procedure

- Before attempting intubation briefly ventilate and oxygenate the patient with a bag-valve mask device.
- Place the patient supine in the clear airway

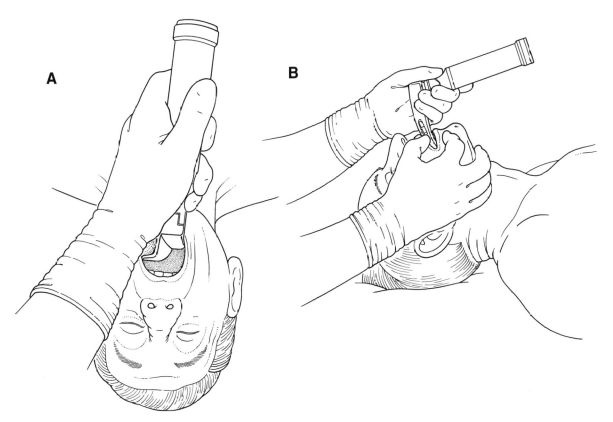

FIG. IOA—F. Tracheal intubation. Tracheal intubation provides the definitive clear and secure airway through which ventilation and oxygenation can be provided during a cardiorespiratory arrest. A and B: Using the left hand, the laryngoscope is inserted into the right-hand corner of the mouth.

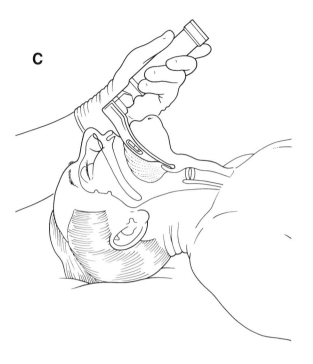

FIG. IOC. The tip of the laryngoscope is passed into the vallecula.

FIG. IOD. View of the larynx at laryngoscopy.

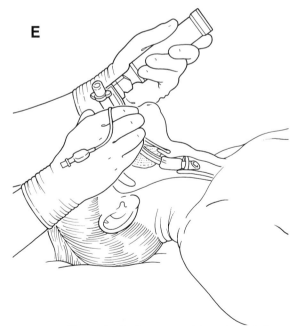

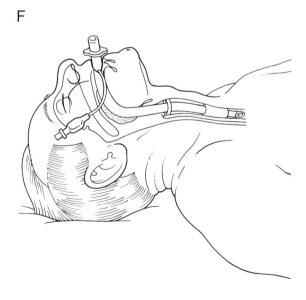

FIG. IOE. The tracheal tube is passed from the right-hand corner of the mouth and through the vocal cords under direct vision

FIG. IOF. The tracheal tube cuff should lie just below the glottic opening

position with one pillow under the head thus flexing the lower cervical spine and extending at the atlanto-occipital junction (the "sniffing the morning air" position).

- Using the left hand to hold the laryngoscope handle, insert the laryngoscope blade into the right hand corner of the mouth ensuring that the lower lip is not caught between the blade and the lower teeth (Fig. 10A and B).
- Slide the laryngoscope blade towards the posterior pharyngeal wall, aiming for the midline at laryngeal level and displacing the body of the tongue towards the left hand side of the mouth.
- When the laryngoscope tip reaches the larynx, lift the laryngoscope handle forwards and upwards (towards the junction of the ceiling and the opposite wall) and observe the tip of the laryngoscope blade.
- If using the curved laryngoscope blade, slide the tip of the blade between the back of the tongue and the base of the epiglottis (the vallecula), maintaining head tilt by occipital pressure with the right hand (Fig. 10C). If using a straight laryngoscope blade, place the tip of the blade beneath the epiglottis.
- Adjust the tip of blade to improve the view of the cords (Fig. 10D). Pressure on the cricoid cartilage may improve the view and reduces the possibility of gastric regurgitation.
- Pass the tracheal tube through the right hand corner of the mouth and between the vocal cords under direct vision (Fig. 10E). If necessary rotate the tube 90° counterclockwise to ease the passage through the glottic opening.
- If the view is restricted to only the epiglottis or arytenoids, use a gum elastic bougie. The distal end of the bougie is angled to 45° and, if passed directly behind the epiglottis it will usually pass through the vocal cords into the trachea. Tracheal placement of the bougie is confirmed if the bougie is felt to "click" across the tracheal rings or when it is "held up" in the bronchial tree. Leaving the laryngoscope in the mouth, railroad the tracheal tube over the bougie into the trachea.
- Once the tube has passed between the vocal cords, it should be advanced so that the cuff lies just below the glottic opening (Fig. 10F).
- Inflate the cuff through the pilot tube until the audible leak associated with positive pressure ventilation ceases. Suspect an incorrectly placed tube in the oesophagus if cuff inflation volumes of more than 10–15 ml are required.
- Keep hold of the tube and withdraw the bougie.
- Check that the tube is in the trachea by observing bilateral chest movement and auscultate breath sounds over both upper lobes in the axillae. Listen over the epigastrium; gurgling sounds suggest oesophageal placement. If an oesophageal detector device is available, connect to the tracheal tube and attempt to aspirate air. Easy aspiration of air and no return of the plunger confirms correct tracheal placement. Difficulty in aspirating air and the generation of a negative pressure suggests oesophageal placement. The detection of end tidal CO_2 by capnometry can be a useful adjunct for confirming tracheal intubation. End-tidal CO_2 levels during CPR may be very low but usually not zero. If no CO_2 is detected, tube placement should be carefully re-evaluated by another reliable method.
- Secure the tube in place with a tie or tape and recheck tube placement.
- During cardiopulmonary resuscitation allow no more than 30 s for the intubation attempt. If the attempt has failed after this time, remove the laryngoscope and tube, and ventilate with oxygen via the bag-valve-mask device for 1–2 min before trying again.

Additional notes

1. Tracheal intubation can, with practice, also be performed with the patient in the lateral position if it is not possible or safe to turn him into the supine position.
2. If the patient is lying on the ground the rescuer should ideally also lie on the ground at the head of the patient with elbows placed either side of the patient's head.

Hazards

- Unrecognised oesophageal intubation;
- Failed intubation;
- Laryngoscopy in the semiconscious patient may provoke regurgitation;
- Intubation of a single bronchus;
- Trauma to teeth, lips, tongue and structures in the pharynx or larynx; and
- Kinking of the tracheal tube in the pharynx or mouth.

Precautions

- Prolonged attempts at intubation will cause significant hypoxia. If the attempt has not been successful after 30 s, ventilate the patient with 100% oxygen via a bag-valve-mask (4–5 breaths of approximately 500 ml before trying again).
- Overinflation of the cuff may obstruct the lumen of the tube.

Limitations

- Laryngoscopy will be very difficult if the patient is not deeply unconscious.
- Direct oral intubation is a skill that has to be acquired and maintained. If the skill is not used regularly, the success rate will deteriorate.

Modifications for infants and children

ANATOMICAL AND PHYSIOLOGICAL
CONSIDERATIONS

The neonate is an obligate nose breather, thus nasal obstruction is immediately life threatening. An infant's head is larger in relation to their body in comparison with an adult. In the supine position the neck tends to be flexed, and increasing this degree of flexion by using a pillow may worsen the view of the larynx. Children have large tongues in relation to the size of the oral cavity; large tonsils and adenoids increase the risk of upper airway obstruction and may inter-fere with laryngoscopy. At laryngoscopy the larynx is more anterior and the epiglottis tends to be a large U or V shaped, floppy structure. The neonate's trachea is only 4–5 cm long which increases the risk of endobronchial intubation. Up to the age of 8–10 years (around puberty) the cricoid cartilage is the narrowest part of the upper airway (in the adult the narrowest point is at the vocal cords); mucosal ischaemia and trauma at this level is associated with subglottic stenosis, therefore uncuffed tracheal tubes are used. Oxygen consumption is much higher in the child because of the high metabolic rate. This results in a high minute ventilation, manifested as a high ventilatory rate. The increased oxygen consumption coupled with the reduced oxygen reserve results in rapid arterial oxygen desaturation, in the presence of upper airway obstruction or apnoea. In infants the lung functional residual capacity (FRC) is small and the closing volume of the airways is relatively large; to avoid airway closure in the obtunded or anaesthetised child, continuous positive airway pressure is beneficial.

MODIFICATIONS TO PROCEDURE

- Because of the anatomical differences discussed above it is often preferable to use a straight bladed laryngoscope in children below 2 years of age. The straight blade should be passed behind the epiglottis (not in front, as with the curved blade).
- The size of the tracheal tube is critical, there must be a leak to prevent the possible complication of subglottic stenosis associated with prolonged intubation. A slight leak during positive pressure ventilation is acceptable. Use an uncuffed tube for children under the age of 10 years. The correct internal diameter and length can be calculated for children from 1–16 years of age using the following formulae:

Internal diameter (mm) = (Age of child/4) + 4

Length (cm) = (Age of child/2) + 12 (add 1–3 cm for nasal tubes)

6.4.1.3. Cricoid pressure

Cricoid pressure was introduced by Sellick [34] in an effort to reduce the incidence of aspiration of gastric contents during the induction of anaesthesia and has also been advocated during CPR [35,36]. The efficacy of cricoid pressure has been demonstrated by Lawes [37] who showed that even "gentle" inflation pressure produced risk of gastric inflation and that cricoid pressure, correctly applied, would prevent gastric insufflation even when inflation pressures of up to 60 cmH$_2$O were used [38], In view of the high incidence of pulmonary aspiration in connection with cardiac arrest [38] it would seem prudent to endorse the value of cricoid pressure in both basic and advanced life support until the airway is secure (Fig. 11).

Technique

Backward pressure should be applied with the finger and thumb on either side of the cricoid cartilage to obstruct the lumen of the oesophagus lying posteriorly. Counterpressure may be applied at the back of the neck.

Precautions

Release cricoid pressure and place the patient in the lateral position immediately if the patient starts to vomit actively.

6.4.1.4. The laryngeal mask airway (LMA)

This airway consists of a wide bore tube with an elliptical inflation cuff at the distal end which is designed to seal the hypopharynx around the laryngeal opening leaving the tube orifice in close proximity to the glottic opening [39]. It was first introduced into clinical anaesthetic practice in 1988. The advantage of the LMA is that it can provide a clear and secure airway without the skill required for laryngoscopy and tracheal intubation [40,41]. Furthermore, ventilation is more efficient and easier compared with a bag-valve-

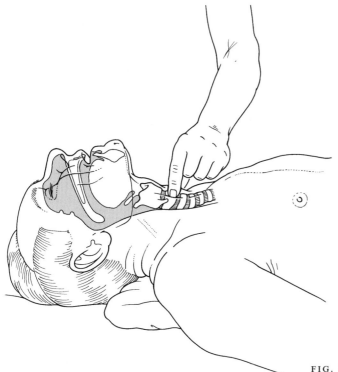

FIG. 11. Cricoid pressure or Sellick's manoeuvre.

mask device [42,43]. While not guaranteeing absolute protection of the airway in every case [44], the LMA offers greater security and convenience than most other airways except the endotracheal tube [45–48]. It can be used when there is the possibility of unstable neck or access with a laryngoscope is limited or intubation proves difficult [49–52]. Carefully applied intermittent positive pressure ventilation may be provided via the LMA which incorporates a standard connector to join directly to a self-inflating bag valve (Fig. 12).

The technique can easily be taught to nurses, paramedics and nonspecialist doctors [40–43, 53]. The LMA has been used successfully by nurses in the management of cardiac arrest [46,47]. It offers a method of establishing a clear airway in the profoundly unconscious patient before tracheal intubation skills and equipment are available. The LMA may be inserted during the application of cricoid pressure, albeit with some increasing difficulty [54–57].

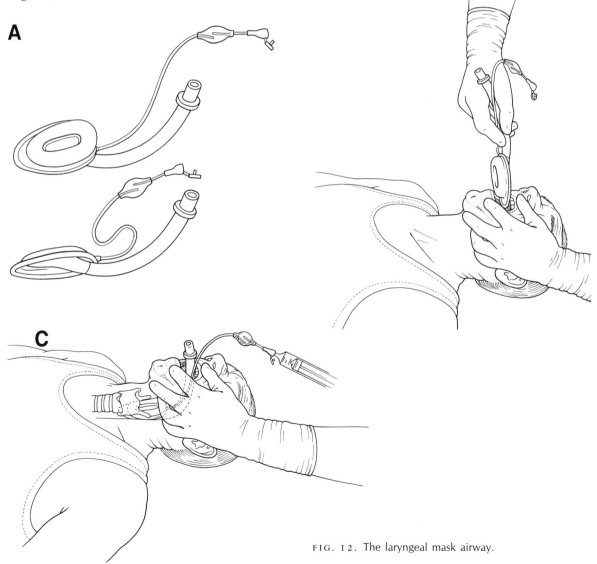

FIG. 12. The laryngeal mask airway.

TABLE 4. Sizing and cuff inflation volume for the LMA.

Size	Patient	Cuff volume (ml)
1	Neonates/infants up to 6.5 kg	2–4
2	Infants/children	10
2.5	Children 15–30 kg	15
3	Small adults/children 30–35 kg	20
4	Normal adults	30
5	Large adults	40

The LMA is manufactured in a range of sizes suitable for infants to large adults in both standard and flexible reinforced materials (Table 4).

Indications

- An unconscious patient with absent glossopharyngeal and laryngeal reflexes at risk of airway obstruction and who may need artificial ventilation when intubation is precluded by lack of available expertise or equipment.
- Known or unexpected difficult intubation.

Relative contraindications

- Chronic obstructive pulmonary disease or a requirement for high inflation pressures;
- Severe oropharyngeal trauma; and
- Known full stomach.

Equipment

- LMA of appropriate size;
- Lubricating jelly;
- 50 ml syringe to inflate cuff;
- Suction apparatus; and
- Facility to ventilate the lungs.

Procedure

- Lubricate the back and sides of the completed deflated cuff.
- Place the patient in the supine position with the head and neck aligned in the clear airway protection. (Care should be taken with patients with suspected cervical spine injury.)

- Holding the tube like a pen introduce the LMA into the mouth with the distal aperture facing caudad.
- Advance the tip, applying it to the surface of the palate until it reaches the posterior pharyngeal wall.
- Now move the operating hand to the proximal end of the tube and press the mask into position until the resistance is felt as it locates in the back of the hypopharynx.
- The black line on the tube should be aligned with the nasal septum.
- Inflate the cuff with the appropriate amount of air. The tube rises out of the mouth 1–2 cm and the larynx is pushed forward.
- Confirm that a clear airway exists by gently inflating the lungs with a bag attached to the tube and note inflation pressure, chest movement, bilateral breath sounds and leakage around the cuff.
- Insert a bite block or oropharyngeal airway alongside the tube and secure it with a tie or tape.

Hazards

- Rejection, coughing, straining and laryngeal spasm in patients with active reflexes.
- Incorrect placement due to folding of the tip of the cuff during insertion. Withdraw, ensure that the tip is flat and reinsert.
- Airway obstruction due to downfolding of the epiglottis. Withdraw the tube, deflate the cuff and reinsert applying the mask to the palate during introduction.
- Persistent leakage around the cuff may be due to incorrect sizing, inadequate cuff inflation, excessive lung inflation pressure or poor lung compliance.

Positive inflation pressures should not exceed 20 cmH_2O. In the majority of patients adequate ventilation can be achieved within this limit by reducing the inspiratory flow rate and allowing a reasonable expiratory time.

6.4.1.5. The intubating laryngeal mask

A modification of the standard laryngeal mask is currently undergoing evaluation [58–60]. This device makes it possible to insert a cuffed tube through the laryngeal mask and into the trachea. In anaesthetised patients intubation is successful, within three attempts, in 95% of cases [61]. Its role in CPR has yet to be determined.

6.4.1.6. The Combitube

The Combitube is a double lumen tube which is introduced blindly into the mouth and is designed to ventilate the patient's lungs whether the tube enters the trachea or the oesophagus [62]. The "tracheal" channel has an open distal end and the "oesophageal" channel has a blind end with openings at supraglottic level. There is a small volume distal cuff and a high volume (100 ml) cuff designed to occupy the hypopharynx. If the tube enters the oesophagus the patient is ventilated through the "oesophageal" channel through the openings just above the glottic opening. The inflating gas is prevented from passing anywhere else by the distal and hypopharyngeal cuffs. If the tube enters the trachea ventilation it should be via the "tracheal" port. The hypopharyngeal cuff is redundant (Fig. 13).

The Combitube has been used successfully as an airway adjunct during cardiorespiratory arrest [63–65]. The device has been evaluated for use by ICU nurses and by paramedics in the prehospital field [66]. It has also been reported to be an effective substitute for endotracheal intubation in cases of difficulty.

Indications

An unconscious patient with absent glossopharyngeal and laryngeal reflexes at risk of airway obstruction and who may need artificial ventilation where endotracheal intubation is precluded by lack of available expertise or equipment.

Contraindications

- Severe oropharyngeal trauma; and
- Small mouth.

Equipment

- Combitube;
- Lubricating jelly;
- 50 and 20 ml syringes to inflate cuffs;
- Suction apparatus; and
- Facility to ventilate the lungs.

Procedure

- Place the patient in the supine position with the head and neck aligned in the clear airway position.
- Lubricate the Combitube.
- Pass the tube to a distance of approximately 24 cm.
- Inflate the distal cuff.
- Check for tube placement in the trachea by inflation through the "tracheal" tube and by auscultation and observation of chest movement.
- If the tube is placed in the trachea, continue ventilation through the "tracheal" port.
- If the tube is placed in the oesophagus inflate the hypopharyngeal cuff and ventilate through the "oesophageal" port.

Hazards

- The device is relatively bulky and may be difficult to introduce in patients with small mouths.
- The cuffs may be damaged by sharp teeth during insertion.
- Further damage to soft tissues in patients with oropharyngeal injures may occur.
- Inflation of the stomach may occur if ventilation is applied to the wrong tube located in the oesophagus.

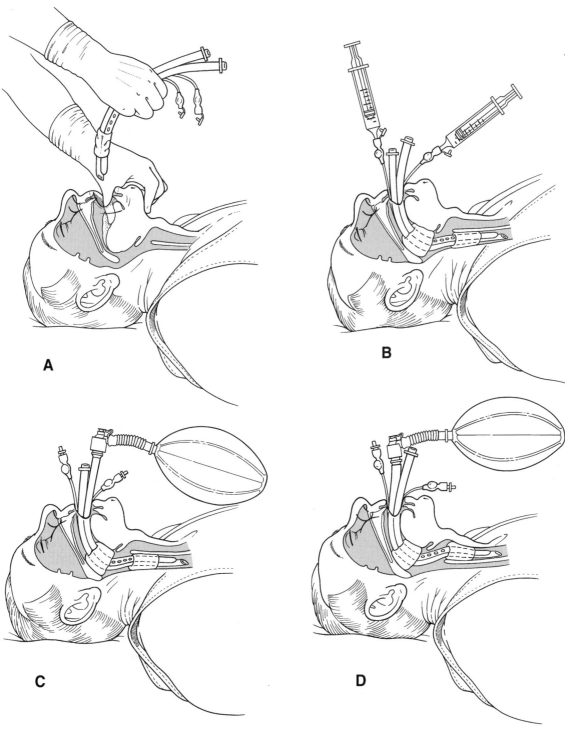

FIG. 13. The Combitube.

6.4.2. Managing the Airway Via the Cricothyroid Membrane

Introduction

Provided that personnel who are skilled at difficult airway management and tracheal intubation are available, resorting to the surgical airway is very rarely necessary in patients with cardiac arrest except when trauma to the head and neck are involved. In patients with actual or impending cardiac arrest, direct surgical access to the trachea should be made through the cricothyroid membrane unless there is severe trauma in this region. Tracheostomy in the emergency situation is extremely difficult and is usually hampered by extensive bleeding from the thyroid vessels. It will not be discussed further because it has virtually no place in airway management during cardiac arrest.

There are a number of methods of gaining access to the airway through the cricothyroid membrane. These include:

- Needle cricothyroidostomy,
- Surgical cricothyroidotomy, and
- Various specially designed cannulae that can be inserted after a "stab" incision with or without a Seldinger wire.

All of these methods are difficult and hazardous in the emergency situation. They should be undertaken only where there is no other option and then only by trained and practised operators.

6.4.2.1. Needle cricothyroidostomy technique

- A 14-G (2.0 mm) intravenous cannula directed slightly caudally to avoid damage to the vocal cords is introduced through the cricothyroid membrane with an attached 20-ml syringe aspirating continually until a free flow of air is obtained (Fig. 14).
- The needle is then withdrawn leaving the cannula in situ.
- Correct placement of the cannula is reconfirmed by free aspiration of air.
- A 14-G cannula is of insufficient diameter to allow any significant spontaneous ventilation

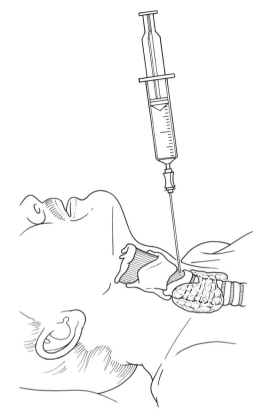

FIG. 14. Needle cricothyroidostomy.

to occur. Positive pressure ventilation must be provided using a self-inflating bag attached to connector designed for a 3.0-mm tracheal tube which will fit a Luer I.V. connection. Ventilation provided by this method is marginal and sufficient only to buy a few minutes time until an alternative is available. Better results are obtained with a 4.0-mm venous cannula from the Arrow Central Emergency Fluid Resuscitation Device. or better still a 4.0-mm kink resistant cannula made by Cook Critical Care and designed specifically for the purpose.

- Effective ventilation can be provided through noncompliant tubing using a high-pressure jet injector system generated directly from the oxygen cylinder fitted with a regulator to produce a pressure in the region of 400 kPa.
- Inflation may be produced by a finger intermittently occluding a hole in the oxygen tub-

ing or a specially designed system with a manually operated trigger which produces inflation when depressed.

- Each inflation must be very carefully observed and the trigger released immediately when normal chest expansion occurs otherwise lung barotrauma will occur.
- Ample time must be left for lung deflation and for the technique to be safe there must be a clear route through the larynx and mouth for the expired gases to escape otherwise lung barotrauma will occur immediately with life-threatening subcutaneous and mediastinal emphysema.

6.4.2.2. Surgical cricothyroidotomy (Fig. 15)

A number of institutions have reviewed their series of emergency cricothyroidotomies [67–77] but most of these are in trauma patients; some of these included cases of cricothyroidotomy performed during CPR.

Technique

- A 2–3 cm transverse or longitudinal incision

is made in the skin over the cricothyroid membrane.

- The subcutaneous tissues down to the membrane are dissected using blunt artery forceps and a self-retaining retractor inserted to expose the membrane.
- The membrane is incised 1 cm transversely and the handle of the scalpel inserted into the incision and rotated through 90° to achieve an airway.
- Alternatively a pair of double-pointed scissors can be used for subcutaneous dissection, incision of the membrane and retraction of the incision prior to insertion of the tube. This technique may be safer than the use of a scalpel.
- A 6.5–7.0 mm lubricated tracheostomy or tracheal tube is inserted through the incision and directed towards the lower trachea.
- The cuff is inflated and the tube is secured with a tape and connected to the ventilating apparatus.

Hazards and Precautions

It seems likely that surgical cricothyroidotomy

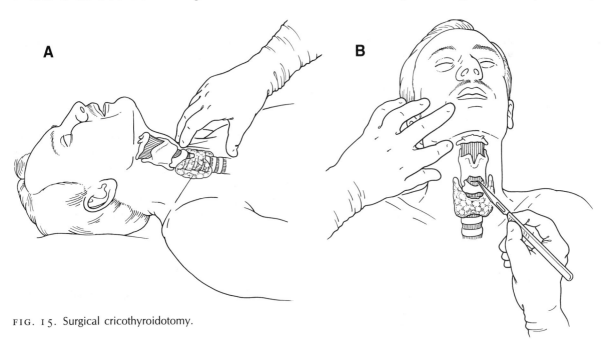

FIG. 15. Surgical cricothyroidotomy.

provides the best surgical airway in cardiac arrest patients. However, there are no good prospective studies; the complication rate, even if much less than surgical tracheostomy, is far from negligible including total failure (up to 12%) delayed success and late complications [72]. Several precautions should be taken during surgical cricothyroidotomy. The incision in the skin and cricothyroid membrane should not extend too far laterally or inferiorly, to avoid arteries, jugular veins or the thyroid gland. The incision should be made in the inferior part of the cricothyroid membrane in an attempt to miss the cricothyroid arteries. Transection of the cricoid cartilage or tracheal rings causes late complications such as subglottic stenosis. Directing the scalpel towards the head risks damaging the vocal cords.

Indications and Contraindications

Surgical cricothyroidotomy is indicated in patients with life-threatening upper airway obstruction when oral or nasal intubation is contraindicated or impossible and the airway cannot be secured by other means. Persistent unsuccessful attempts at tracheal intubation result in an inordinate delay in airway control and oxygenation [78]. However, the incidence of complications in cricothyroidotomy is relatively high. Contraindications include situations where endo-tracheal intubation can be accomplished easily and quickly, and acute laryngeal disease or injury. The procedure is relatively contraindicated in children under 10 years of age unless the airway cannot be secured by any other means.

6.4.3. Advanced Management of Ventilation

6.4.3.1. Oxygen-powered resuscitators

Oxygen-powered resuscitators have been designed to take over from the self-inflating bag. They are driven directly from a high pressure (400 kPa) oxygen source so are valuable in contaminated atmospheres. The devices may be connected to a face mask, laryngeal mask, Combitube, tracheal tube and tracheostomy tube. An FiO_2 of 1.0 is assured.

Two types of oxygen-powered resuscitators are available:
- Manually triggered resuscitators; and
- Automatically triggered resuscitators.

Manually triggered resuscitators

These devices are triggered by manually pressing a lever or button at the patient valve. Both hands are free to ensure an airtight fit and maintain airway alignment if a face mask is used, but there is a lack of direct "feel" compared with a self-inflating bag during the inspiratory phase which may increase the risk of gastric inflation associated with imperfect airway alignment. Unlike the automatic resuscitator, one operator is tied to providing ventilation exclusively, even when a tracheal tube is in place. Some models have a triggered demand valve to provide assisted ventilation in time with the patient's own inspiratory efforts.

Design requirements

- Compact, robust, lightweight, ergonomic design.
- Conveniently located trigger which can be operated while both hands hold the face mask.
- 15/22 mm connectors should be fitted.
- Capable of delivering 100% oxygen at a flow rate no greater than 40 l/min.
- Should incorporate an excess inspiratory pressure relief valve operating at pressures above 60 cmH$_2$O which triggers an audible warning.
- Should incorporate a demand flow system responsive to spontaneous respiratory efforts.
- Should operate satisfactorily under all environmental conditions and climatic temperature ranges.

Automatic resuscitators

Automatic resuscitators are in extensive use and there have been many reports of their performance [79–84]. These resuscitators cycle between inspiration and expiration using a fluid logic system or by electronic control. For work in the emergency setting, cycling should be related to volume and time, not to pressure. The automatic resuscitator provides consistent automatic ventilation at the preset tidal volume, rate and respiratory pattern. If a tracheal, Combitube or laryngeal mask is in place, the rescuer is free to attend to other tasks, e.g., venous cannulation. Automatic resuscitators vary in versatility in terms of variation of the inspiratory and expiratory pattern. Some models have the option of ventilation with air/oxygen mixtures to conserve oxygen supplies and some incorporate a demand valve to synchronise with the patient's own inspiratory efforts. Models with a low inspiratory flow rate and a blow off valve with audible warning are most satisfactory. They are said to carry less danger of gastric inflation when used with a face mask than a self-inflating bag.

Design requirements

- Compact robust lightweight and portable design. Overall dimensions should be of the order of $20 \times 10 \times 20$ cm and the weight should not exceed 5 kg.
- 15/22 mm connectors should be used.
- Capable of delivering 100% oxygen at flow rates up to 40 l/min.
- Capable of delivering a tidal volume of 600 ml at a compliance of 20 ml/cmH$_2$O and a resistance of 20 cmH$_2$O/l/s using an inspiratory/expiratory ratio of 1:2 and a respiratory rate of 20/min.
- Should use a volume/time triggering arrangement with a triggering pressure of 1–2 cmH$_2$O.
- Should provide a volume constant operation.
- Should incorporate an excess inspiratory pressure relief valve with an audible warning operating at pressures above 60 cmH$_2$O.
- Should incorporate a demand system responsive to spontaneous respiratory efforts.
- Should operate satisfactorily under all environmental conditions and climatic temperature ranges.

Other valuable optional design requirements include:

- Variable air mix facilities to allow FiO$_2$ to range from 1.0–0.4 and conserve oxygen;
- PEEP valve up to +10 cmH$_2$O;
- Potential manual triggering arrangement;
- Disconnect alarm;
- Variable inspiratory slow rates and I/E ratios; and
- Pressure monitoring facility.

6.4.3.2. Monitoring of ventilation

Lung compliance falls during cardiac arrest, and venous arterial shunting and pulmonary oedema also occur. All transpire to produce hypoxia which is difficult to overcome even with optimal ventilation [85]. PEEP may help but at the expense of carotid blood flow [86].

The following ventilation parameters should be monitored during CPR:
- End tidal carbon dioxide,
- Pulse oximetry,
- Inspiratory pressure, and
- Acid base status.

End tidal carbon dioxide

End tidal CO$_2$ remains low during cardiac arrest mainly due to the fact that little CO$_2$ is presented to the lungs [87]. As cardiac output increases as a result of resuscitation or return of spontaneous circulation, the end tidal CO$_2$ rises logarithmically [88] and then becomes a measure of adequacy of ventilation volume (assuming little pulmonary ventilation/perfusion mismatch) and, indirectly, a measure of cardiac output and tissue perfusion.

Pulse oximetry

Pulse oximetry has limited application during cardiac arrest but is a useful monitor of oxygen saturation and pulsatile flow once there is a return of spontaneous circulation. It is inaccurate in low flow states (systolic blood pressure < 50 mmHg) [89] and does not, of course, have a linear relationship with arterial oxygen tension.

Summary

- Airway control and ventilation are essential components of cardiopulmonary resuscitation.
- Basic manoeuvres alone are often enough to provide adequate oxygenation and ventilation.
- With appropriate training airway adjuncts may improve the reliability of these basic techniques.

6.5. REFERENCES

1. Baskett PJF et al. Guidelines for the basic management of the airway and ventilation during resuscitation. Resuscitation 1996;31:187–200.
2. Baskett PJF et al. Guidelines for the advanced management of the airway and ventilation during resuscitation. Resuscitation 1996;31:201–230.
3. Gabbott DA, Baskett PJF. Management of the airway and ventilation during resuscitation. Br J Anaesth 1997;79:159–171.
4. Safar P. Ventilatory efficiency of mouth to mouth respiration: airway obstruction during manual and mouth to mouth artificial ventilation. JAMA 1958;167:335.
5. Safar P, Aguto Escarraga L, Chang F. A study of upper airway obstruction in the unconscious patient. J Appl Physiol 1959;14:760.
6. Elam JO, Greene OG, Schneider MA et al. Head tilt method of oral resuscitation. JAMA 1960;172:812–815.
7. Morikawa S, Safar P, De Carlo J. Influence of head position on upper airway patency. Anesthesiology 1961;22:265–270.
8. Ruben HM, Elam JO, Ruben AM. Investigation of upper airway problems in resuscitation. Anesthesiology 1961;22:271–279.
9. Greene DG, Elam JO, Dobkin AB et al. Cinefluorographic study of hyperextension of the neck and upper airway patency. JAMA 1961;176:570–573.
10. Committee on Trauma of the American College of Surgeons. Advanced Trauma Life Support Instructor Manual, Chicago. American College of Surgeons 1997.
11. Nolan JP, Parr MJA. Aspects of resuscitation in trauma. Br J Anaesth 1997;79:226–240.
12. Elam JO, Brown ES, Elder JD. Artificial respiration by the mouth to mouth method. A study of the respiratory gas exchange in paralysed patients ventilated by the operator's expired air. N Engl J Med 1954;150:749–753.
13. Elam JO, Greene DG, Brown ES et al. Oxygen and carbon dioxide exchange and energy cost of expired air resuscitation. JAMA 1958;167:328.
14. Safar P, Aguto Escarraga L, Elam JO. A comparison of the mouth to mouth and mouth to airway methods of artificial respiration with the chest-pressure arm-lift methods. N Engl J Med 1958;258:671.
15. Elam JO, Greene DG. Mission accomplished: successful mouth to mouth resuscitation. Anesth Analg 1961;40:440,578,672.
16. Thomas AN, O'Sullivan K, Hyatt J, Barker SJ. A comparison of bag mask and mouth mask ventilation in anaesthetised patients. Resuscitation 1993;26:13–21.
17. Johannigmann JA, Branson RD, Davis KRRT, Hurst JM. Technique of emergency ventilation: A model to evaluate tidal volume, airway pressure and gastric inflation. J Trauma 1991;31:93–98.
18. Stahl JM, Cutfield GR, Harrison GA. Alveolar oxygenation and mouth-to-mask ventilation: effects of oxygen insufflation. Anaesth Intens Care 1992;20:177–186.
19. Palmisano JM, Moler FW, Galura C, Gordon M, Custer JR. Influence of tidal volume, respiratory rate and supplementary oxygen flow on delivered oxygen fraction using a mouth ventilation device. J Emerg Med 1993;11:685–689.
20. Carden E, Bemstein M. Investigation of the nine most commonly used resuscitator bags. JAMA 1970;212:4:589–592.
21. Johnstone RE, Smith TC. Rebreathing bags as pressure-limiting devices. Anesthesiology 1973;38:192–194.
22. Kissoon N, Nykanen D, Tiffin N, Frewen T, Brasher P. Evaluation of performance characteristics of disposable bag-valve resuscitators. Crit Care Med 1991;19:102.
23. Le Bouef LL. Assessment of eight adult manual resuscitators. Respir Care 1980;25:1136–1142.
24. Lindell DW, Bortle Ch, Cohen SB, Cone DC, Davidson SJ. Emergency ventilation volumes: a comparison of commonly used ventilators during two-person cardiac resuscitation. Prehosp Dis Med 1994;S63.
25. Baskett PJF. Resuscitation Handbook, 2nd Edition. London: Mosby Europe, 1993;37–39.
26. Lotz P, Dick W, Ahnefeld FW, Wyrwoll K, Becker M. Vergleichende Untersuchungen von Handbeatmungsgeraten. Teil 1: Prinzipielle Aspekte, Testkritenen – allegmeine Eigenschaften der untersuchten Gerate. Notfallmedizin 1983;9:745–763.
27. Lotz P, Dick W, Ahnefeld FW, Wywroll K, Becker M. Vergleichende Untersuchungen von Handbeatmungsgeraten Teil I 1: MeBergebnisse. Notfallmedzin 1983;9:825–844.
28. Lotz P, Schlipf M, Ahnefeld FW, Dick W. Ver-

gleichende Untersuchungen von Handbeatmungsge-raten. Teil IV: Der Ubergangsbereich zwischen Kinder – und Erwachsenen-Geraten am Beispiel von Ambu-Baby, Ambu Mark III und Weinmnann-Combi-Bag. Notfallmedizin 1986;12:396−422.

29. Augustine JA, Seidel DR, McCabe IB. Ventilation per-formance using a self inflating anaesthesia bag: effect of operator characteristics. Am J Emerg Med 1987;5: 267−270.

30. Rosenberg A, Carli P. End tidal CO_2 during pre-hos-pital cardiopulmonary resuscitation. Anesthesiology 1990;73A:531.

31. Idris AH, Banner MJ, Wenzel V, Fuerst RS, Becker LB, Melker RJ. Ventilation caused by external chest com-pression is unable to sustain effective gas exchange during CPR: a comparison with mechanical ventila-tion. Resuscitation 1994;28:143−150.

32. Garnett AR, Ornato JP, Gonzalez ER, Johnson EB. End Tidal carbon dioxide monitoring during cardiopul-monary resuscitation. JAMA 1987;257:512−515.

33. Baskett PJF, Nolan JP, Parr MJ. Tidal volumes per-ceived to be adequate for resuscitation. Resuscitation 1996;31:231−234.

34. Sellick BA. Cricoid pressure to control regurgitation of stomach contents during the induction of anaesthesia. Lancet 1961;ii:404.

35. Bircher NG. Wolf Creek III. A time to look forward, a time to look back. Crit Care Med 1985;13:950.

36. Melker RJ, Banner MJ. Ventilation during CPR two rescuer standards re-appraised. Ann Emerg Med 1985;14:197.

37. Lawes EG, Campbell I, Mercer D. Inflation pressure, gastric insufflation and rapid sequence induction. Br J Anaesth 1987;59:315−318.

38. Lawes EG, Baskett PJF. Pulmonary aspiration during unsuccessful cardiopulmonary resuscitation. Intens Care Med 1987;13:379−382.

39. Brain AIJ. The laryngeal mask – a new concept in airway management. Br J Anaesth 1983;55:801−805.

40. Pennant JH, Walker MB. Comparison of the endotra-cheal tube and laryngeal mask in airway management by paramedical personnel. Anesth Analg 1992;74: 531−534.

41. Davies PRF, Tighe SQM, Greenslade GL, Evans GH. Laryngeal mask airway and tracheal tube insertion by unskilled personnel. Lancet 1990;336:977−979.

42. Alexander R, Hodgson P, Lomax D, Bullen C. A com-parison of the laryngeal mask airway and Guedel air-way, bag and facemask for manual ventilation. Anaes-thesia 1993;48:231−234.

43. Martin PD, Cyna AM, Hunter WAH, Henry J, Ramayya GR. Training nursing staff in airway manage-ment for resuscitation. Anaesthesia 1993;48:133−137.

44. Owens MT, Robertson P, Twomey C, Doyle M, McDonald N, McShame A. The incidence of gastro-

esophageal reflux using the laryngeal mask: A com-parison with the face mask using esophageal lumen pH electrodes. Anesth Analg 1995;80:980−984.

45. Brimacombe IR, Berry A. The incidence of aspiration associated with the laryngeal mask airway: A meta-analysis of published literature. J Clin Anaesth 1995; 7:297−305.

46. Leach A, Alexander CA, Stone B. The laryngeal mask in cardiopulmonary resuscitation in a district general hospital: a preliminary communication. Resuscitation 1993;25:245−248.

47. Baskett PJF. The use of the laryngeal mask airway by nurses during cardiopulmonary resuscitation. Results of a multicentre trial. Anaesthesia 1994;49:3−7.

48. Kokkinis TI. The use of the laryngeal mask airway in CPR. Resuscitation 1994;271:9−12.

49. Brain AII. Three cases of difficult intubation overcome by the laryngeal mask airway. Anaesthesia 1985:40: 353−355

50. Brain AIJ. The laryngeal mask airway − a possible new solution to airway problems in the emergency situation. Arch Emerg Med 1984;1:229−232.

51. Calder I, Ordman AJ, Jackowski A, Crockard HA. The brain laryngeal mask airway. An alternative to emer-gency tracheal intubation. Anaesthesia 1990;45:137−139.

52. Greene MK, Roden R, Hinchley G. The laryngeal mask airway. Two cases of prehospital trauma care. Anaesthesia 1992;47:688−689.

53. Samarkandi AH, Seraj MA, El Dawlathy A, Mastan M, Bahamces HB. The role of the laryngeal mask airway in cardiopulmonary resuscitation. Resuscitation 1994; 28:103−106.

54. Ansermino JM, Blogg CE. Cricoid pressure may pre-vent insertion of the laryngeal mask airway. Br J Anaesth 1992;69:465−467.

55. Brimacombe J. Cricoid pressure and the laryngeal mask airway. Anaesthesia 1991;46:986−987.

56. Brimacombe J, White A, Berry A. Effect of cricoid pressure on ease of insertion of the laryngeal mask airway. Br J Anaesth 1993;71:800−802.

57. Strang TI. Does the laryngeal mask airway compro-mise cricoid pressure? Anaesthesia 1992;47:829−831.

58. Brain AIJ, Verghese C, Addy EV, Kapila A. The intu-bating laryngeal mask I: development of a new device for intubation of the trachea. Br J Anaesth 1997;79: 699−703.

59. Brain AIJ, Verghese C, Addy EV, Kapila A, Brima-combe J. The intubating laryngeal mask II: a prelimi-nary clinical report of a new means of intubating the trachea. Br J Anaesth 1997;79:704−709.

60. Kapila A, Addy EV, Verghese C, Brain AIJ. The intu-bating laryngeal mask airway: an initial assessment of performance. Br J Anaesth 1997;79:710−713.

61. Baskett PJF et al. The intubating laryngeal mask:

results of a multicentre trial with experience of 500 cases (In press).

62. Frass M, Rodler S, Frenzer, Ilias W, Leithner C, Lackner E. Esophageal tracheal Combitube, endotracheal airway and mask: comparison of ventilatory pressure curves. J Trauma 1989;29:1476—1479.

63. Frass M, Frenzer R, Rauscha R, Weber H, Pacher R, Leithner C. Evaluation of the oesophageal tracheal Combitube in cardiopulmonary resuscitation. Crit Care Med 1987;15:609—611.

64. Frass M, Johnson JC, Alherion GL, Fruhwald FX, Traindl O, Schwaighofer B, Leithner C. Esophageal tracheal Combitube (ETC) for emergency intubation: an anatomical evaluation of ETC placement by radiography. Resuscitation 1989;18:95—102.

65. Staudinger T, Brugger S, Watschinger B, Roggla M, Dielacher C, Lobl T, Fink D, Klauser R, Frass M. Emergency intubation with the Combitube: comparison with the endotracheal airway. Ann Emerg Med 1993;22:1573—1575.

66. Atherton G, Johnson JC. Ability of paramedics to use the Combitube in prehospital cardiac arrest. Ann Emerg Med 1993;22:1263—1268.

67. Boyd A, Conlan A. Emergency cricothyrotomy: Is its use justified? Surg Round 1979;2:19—23.

68. DeLaurier G, Hawkins M, Treat R, Mansberger A Jr. Acute airway management: Role of cricothyroidotomy. Am Surg 1990;56:12—15.

69. Erlandson M, Clinton J, Ruiz E et al. Cricothyroidotomy in the emergency department revisited. J Emerg Med 1989;7:115—118.

70. McGill J, Clintin J, Ruiz E. Cricothyroidotomy in the emergency department. Ann Emerg Med 1982;11:36—364.

71. Miklus R, Elliot C, Snow M. Surgical cricothyrotomy in the field: Experience of a helicopter transport team. J Trauma 1989;29:506—508.

72. Spaite D, Joseph M. Prehospital cricothyrotomy: An investigation of indications, technique, complications and patient outcome. Ann Emerg Med 1990;19:279—285.

73. Nugent W, Rhee K, Wisner D. Can nurses perform surgical cricothyrotomy with acceptable success and complication rates. Ann Emerg Med 1991;20:367—370.

74. Salvino C, Dries D, Gamely R, Murphy-Macabobby M, Marshall W. Emergency cricothyroidotomy in trauma victims. J Trauma 1993;34:503—505.

75. Boyle MF, Hatton D, Sheets C. Surgical cricothyrotomy performed by air ambulance flight nurses: a 5-year experience. J Emerg Med 1993;11:41—45.

76. Hawkins ML, Shapiro MB, Cue JI, Wiggins SS. Emergency cricothyrotomy: a reassessment. Am Surgeon 1995;61:52—55.

77. Jacobson LE, Gomez GA, Sobieray RJ, Rodman GH, Solotkin KC, Misinski ME. Surgical cricothryoidotomy in trauma patients: analysis of its use by paramedics in the field. J Trauma 1996;41:15—20.

78. Mace S. Cricothyrotomy. J Emerg Med 1988;6:309—319.

79. Dick WE. Respiratorische Norfalle: aerate für die Diagnostik, Therapie und Uberwachung. Notfallmedizin 1989;15:253.

80. Adams AP, Henville JD. A new generation of anaesthetic ventilators. Anaesthesia 1977;32:34—40.

81. Baskett PJF. Advances in cardiopulmonary resuscitation. Br J Anaesth 1992;69:182—193.

82. ISO. Resuscitators intended for use with humans: International Organisation for Standardisation 1986. ISO/Dis 8382.

83. Nolan JP, Baskett PJE. Gas powered and portable ventilators: An evaluation of six models. Prehosp Dis Med 1992;7:25—34.

84. World Federation of Societies of Intensive and Critical Care Medicine: Committee of Ventilator Technology — Classification and minimal requirements of ventilators. Int Crit Care Digest 1993;12:29—30.

85. Ornato JP, Bryson BL, Donovan PJ, Farquharson RR, Jaeger C. Measurement of ventilation during cardiopulmonary resuscitation. Crit Care Med 1983;11:79—82.

86. Hodgkin BC, Lambrew CT, Lawrence FH, Angelakos ET. Effects of PEEP and of increased frequency of ventilation during CPR. Crit Care Med 1980;8:123—126.

87. Garnett AR, Ornato JP, Gonzalez ER, Johnson EB. End tidal carbon dioxide monitoring during cardiopulmonary resuscitation. JAMA 1987;257:512—515.

88. Ornato JP, Garnett AR, Glauser FL. Relationship between cardiac output and the end tidal carbon dioxide tension. Ann Emerg Med 1990;19:1104—1106.

89. Severinghaus JW, Spellman MJ. Pulse Oximetry failure thresholds in hypotension and ischaemia. Anesthesiology 1990;73:532—537.

7. Periarrest Arrhythmias: Management of Arrhythmias Associated With Cardiac Arrest

A statement by the Advanced Cardiac Life Support Committee of the European Resuscitation Council, 1994 [1], Updated 1996 [2] and 1998.

Writing Subcommittee: Douglas Chamberlain, Richard Vincent (co-opted), Peter Baskett, Leo Bossaert, Colin Robertson (co-opted), Rudolf Juchems and Karl Lindner

CONTENTS:

7.1. INTRODUCTION

The essentials of a successful strategy to reduce the toll of cardiac arrests should include measures to prevent fatal arrhythmias, optimal management of these arrhythmias, and stabilisation of the patient after the return of spontaneous circulation. The European Resuscitation Council produced guidelines for the management of cardiac arrest in 1992 [3] and these have now been revised in 1998 [4]. But prevention – when possible – and stabilisation of the patient to prevent recurrence must include management of rhythm disorders that are of prognostic importance. Ventricular fibrillation in vulnerable patients is, for example, often triggered by tachyarrhythmias [5], especially in the prehospital setting, whilst any patient may have arrhythmias in the first phase of a return of coordinated rhythm, or during the postarrest phase.

The first responders with advanced cardiac life support skills who manage cardiac arrest are not usually cardiologists. The European Resuscitation Council therefore considers it important to provide guidelines for the initial management of the various arrhythmias associated with cardiac arrest. These guidelines must, necessarily, be simple and – as far as possible – applicable in all European countries notwithstanding different traditions of antiarrhythmic therapy. An important component of the algorithms must be advice on when expert help might reasonably be requested. Help will not always be available immediately. The algorithms therefore show the treatment modalities most likely to be appropriate as guidance for continued management.

The guidelines that follow were drawn up by a subgroup of the Advanced Life Support Committee of the European Resuscitation Council with two co-opted members. The subgroup also benefitted from informal advice from designated members of the Arrhythmia Working Group of the European Society of Cardiology. The first version of the document was updated in 1996 primarily to bring the doses of amiodarone in line with the data sheets. This second minor update includes additional considerations in relation to atrial fibrillation.

The guidelines are presented as three algorithms: for bradyarrhythmias and intracardiac blocks, for broad complex tachycardias which can be equated under resuscitation conditions to ventricular tachycardia (under these conditions the distinction from less common varieties of supraventricular tachycardia may be impracticable), and for narrow complex tachycardias that can be equated with supraventricular tachycardia or atrial fibrillation.

Three important reservations must be stressed in relation to the algorithms. First they cannot encompass all situations that might arise: there are important variables relating to the heart rhythm, to the haemodynamic state, to patient characteristics, and to local traditions and circumstances – all of which might appropriately call for measures different from those suggested here. Secondly, the advice to call for help is conditional upon the individual already involved believing that he or she does not have the expertise necessary for definitive management. Such skills may be possessed by any medical practitioner and not only those who are arrhythmia specialists. Thirdly, some drugs are not available in all European countries and some have alternatives that find favour within distinct geographical areas. Whilst common variations have been included in the algorithms, not all can be accommodated without undue expansion and complexity. The special situations relating to toxins and drug overdoses are not included: for these expert help is mandatory. National versions of the guidelines may be produced under the auspices of the European Resuscitation Council with clear indicators of where they vary from those more generally applicable.

Two hazards must also be stressed. First, all antiarrhythmic strategies – physical manoeuvres [6], drugs [7], or electrical treatment [8] – can also be proarrhythmic [6] so that clinical deterioration may occur as a result of treatment rather than a consequence of lack of effect. Secondly, the use of multiple antiarrhythmic drugs or high doses of a single drug can cause myocardial depression and hypotension. The serious consequences may include deterioration in cardiac rhythm. Clinical decisions must be made judiciously especially in refractory cases.

7.2. THE ALGORITHMS

These are shown in Figs. 1–3.

Oxygen is recommended in all algorithms in recognition that this treatment is usually appropriate in a setting that threatens or follows cardiac arrest.

7.2.1. Bradycardias and Blocks

The algorithm is shown in Fig. 1. The apparent complexity represents the management principles that are in fact simple and may be summarised thus: *if there is a risk of asystole, pace immediately; if there is no perceived risk of asystole but the haemodynamic state of the patient is poor, give atropine and pace only if this is ineffective; if there is no perceived risk of asystole and the patient is not compromised haemodynamically to an important degree then only observation is required.* The algorithm, however, provides

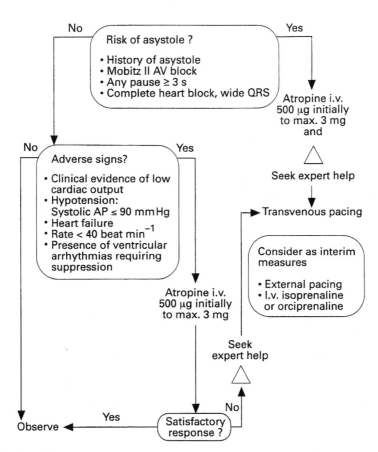

Bradycardia

If not already done, give oxygen and establish i.v. access
Doses based on adult of average body weight

FIG. 1. Algorithm for bradycardia.

more information around this framework.

No precise definition is called for beyond recognition that the heart rate is either abnormally slow in absolute terms or too slow for the haemodynamic state of the patient (relative bradycardia). A heart rate of 65 beats per minute, for example, may be inappropriately slow for a patient with clinical evidence of a critical low output state.

The recommendations for the bradycardias and blocks depend on whether or not there is a recognisable appreciable risk of asystole with four possible determinants listed. It will be noted that complete third degree heart block with a narrow QRS is not in itself an indication for treatment because atrioventricular junctional ectopic pacemakers (with a narrow QRS) often provide a reasonable and stable heart rate.

If asystole is held to be a definite risk, the responder who is not an expert in arrhythmia management may wish to do no more than establish intravenous access and give atropine before seeking help from others with the necessary specific skills for the transvenous pacing. If a patient's condition is too critical to wait for placement of a transvenous ventricular pacing wire, external pacing [9] may be appropriate (after sedation if necessary). Judicious use of isoprenaline is an alternative strategy, with the usual starting dose of approximately 1 μg/min. A suitable solution is obtained by dissolving 2.5 mg in 500 ml of a carrier solution, administered with an infusion pump initially at 0.2 ml/min (with appropriate adjustments to solution strengths and infusion rate if a conventional drip set has to be used). The dose may be increased rapidly (to a maximum which cannot be specified if the emergency is a desperate one, but may be 10 or 20 times greater than was used initially) – but regard should be paid to the risk of precipitating or worsening ventricular arrhythmias and increasing myocardial oxygen consumption. Isoprenaline for infusion is not available in all European countries and orciprenaline is an appropriate alternative.

If there is no perceived risk of asystole, a further question must be asked: are adverse clinical signs evident? Suggested indicators are shown in the algorithm that relate to severe impairment of myocardial function, very slow absolute heart rate, or the progression of emerging ventricular tachyarrhythmias that require suppression. Without such signs only observation may be required. But if one or more signs are present atropine should be administered with an initial dose of 500 μg by slow intravenous injection. Increments of 500 μg or 1 mg can be given at intervals of a few minutes up to a total dose of 3 mg. Higher doses will not be beneficial but may add to unwanted effects. After a satisfactory response only observation may be needed, but failure to respond to atropine in the presence of adverse signs calls for expert help (if needed) with a view to transvenous pacing – and the possibility of interim measures as previously defined. Doses of atropine may produce a beneficial effect that is evanescent: if large doses have to be repeated, and certainly if they are required more frequently than every few hours, then expert help may be necessary with the likelihood that transvenous pacing will be needed for more long-lasting stabilisation.

7.2.2. Broad Complex Tachycardia (Fig. 2)

The algorithm is shown in Fig. 2, and can be summarised into three possible treatment policies. *If there is no pulse as a result of the arrhythmia the condition should be treated as cardiac arrest using the ventricular fibrillation/ventricular tachycardia protocol for cardiac arrest. If there is a pulse but inadequate perfusion then cardioversion is required as soon as possible. If there is a broad complex tachycardia without adverse haemodynamic disturbance then routine antiarrhythmic therapy should be used, with cardioversion only if this fails.* The algorithm provides further information around this framework.

Although broad complex tachycardias maybe supraventricular with aberrant intraventricular conduction, the distinction can be subtle and – particularly in the context of resuscitation – the default position [10] must be an assumption that

Broad complex tachycardia

(Sustained ventricular tachycardia)
If not already done, give oxygen and establish i.v. access
Doses based on adult of average body weight

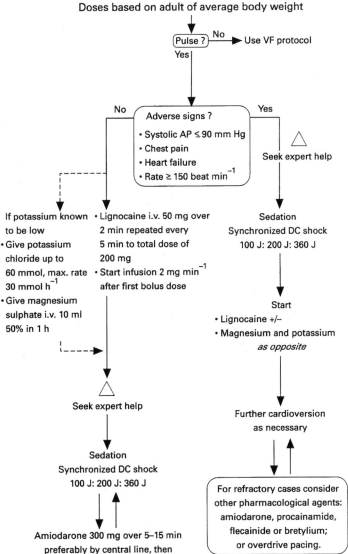

FIG. 2. Algorithm for broad complex tachycardia.

such complexes are of ventricular origin. Little harm results if a supraventricular tachycardia is treated as a ventricular one, whereas very serious consequences can follow from the opposite error.

With a broad complex tachycardia, the first determinant of management is whether or not there is a palpable pulse. Pulseless ventricular tachycardia is a rhythm akin to ventricular fibrillation, and the patient will be unconscious due to inadequate cerebral perfusion. The treatment then follows the guideline for ventricular fibrillation and pulseless ventricular tachycardia [4]. Once this distinction has been made and a palpable pulse located then oxygen is administered, intravenous access established if a line is not already in situ, and then – with the proviso mentioned above – expert help may be sought. This help may not, of course, be available immediately.

The question must then be asked whether or not adverse signs are present, and the algorithm shows four suggested determinants for this decision to be made. If there are adverse signs then the arrhythmia can be regarded as an emergency, and in most cases synchronised DC shock will be considered appropriate after any necessary sedation has been given. If this does not immediately resolve the situation lidocaine should be administered. If the plasma potassium concentration is known to be less than 3.6 mmol/l, especially in the presence of recent infarction [11], most authorities would recommend starting infusions of potassium and magnesium [12] whilst the patient is prepared for further cardioversion.

Other pharmacological agents that might be considered for refractory cases include procainamide [13], flecainide [14], propafenone [15], bretylium tosylate [16], and amiodarone [17] which can have a rapid action that depends on the plasma concentrations of the drug. Overdrive pacing [18] may also be considered if the expertise is available.

In the absence of adverse signs lidocaine can be administered in conventional doses, and if the potassium level is known to be low an infusion of potassium and magnesium is recommended to help prevent recurrent disturbances of rhythm. If lidocaine is ineffective then synchronised DC shock should be considered as for the symptomatic patient. For refractory cases without adverse signs amiodarone should be given by slow intravenous injection followed by an infusion, with another attempt at synchronised cardioversion after a period of up to 1 h has elapsed for this antiarrhythmic drug to produce a powerful pharmacological effect.

7.2.3. Narrow Complex Tachycardia (Fig. 3)

The algorithm shown in Fig. 3 can be sum-marised as follows. *For regular arrhythmic supraventricular tachycardias (that almost always have heart rates faster than 140 per minute), vagal manoeuvres or adenosine may be tried first, but if these are not successful in the presence of adverse signs the recommended strategy is cardioversion. Without adverse signs there is a choice of routine antiarrhythmics that include a short acting β blocker, digoxin, verapamil, and amiodarone.* Atrial fibrillation is a special case: rigid guidelines cannot readily be applied, and expert help may be prudent when the rate is persistently over 130 beats per minutes (see below). The algorithm adds further details to this outline.

Narrow complex tachycardia will almost always be supraventricular in origin and is somewhat less hazardous than broad complex tachycardia (though supraventricular tachycardias are a recognised trigger for ventricular fibrillation in critical situations [5]. Atrial fibrillation is a relatively common periarrest arrhythmia. It may cause serious haemodynamic disturbance not only because the rate may be rapid, but also because it tends to be associated with myocardial impairment, there is no atrial transport, and the irregularity may itself carry a haemodynamic penalty [19].

As for other arrhythmias in the context of resuscitation oxygen should be administered and intravenous access secured. Sinus tachycardia – which is likely to be regular with a rate less than 140 per minute – may cause diagnostic confusion and should be excluded. Its causes include pain and cardiogenic shock that should be treated appropriately.

The possibility of vagal manoeuvres (in particular a Valsalva manoeuvre or carotid sinus massage) must always be considered for supraventricular tachycardias, but in the context of resuscitation there are hazards that must be emphasised. In particular, strong vagal manoeuvres that cause sudden bradycardia may trigger ventricular fibrillation in the context of acute ischaemia or digitalis toxicity. Elderly patients are also vulnerable to plaque rupture [20] with cerebrovascular complications following carotid massage.

Narrow complex tachycardia

(Supraventricular tachycardia)
If not already done, give oxygen and establish i.v. access
Doses based on adult of average body weight

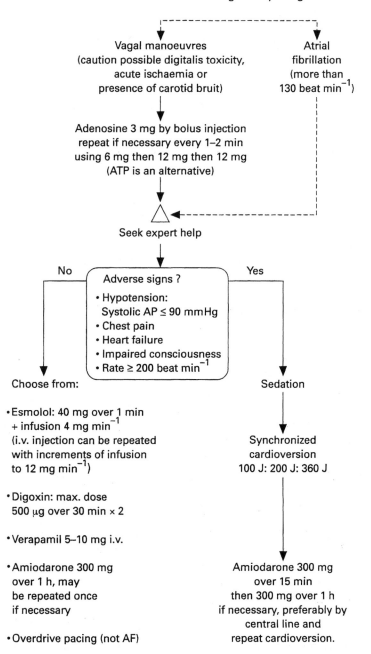

Vagal manoeuvres
(caution possible digitalis toxicity,
acute ischaemia or
presence of carotid bruit)

Atrial
fibrillation
(more than
130 beat min^{-1})

Adenosine 3 mg by bolus injection
repeat if necessary every 1–2 min
using 6 mg then 12 mg then 12 mg
(ATP is an alternative)

Seek expert help

No

Adverse signs ?

• Hypotension:
Systolic AP ≤ 90 mmHg
• Chest pain
• Heart failure
• Impaired consciousness
• Rate ≥ 200 beat min^{-1}

Yes

Choose from:

Sedation

• Esmolol: 40 mg over 1 min
+ infusion 4 mg min^{-1}
(i.v. injection can be repeated
with increments of infusion
to 12 mg min^{-1})

Synchronized
cardioversion
100 J: 200 J: 360 J

• Digoxin: max. dose
500 μg over 30 min × 2

• Verapamil 5–10 mg i.v.

• Amiodarone 300 mg
over 1 h, may
be repeated once
if necessary

Amiodarone 300 mg
over 15 min
then 300 mg over 1 h
if necessary, preferably by
central line and
repeat cardioversion.

• Overdrive pacing (not AF)

FIG. 3. Algorithm for narrow complex tachycardia.

The pharmacological treatment of choice for regular supraventricular tachycardias is adenosine [21]. Although this causes unpleasant side effects (particularly nausea,flushing, and chest discomfort) these are very brief and well tolerated if the patient is informed of their nature and duration before the injection is given. The recommendation in the algorithm predicates the initial use of a small dose of 3 mg. This will be effective only in a minority of cases, but increments can be given every 1–2 min with at least two injections of 12 mg if necessary. Adenosine is not available in some European countries, but adenosine triphosphate is an alternative. (In a few European countries neither preparation is available and one of the drugs lower in the algorithm will be favoured locally.)

If adenosine is not successful in establishing a satisfactory rhythm, or if atrial fibrillation at greater than 130 beats per minute is encountered, then expert help should be sought if appropriate. At this point management will depend upon whether or not adverse signs are present with determinants similar to those for broad complex tachycardia.

In the presence of adverse signs the treatment is synchronised DC shock after any necessary sedation. If this is unsuccessful it should be repeated after a slow intravenous injection followed by an infusion of amiodarone. If there is no perceived need for urgency then up to 1 h may elapse before further shocks are attempted, but of course circumstances may dictate that cardioversion is attempted after a shorter interval.

In the absence of adverse signs no one recommendation can be made because of different traditions of treatment between and within European countries. The suggestions that are offered include a short-acting β blocker (e.g., esmolol) [22], digoxin, verapamil, and amiodarone. Overdrive pacing can also be successful if the appropriate expertise is available, but is not an appropriate modality for the treatment of atrial fibrillation. Digoxin slows the ventricular rate relatively slowly [23] and may not be the best option if rate control is considered urgent.

A word of caution is necessary in relation to verapamil. This is a widely used and usually very successful agent in this situation, but there are circumstances in which verapamil is hazardous. These include arrhythmias associated with Wolff-Parkinson-White syndrome [24], tachycardias that are in fact ventricular in origin and not supraventricular [25], and some of the supraventricular arrhythmias of childhood [26]. The potentially serious interaction between verapamil and β blocking drugs should also be remembered [27]: this is particularly dangerous if both drugs have been administered intravenously.

ACKNOWLEDGEMENTS

We are grateful to Prof RWF Campbell, Dr Nina Rehnqvist, and Prof Stuart Cobbe for their helpful advice in the preparation of the original document.

7.3. REFERENCES

1. Chamberlain D, Vincent R, Baskett P, Bossaert L, Robertson C, Juchems R, Lindner K. Peri-arrest Arrhythmias (Management of arrhythmias associated with cardiac arrest). A statement by the Advanced Life Support Committee of the European Resuscitation Council. Resuscitation 1994;28:151-159.
2. Chamberlain D, Bossaert L et al. Peri-arrest arrhythmias: notice of 1st update. Resuscitation 1996;31:281.
3. Advanced Life Support Working Party of the European Resuscitation Council. Guidelines for advanced life support. Resuscitation 1992;24:111–21.
4. Advanced Life Support Working Party of the European Resuscitation Council. The 1998 European Resuscitation Council guidelines for adult advanced life support. Resuscitation 1998;17(2):(In press) (See also this volume Chapter 3.1, pp. 36–47).
5. Hayes LJ, Lerman BB, DiMarco JP. Nonventricular arrhythmias as precursors of ventricular fibrillation in patients with out-of-hospital cardiac arrest. Am Heart J 1989;118:53–57.
6. Sclarovsky S, Kracoff OH, Agmon J. Acceleration of ventricular tachycardia induced by a chest thump. Chest 1981;80:596–599.
7. Horowitz LN, Zipes DP (eds). A symposium: Perspectives on proarrhythmia. Am J Cardiol 1987;59:1E–56E.
8. Desilva RA, Graboys TB, Podrid PJ, Lown B. Cardioversion and defibrillation. Am Heart J 1980;100:881–895.

9. Falk RH, Zoll PM, Zoll RH. Safety and efficacy of noninvasive pacing. N Engl J Med 1983;309:1166–1168.

10. Griffith MJ, Garratt CJ, Mounsey P, Camm AJ. Ventricular tachycardia as default diagnosis in broad complex tachycardia. Lancet 1994;343:386–388.

11. Nordrehaug JE, von der Lippe G. Hypokalaemia and ventricular fibrillation in acute myocardial infarction. Br Heart J 1983;50:525–529.

12. Tzivoni D, Keren A. Suppression of ventricular arrhythmias by magnesium. Am J Cardiol 1990;65:1397–1399.

13. Lima JJ, Goldfarb AL, Conti DR, Golden LH, Bascomb BL, Benedetti GM, Jusko WJ. Safety and efficacy of procainamede infusions. Am J Cardiol 1979;43:98–105.

14. Roden DM, Woosley RL. Drug therapy: flecainide. N Engl J Med 1986;315:36–41.

15. Oates JA, Wood AJ. Propafenone. N Engl J Med 1990;322:518–525.

16. Bacaner MB. Treatment of ventricular fibrillation and other acute arrhythmias with bretylium tosylate. Am J Cardiol 1968;21:530–543.

17. Schützenberger WM, Leisch F, Kerschner K, Harringer W, Herbinger W. Clinical efficacy of intravenous amiodarone in the short term treatment of recurrent sustained ventricular tachycardia and ventricular fibrillation. Br Heart J 1989;62:367–371.

18. Wellens HJJ, Schuilenburg RM, Durrer D. Electrical stimulation of the heart in patients with ventricular tachycardia. Circulation 1972;46:216–226.

19. Clark DM, Plumb VJ, Epstein AE, Kay GN. Hemodynamic effects of an irregular sequence of ventricular cycle lengths during atrial fibrillation. JACC 1997;30:1039–1045.

20. Bastuli JA, Orlowski JP. Stroke as a complication of carotid sinus massage. Crit Care Med 1985;13:869.

21. Camm AJ, Malcolm AD, Garratt CJ. Adenosine and cardiac arrhythmias. The preferred treatment for supraventricular tachycardia. Br Med J 1992;305:3–4.

22. Turlapaty P, Laddu A, Murthy S, Singh B, Lee R. Esmolol: a titratable short-acting intravenous beta blocker for acute critical care settings. Am Heart J 1987;114:866–885.

23. Jordaens L, Trouerbach J, Calle P, Tavernier R, Derycke E, Vertongen P, Bergez B, Vandekerckhove Y. Conversion of atrial fibrillation to sinus rhythm and rate control by digoxin in comparison to placebo. Eur Heart J 1997;18:643–648.

24. Gulamhusein S, Ko P, Klein GJ. Ventricular fibrillation following verapamil in the Wolff-Parkinson-White syndrome. Am Heart J 1983;106:145–147.

25. Rankin AC, Rae AP, Cobbe SM. Misuse of intravenous verapamil in patients with ventricular tachycardia. Lancet 1987;ii:472–474.

26. Porter CJ, Gillette PC, Garson A, Hesslein PS, Karpawich PP, McNamara DG. Effects of verapamil on supraventricular tachycardia in children. Am J Cardiol 1991;48:478–491.

27. Lander R. Verapamil/beta-blocker interaction. A review. Mo Med 1983;80:626–629.

8. The Prehospital Management of Acute Heart Attacks

Recommendations of a Task Force of the European Society of Cardiology and The European Resuscitation Council*

CONTENTS:

*Members of Task Force in alphabetical order: Dr Hans-Richard Arntz (ESC); Prof Leo Bossaert (ERC); Prof Pierre Carli (ERC); Prof Douglas Chamberlain (ERC); Prof Michael Davies (Co-opted); Dr Mikael Dellborg (ESC); Prof Wolfgang Dick (ERC); Prof T Haghfelt (ESC); Dr Svein Hapnes (ERC); Prof Rudolf Juchems (ERC); Dr Hannelore Loewel (Co-opted); Dr Rudy Koster (ESC); Dr Alain Leizorovicz (ESC); Prof Mario Marzilli (ESC); Dr John Rawles (ESC); Dr Colin Robertson(ERC); Dr Miguel Ruano (ERC).

8.1. INTRODUCTION

In 1996, the European Society of Cardiology published guidelines on the prehospital and in-hospital management of myocardial infarction [1]. These relate primarily to clinical management specifically of this one condition from the onset of symptoms to the phase of secondary prevention and rehabilitation. The problem of acute heart attacks from a community perspective is, however, more complex and many aspects were not within the remit of this earlier document.

Although "Heart Attack" has no strict medical definition, it is commonly used to indicate a sudden and potentially life-threatening abnormality of heart function. We have chosen to use it as a convenient umbrella term to cover the same spectrum of conditions that most frequently elicits its use by lay people. These are chest pain from prolonged myocardial ischaemia, severely symptomatic cardiac arrhythmias, acute breathlessness of cardiac origin, and – most importantly of all – sudden cardiac death and cardiac arrest. There are advantages in considering the underlying conditions as a group for the purposes of the document for three principal reasons: first, they may all have the same underlying cause and one can lead to another; secondly, the strategies to counteract them have much in common; thirdly, in the earliest stage of a cardiac illness during the prehospital phase categorisation under a specific diagnostic label may be impossible.

The majority of deaths from coronary disease occur in the prehospital phase and most victims do not survive long enough to receive medical help. Despite these two challenging facts, inadequate attention and resources have been devoted to emergency systems in most European countries. Thus patterns of care available to heart attack victims in the initial hour or so have changed little in recent decades and speed of response does not usually match the urgency of sudden attacks. Treatment strategies even for recognised ischaemic syndromes need some modification to address the special problems of unstable patients often in the evolving phase of the acute attack

who face a journey to hospital under circumstances that may be less than ideal. Other diagnoses may be responsible for sudden cardiac death particularly in the younger and older age groups and may require some modification of routine resuscitation procedures. For all these reasons the encouraging reduction in hospital mortality has not been reflected in community mortality. New strategies are needed if any impact is to be made. This report was therefore commissioned by the European Society of Cardiology and the European Resuscitation Council to supplement the existing advice available on the management of myocardial infarction and other forms of acute heart attack, with special reference to the prehospital phase.

A decision was made to include the early in-hospital phase – within the emergency department – as part of our remit. The reasons are 3-fold. Firstly, we wish to emphasise the need for continuity of care as the patient leaves the ambulance and enters the hospital. Secondly, we are aware that failures of communication between these care modalities often delay important treatments. Thirdly, in many centres specialist advice and treatment become available only after patients reach the cardiac (coronary) care unit or investigational areas.

The Task Force was set up by the European Society of Cardiology and the European Resuscitation Council. It was the first to be set up jointly by the two organisations, an appropriate innovation for a logistical challenge that is multidisciplinary, involving ambulance services, general practitioners, emergency physicians, intensivists, anesthesiologists, internists, and of course cardiologists in all European countries.

8.2. THE EPIDEMIOLOGY OF ACUTE MYOCARDIAL INFARCTION AND SUDDEN CARDIAC DEATH

Much of our knowledge of the epidemiology of heart attacks derives from the WHO MONICA Project [2]. In European countries around 40% of all cause mortality before the age of 75 years is due to cardiovascular diseases, independent of the different levels of total mortality [3]. The high variation of ischaemic heart disease mortality is a function of both the incidence of acute heart attacks (probable myocardial infarction) and the case fatality rate (number of fatal cases per 100 total cases). In 29 MONICA populations (age 35–64 years) the mean 28-day case fatality rate from episodes thought to be due to acute myocardial infarction is formidably high, at 49% for men and 51% for women [2], increasing with age.

Despite the international mortality differences, the proportion of case fatalities at different stages during the acute event are very similar in all centres. On average, one-third of all cases of myocardial infarction are fatal before hospitalisation [2,3], most of them within the first hour after onset of acute symptoms. The *proportion* of deaths occurring out of hospital is very high, particularly in younger people. Norris has recent-

ly presented data derived from three British cities [4] in which the ratio of out-of-hospital deaths to in-hospital deaths from acute coronary events (which excludes heart failure) ranged from 15.6:1 in the youngest cohort aged less than 50 to 2:1 for the oldest group who were aged 70 to 74. A similar trend has been observed in data derived from the population-based MONICA Augsburg Myocardial Infarction Register, although in that city and the two surrounding rural districts the ratios were somewhat less striking (Table 1a and 1b). If this represents a failure of prehospital care, the failure is particularly notable in the young and middle aged.

A more detailed account of the sequence of events in the first few hours after acute myocardial infarction is obtained from the MONICA register from Augsburg, one of the MONICA collaborating centres [5] (Fig. 1). This register includes

TABLE IA. Ratio of out-of-hospital to in-hospital deaths from acute manifestations of coronary heart disease (deaths from heart failure are not included).

Age (years)	Out-of-hospital fatal events	In-hospital fatal events	Ratio out-of-hospital:in-hospital fatal events
< 50	78	5	15.6
50–54	67	10	6.7
55–59	115	28	4.1
60–64	202	65	3.1
65–69	313	114	2.7
70–74	397	195	2.0

Derived from [4]; Norris RM for United Kingdom Heart Attack study collaborative group.

TABLE IB. Ratio of out-of-hospital to in-hospital deaths from acute manifestations of coronary heart disease (MONICA category "nonclassifiable sudden cardiac deaths" are included).

Age (years) (men and women)	Out-of-hospital fatal events	In-hospital fatal events	Ratio out-of-hospital:in-hospital fatal events
25–34	22	6	3.7
35–44	109	43	2.5
45–54	386	176	2.2
55–64	942	582	1.6
65–74	1811	1508	1.2
All	**3270**	**2315**	**1.4**

Unpublished, derived from population-based MONICA Augsburg Myocardial Infarction Register 1985–1994.

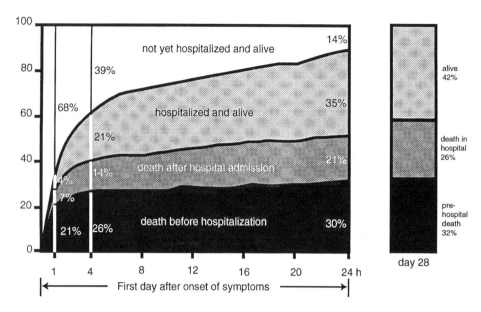

FIG. I. Survival in the 1st day after acute myocardial infarction. Updated English version of original Fig. 3 from [5].

25- to 74-year-old cases and collects specific information on the prehospital phase, additional to the MONICA core design. The Augsburg data highlight the logistical difficulties facing those who seek to improve the prognosis. The 28-day case fatality rate in 3,729 cases of acute myocardial infarction of both sexes and all the age groups was 58%. No less than 28% of the total number had died within 1 h of the onset of symptoms, 40% in 4 h, and 51% in 24 h. Sixty percent of all deaths occurred outside hospital, 30% in hospital on day 1, and 10% on days 2–28. Only 10% of prehospital death cases were seen alive by a doctor and nearly 60% died unwitnessed.

Patients with acute myocardial infarction who survive long enough to enter hospital undoubtedly benefit from new treatments introduced into routine practice within the last decade or so. These have resulted in a fall in hospital mortality [6], and improved long-term survival [7]. Unfortunately the impact on community mortality rates is influenced only marginally by this success, as a relatively small proportion of potential victims reach hospital to benefit from recent advances. Indeed, no detectable fall in the case

fatality rate has been observed in MONICA centres during the years 1985–94 in Augsburg [8] or during the years 1985–91 in Glasgow [9]. A greater investment in hospital treatments (e.g., primary PTCA; or newer, more expensive, and marginally more effective thrombolytic agents) is therefore unlikely to result in any appreciable fall in total mortality. These technological developments should not be discounted. They are valuable to individuals who reach hospital both in terms of early and later case fatality. However, improvement in current strategies and the development of new ones are needed to influence the larger number of prehospital deaths. Improvements in existing services could prevent many of the 12% of deaths which occur between 1 and 4 h from symptom onset and the additional 11% who die between 4 and 24 h [5]. The even larger attrition of the 1st hour calls for initiatives that are not available in most of Europe at present, but the greatest bar is complacency rather than cost. The mechanism of deaths within 4 h will often be ventricular fibrillation, and in the later ones cardiogenic shock: both could be influenced by the energetic application of prompt defibrillation and reperfusion therapy. Thus epidemiological data suggests that greater deployment of resources for prehospital care has more potential for reducing the case fatality rate of acute myocardial infarction than has the intensification of treatment in hospital.

8.3. PATHOPHYSIOLOGY WITH SPECIAL REFERENCE TO THE INFLUENCE OF TIME

8.3.1. Muscle Jeopardy and Necrosis in Acute Coronary Syndromes

Acute myocardial infarction is caused by a sudden and prolonged reduction of coronary blood flow that in turn is the consequence of the abrupt compromise of a major coronary artery or branch. Thrombus formation over a plaque is the major mechanism causing vessel closure but spasm and embolisation of thrombotic material into the intramyocardial vascular bed may contribute. Angiographic studies show that vessels occlude at the sites of mild to moderate stenosis in about 70% of cases [10]. Angiography has no predictive value for the site of a future occlusion.

Abrupt coronary obstruction leads to transmural ischaemia within the area at risk determined by the coronary anatomy. The jeopardized myocardium develops irreversible changes starting in the subendocardium and progressing outwards. This progression of necrosis has been termed the "wavefront phenomenon" [11]. In anaesthetized dogs infarct size increases with duration of coronary occlusion for up to 6 h. After 6 h, reperfusion has no effect on infarct size. The temporal and spatial progression of necrosis across the ventricular wall represents a fundamental pathophysiological phenomenon. The most significant implication of these experimental observations is that the salvage of tissue is a time-dependent phenomenon. There is no reason to believe humans differ in regard to time dependency. Indirect evidence suggests that in humans average infarct size without reperfusion therapy is about 20% of the left ventricle. If thrombolytic treatment is started 1 h after onset, 70% of jeopardized myocardium is salvaged, but myocardial salvage is 0% for thrombolysis initiated 5 h after onset [12,13].

In man several circumstances can change the time course of myocardial necrosis, including preexisting collaterals, ischaemic preconditioning, and age.

Preexisting collateral circulation which may limit infarct size [14] can be visualised at angiography in about one-third of the cases of acute myocardial infarction [15]. Collaterals developing after infarction do not affect infarct size but may mitigate left ventricular remodelling and reduce the possibility of cardiac failure. Preexisting collaterals may also extend the benefit of reperfusion to patients treated after 6 h [16]. In animal models, brief periods of coronary occlusion increase tissue tolerance to subsequent prolonged vessel closure – the so-called "preconditioning" phenomenon. In man, patients with a history of preinfarction angina tend to have less myocardial damage, less cardiac failure, and therefore lower mortality with better left ventricular function at follow-up [17]. Advanced age seems to be associated with increased susceptibility to myocardial injury [18]. Elderly patients may have appreciable damage in the affected zone with commensurate mortality despite sustained arterial patency, possibly because of a greater susceptibility to calcium mediated or oxidative damage. This increased risk may be seen from the decade 65–74 years and is most pronounced in those older than 75 years.

Chest pain is variable and subjective and its onset may not coincide with coronary occlusion. Limited benefit following myocardial reperfusion in acute myocardial infarction may result from an underestimation of occlusion time. On the other hand, coronary occlusion may be intermittent despite the presence of continuous pain. Intermittent spontaneous reperfusion may prevent or limit myocardial damage and benefit may then follow from relatively late therapeutic interventions [19].

The following summarises the available data on the progression of myocardial necrosis that have practical implications for clinical management:

• Although there is variation between species, animal experiments have shown that after 6 h of persistent coronary occlusion only

10–15% of ischaemic myocardium is still viable. Reperfusion beyond 3–4 h is then unlikely to result in the salvage of any significant amount of myocardial muscle.

- In humans a very similar time course usually exists for true salvage. Benefits from reperfusion after this time window must be attributed to different mechanisms.

- Several factors, including thrombus dimensions and structure, can substantially influence the time-window for effective reperfusion in an individual patient. The time window is shortest in previously healthy individuals who abruptly occlude an artery. Previous exertional angina through induction of collateral growth or recruitment of preexisting collaterals, may limit infarct size, and in some cases ischaemic preconditioning may also be protective.

- Intermittent anginal pain at rest as a prodromal symptom characterises a patient with intermittent occlusion and intramyocardial emboli of activated platelets [19]. Such patients develop infarction by coalescing small focal areas of necrosis of differing ages and the time window for intervention is extended.

8.3.2. Malignant Arrhythmias in Acute Coronary Syndromes

Despite the reduction in mortality from ischaemic heart disease in most Western European countries, sudden cardiac death remains a major medical and social problem. More than half the patients with known ischaemic heart disease die suddenly [20,21]. Of those who come to the attention of clinicians, sudden death is the initial presenting event in nearly one-third and is associated in the majority of cases with malignant ventricular arrhythmias, usually ventricular tachycardia or ventricular fibrillation.

The incidence of primary ventricular fibrillation (i.e., in the absence of severe haemodynamic compromise) is highest during the very early stages of acute ischaemia, and even with established infarction is rare after the first 4 h [22].

Ventricular tachycardia usually occurs later than 4 h after symptom onset [23] but is not a stable rhythm. Degeneration of ventricular tachycardia is a frequent cause of ventricular fibrillation that appears more than 1 day after the onset of infarction. Asystole may be a primary arrhythmia or the end result of ventricular fibrillation that has degenerated to an imperceptible amplitude.

8.3.3. Primary Sudden Death

Up to 20% of patients who suffer sudden cardiac death have no detectable heart disease [24]: the mechanism often remains unknown. Recurrence rate is high after aborted sudden death that was not associated with myocardial infarction [25]. Thus the long-term prognosis after primary sudden death is worse than for survivors of cardiac arrest secondary to ischaemic heart disease.

8.4. ACCESS TO CARE

From a practical viewpoint, the two most important ways in which heart attacks may present are chest pain due to myocardial infarction and cardiac arrest due to ventricular fibrillation. Appropriate treatments are respectively coronary reperfusion and early defibrillation. Both require rapid access to the Emergency Medical System (EMS) but with different priorities. For a patient with cardiac arrest, the need is for a witness only to recognise that an emergency has occurred that requires immediate attention, and for the availability of appropriate first aid followed by rapid defibrillation: speed and simplicity rather than precision and complexity! For acute myocardial infarction an appropriate response requires greater public knowledge to understand the implications of cardiac pain, with the early availability of a medically competent team to offer accurate diagnosis and reperfusion therapy if indicated. An optimal system must therefore achieve the twin aims of rapid response for cardiac arrest and precision in diagnosis of acute myocardial infarction.

The current situation for meeting these needs in Europe varies widely between countries and within countries, as well as between urban and rural areas. Recommendations for improvements must be made on the basis of what is desirable, yet must also be pragmatic. Where optimal systems cannot be achieved in the foreseeable future, progress can always be made towards the ultimate goal. Many obstacles to progress can be corrected at little or no cost by better organisation and by modifications to outmoded laws and practices. Recommendations will therefore be classed as "basic" which is regarded as the least that is acceptable as an interim standard, and "optimal" which should be attainable as soon as possible (see Section 8.7. Principal Recommendations).

8.4.1. Delays in Providing Treatment for Cardiac Emergencies

Patient decision time

The interval from the onset of symptoms until medical assistance is sought varies widely. Despite widespread public education, reports on patient delays have demonstrated only small trends to shorter time intervals [26]. Decision time is not closely related to knowledge of heart symptoms. Symptoms are often interpreted incorrectly [27] because of psychological defence mechanisms such as denial [28] or displacement and rationalization [29]; but responses are influenced by severity of pain [30], the emotional reactions to it [31], and the degree of left ventricular dysfunction [32].

Doctor decision time

Although call-to-needle times can be very short when general practitioners give thrombolytics prehospital [33], many studies have shown that the involvement of the majority who do not themselves give thrombolytic therapy in the management of myocardial infarction results in substantial delay in definitive treatment given after arrival in hospital [34,35]. Calling a general practitioner alone in response to a cardiac arrest may be even less appropriate in countries where few

are equipped for defibrillation. Little information is available on the potential value of general practitioners playing a supporting role in coordination with the emergency services but there must be many situations in which this can be of value.

Dispatching

The nature of any response to the request for help in the event of chest pain requires clear guidelines. It will be influenced by the training and qualifications of the dispatcher, the way the message is presented, knowledge of any previous medical history, the cost of sending help when a response is not warranted, and the medical and legal consequences of refusing help when in retrospect it may have been justified. A medical background allows some discretion in the interpretation of calls that would not be appropriate for a nonmedical dispatcher. The dispatcher has four decisions to make: first, whether or not to send an ambulance; secondly, if an ambulance is to be sent the type of ambulance to be deployed; thirdly how much urgency is needed; fourthly whether advice should be given to the caller on actions to be taken meanwhile. The first of these is the most difficult even for experienced medical dispatchers, because the quality of information is frequently too poor for any safe decision not to send an ambulance [36]. For this reason and to avert possible legal consequences, dispatchers tend to send vehicles in all but the most obvious trivial circumstances: "better safe than sorry" is a valid principle. In consequence, many ambulances are dispatched to patients whose complaints turn out not to have been urgent [37]. Many ambulance control centres send vehicles in response to all requests for help whilst others use algorithms to assess the urgency and priority of calls. These have been introduced in several places in Europe and the USA, but evaluation so far has been limited [38].

Ambulance response interval

The ambulance response interval (which measures the duration from call to arrival at the patient's side) of the first or only tier is in general the shortest of all the delays. In some countries, a time limit is set whereby 95% of all ambulance journeys must be completed within 15 min and 80% within 10 min. In others, strict time criteria are being set for selected cases based on the information received and using systems of prioritised despatch. Both of these approaches are in line with the concepts of early defibrillation for cardiac arrest and early reperfusion for acute myocardial infarction. When ambulance provision includes defibrillation and drug administration (especially thrombolysis for selected patients), then the coronary care unit is effectively brought to the patient within the community: the delay to treatment ends at that point.

8.4.2. The Chain of Survival for Cardiac Arrest

In no medical emergency is time such a decisive determinant of outcome as in circulatory arrest. The "chain of survival" concept clearly describes the important links involved [39,40]. The chain is usually regarded as having four links:

Early access

Immediate access to an ambulance dispatch centre is a primary requirement because any delay in calling the ambulance service inevitably decreases the prospects of survival. The initial contact should not be with a physician, unless he has the role of first tier in the EMS and has a defibrillator. In most European countries access to the EMS is achieved by means of a single dedicated telephone number. The European Council has agreed that a uniform number "112" should be used throughout Europe by 1997, but this has not been widely implemented nor promoted [41]. The caller's description of the problem should influence the degree of priority that is accorded preferably by the use of one of the evaluated algorithm systems: the dispatcher should be alerted by any suggestion of impaired consciousness and should not be reassured by the statement that the victim is breathing, as

gasping may continue for minutes after circulatory arrest. Convulsion and vaso-vagal collapse may cause confusion.

Early CPR

Investigators in Europe and the USA have demonstrated that bystander CPR extends the period for successful resuscitation, and provides a bridge to first defibrillation. It has been estimated that at any point in time between collapse and first defibrillation, bystander CPR at least doubles the chance of survival [42,43], with the possible exception of the first few minutes [43]. Unfortunately, in most European countries bystander CPR is carried out in only a minority of cases.

Early defibrillation 1

In most instances ventricular fibrillation is the initial rhythm associated with circulatory arrest. As time passes, the waveform of ventricular fibrillation loses amplitude and frequency until no deflections can be detected. Electrical defibrillation is the only effective therapy for ventricular fibrillation, and the interval between the onset of the arrhythmia and the delivery of the first defibrillating shock is the main determinant of successful defibrillation and survival. The possibility of successful defibrillation decreases by more than 5% per minute from the time of collapse. To achieve early defibrillation, it is mandatory that people other than doctors be permitted to defibrillate. In particular, all first tier ambulances should be equipped with defibrillators, and ambulance personnel should be proficient in their use [44]. Nonmedical ambulance personnel can be trained in defibrillation in as little as 8–10 h, provided they have good training in basic life support. The important goal of facilitating early defibrillation, with all emergency personnel responding to cardiac arrest being trained, equipped, and permitted to use the modest skill, is still to be widely implemented in most European countries.

Early defibrillation 2. Automated external defibrillation

The automated external defibrillator (AED) can be employed by persons with a limited training targeted to use of the equipment, but without sufficient knowledge for a reliable diagnosis of ventricular fibrillation [45]. This makes it possible to bring the defibrillator to locations with large crowds such as stadiums, airports, shopping malls, and railway stations, where trained first aid personnel can employ them rapidly and in locations where EMS intervention is almost impossible such as airplanes or cruise ships.

Early defibrillation 3. Immediate defibrillation by first responders

Because a considerable time may elapse between the onset of VF and the arrival of the emergency medical services, immediate defibrillation by individuals who can be classed as "first responders" may implement the ideal of early defibrillation [46]. A first responder may be defined as a trained individual acting independently but within a physician – controlled system. The availability of AEDs makes first responder defibrillation a practicable option. Target groups to deliver immediate defibrillation with an AED could include firefighters [46], police and security personnel [47], lifeguards, and flight attendants [48]. Every working day these personnel encounter many members of the public at risk from heart attacks. Although immediate defibrillation by first responders is the logical step after implementation of defibrillation by ambulance personnel, at present no conclusive evidence can show that bystander defibrillation significantly increases survival rates. A few cases of successful defibrillation in-flight and in a railway station have been recorded, and it has been demonstrated that even small differences in call-to-shock time achieved by equipping policemen with defibrillators are critical determinants in the restoration of spontaneous circulation and discharge alive from the hospital [47]. Implementation of programmes for first responder defibrillation should be care-

fully planned and critically evaluated before wide ranging recommendations can be made. Nevertheless, a recent advisory statement of the International Liaison Committee on Resuscitation (ILCOR) clearly advocates this approach [49].

Early advanced care

In many instances CPR and defibrillation alone do not achieve or sustain resuscitation, and advanced cardiac life support is necessary further to improve the prospect of survival. In some systems endotracheal intubation and intravenous medication are not provided out of hospital, while in others advanced life support is available from the first tier of the ambulance service, or more commonly by a second tier. Transportation to the hospital intensive care unit should not be allowed to interrupt appropriate advanced care.

8.4.3. Emergency Medical Systems in Europe

There is a wide variety of emergency medical systems:

- 1-tier systems delivering only BLS by an EMT;
- 1-tier systems delivering BLS and defibrillation by an EMT-D;
- 1-tier systems delivering BLS and ALS by paramedics, doctors and/or nurses;
- 2-tier systems delivering BLS followed by ALS by doctors, paramedics and/or nurses;
- 2-tier systems delivering BLS and defibrillation, followed by ALS by doctors, paramedics and/or nurses.

The structure and organisation of the emergency medical systems in European countries is summarised in Table 2. In the majority of European countries, doctors have an active role in prehospital emergency medical care as part of the first or of the second tier. In England and Wales all emergency ambulances have at least one paramedic, whilst in parts of Scandinavia paramedics serve as members of the second tier. An experienced nurse is part of the crew of every ambulance in The Netherlands. The availability of phy-

TABLE 2. EMS system in European countries. Figures between brackets indicate local variations in the country.

Country	1st tier	2nd tier	Emergency phone	Who is allowed to defribillate
Austria	emt	md	144	md, emt[a]
Belgium	emt-(d)	md	100	md, rn, emt-d
Bulgaria	md	md	150	members of resuscitation team
Croatia	md	–	94	md
Czechia	emt	md	155	md, pm
Denmark	emt-(d)	(pm)	112	dr, rn, emt-d
Finland	emt-(d)	md	112	everybody trained
France	emt	md	15	md, rn, emt-d
Germany	emt paramedic	md	112	md, pm
Greece	emt	–	166	md
Hungary	emt-(d)	rn/md	104	md, pm, emt-d
Iceland	emt-(d)	md	0112	md, emt[a]
Ireland	emt	–	999	md, rn, pm
Italy	emt	(md)	118	md, rn
Netherlands	rn	–	112	md, rn
Norway	emt-d	md/pm	113	md + assistant in function
Poland	md	md	999	md, emt[a]
Portugal	md	–	115	md, emt[a]
Romania	rn/md	md	06	md, rn
Russia	md	–	03	md/representative
Slovakia	md/pm/rn	md	155	md, rn, emt-d, pm
Slovenia	md	–	94	md, rn, emt-d
Spain	emt/rn/md	–	061	md, rn no law
Sweden	emt-d	pm	112	md, rn, emt-d
Switzerland	emt	(md)	114	md, rn, pm
Turkey	md	–	118	md
UK	emt-(d)	(pm)	999	no law
Yugoslavia	md	md	94	md, rn, emt

Abbreviations: md = medical doctor; rn = nurse; pm = paramedic; emt = emergency medical technician; emt-d = emergency medical technician qualified for use of AED.
[a]In presence of a doctor. For permission to defibrillate, the minimum training level is mentioned.

sicians in the field may be the reason for the legislation delaying the implementation of defibrillation by ambulance personnel in too many countries, yet this practice may still improve the prospects of early defibrillation. The wisdom of such legislation must therefore be questioned.

Some of the wide variety of approaches and organisations are better suited than others for responding to circulatory arrest (Table 2). When a two-tiered system exists, the training level of the first responding ambulance personnel may not permit recognition of ventricular fibrillation and subsequent defibrillation. In this situation the time taken for arrival of the second tier causes an unacceptable delay. Two solutions

should be considered: either improve the training of first responders to enable them to diagnose and treat ventricular fibrillation and carry out defibrillation [44], or introduce automated external defibrillators (AED) within the first tier. The latter solution has been evaluated and proved successful [50] and with recent models easier to use and safe [46]. The situation is least favourable if a single-tier system exists without the possibility of prehospital defibrillation: this must be a priority for change. Best performance, in terms of survival, has been achieved by two-tiered systems with AED availability in the first tier, and well-trained paramedics or emergency physicians in the second tier [51].

8.4.4. Legislation Relating to Basic Life Support and Defibrillation

For historical, organisational, and political reasons, legislation relating to resuscitation and defibrillation varies greatly within European countries. Information about legal regulations was collected from 28 European countries. Throughout most of Europe, providing CPR when indicated is an intrinsic part of the duties of all who respond to cardiac arrests as members of the emergency system. In virtually all European countries, every health care provider and everyone who has been trained in CPR has a moral and sometimes a legal obligation to offer help, according to the legislation relating to "non-assistance to endangered persons". The Belgian law is cited as an example, but other countries have similar legislation [52]. In 21 of the 28 countries that were surveyed, anyone (or anyone who has been instructed) is permitted or at least not forbidden to initiate CPR.

In the majority of European countries, defibrillation is considered to be a medical procedure. This is a reflection of the historical and continuing involvement of doctors in out-of-hospital emergencies and disasters. Delegation to non-medically qualified personnel of acts that are usually performed by doctors is, however, legally possible in many European countries if a doctor is not immediately available. In countries where historically only ambulancemen and paramedics are present in the field, the implementation of early defibrillation by ambulancemen has been readily accepted. In countries where a medical presence is common in the second or even the first tier, the introduction of defibrillation by first attending ambulancemen has progressed slowly. In two of 28 countries the law restricts the act of defibrillation exclusively to doctors. In four countries defibrillation can be delegated only to nurses. In another four countries, ambulance personnel are allowed to defibrillate only in the presence of a doctor. In 16 of 28 countries, defibrillation can legally be delegated to nurses, paramedics, or qualified health care professionals. Two countries have no legal restrictions relating to defibrillation. Thus in at least 10 European countries the law is an obstacle for nationwide implementation of AED programmes by nonphysicians.

8.4.5. Other Approaches for Improving Access and Decreasing Delay

Priority access for high-risk patients

Besides improving existing facilities, some new approaches have been adopted to improve access and early treatment for patients with acute cardiac symptoms or circulatory arrest. Rapid access to the system for selected high risk patients (mostly with previous myocardial infarction) has been reported [53]. Not only may immediate access be ensured, but also arrhythmia analysis can be performed and treatment advised if appropriate. Specialised centres can offer direct access to dispatchers who can draw on computerised histories of their patients and can also compare electrocardiograms transmitted by patients with reference electrocardiograms on file. Results suggest a reduction of the median interval between onset of symptoms and arrival in hospital to 1 h for patients in the system compared with 3 h for the general population and also an improvement in 1-year postinfarction mortality. Controlled scientific evaluation of this concept is not yet available, however.

Telephone CPR

The outcome of resuscitation is consistently better if basic life support is started by bystanders. Currently this is not performed in the majority of cases of circulatory arrest, partly because of ignorance and lack of confidence and training. Telephone guided CPR by people who have had no previous training has proved feasible [54], and evidence of its efficacy is suggestive though not yet convincingly established [55]. The technique requires intensive training of dispatchers who must use strict protocols.

8.5. PREHOSPITAL TRIAGE OF PATIENTS WITH ACUTE CORONARY SYNDROMES AND ARRANGEMENTS FOR CARE

The recognition that recent chest pain is likely to have a cardiac origin always has therapeutic implications, but this is of special importance with evolving myocardial infarction which requires immediate assessment. The diagnosis of acute myocardial infarction becomes certain only with the passage of time, depending on the patient's developing history, the evolution of abnormalities on the ECG, and a characteristic rise and fall of biochemical markers of myocardial damage. Prehospital prediction of the final diagnosis is based only on a snapshot of the clinical history and a single ECG recording, but can be reasonably accurate. With clinical assessment alone, the diagnostic accuracy of experienced clinicians is about 75% [56]. With the addition of the ECG, accuracy may be increased to 90–95% [57,58].

8.5.1. Prehospital Triage for Reperfusion Therapy in Evolving Myocardial Infarction

The decision to start thrombolysis or refer a patient for primary angioplasty is made by an integrated evaluation of the history, physical examination, an ECG, and a careful consideration of the risks and benefits of treatment. Making such a decision takes time, so for the majority of cases without special diagnostic difficulty clinical assessment must be carried out only once and by the person making the therapeutic decision. In the most efficient systems this role is undertaken by an appropriately trained physician who arrives with the ambulance. Where patients are seen before hospital admission by medical personnel who are unable to make such decisions, much time may be lost by carrying out a full clinical assessment which is repeated later. Rapid triage requiring urgent treatment rather than precise diagnosis should be the aim under these circumstances, including a decision – where facilities permit – on whether the patient should be taken directly to a specialised cardiac

unit or to the emergency department. The most important guide is a 12-lead ECG.

8.5.2. The Electrocardiogram (ECG) for Prehospital Triage and Treatment

At present, many ambulance systems cannot record, interpret, or transmit a 12-lead ECG, but the importance of these facilities should not be overlooked. Several different methods may be used.

Telephonic ECG transmission

Ideally an ECG will be recorded and interpreted on site shortly after the first contact with the patient. In the absence of a system for immediate ECG interpretation, the tracing may be transmitted to a hospital for interpretation by a physician [59]. This must be accomplished with speed and without loss of quality. High quality transfer may be possible with standard telephone lines or digitised networks for computerised communication. Mobile phones have been used but the results with analogue systems may not be reliable [60]. It should be noted that digital mobile telephone networks use compression algorithms that may significantly distort the ECG signal. The reliability of this system has not yet been fully established. Telephone transmission is unlikely to be appropriate in urban areas because some delay is almost inevitable.

Computerised ECG interpretation

Most of the computerised interpretation algorithms have been developed for standard 12-lead ECGs in nonacute settings: the sensitivity of the algorithms may be too high for prehospital use. The purpose of prehospital ECG interpretation is to identify relatively obvious infarction. In the prehospital setting diagnostic algorithms should have lower sensitivity and good specificity to reduce the risk of inappropriate thrombolysis.

8.5.3. Personnel Providing Prehospital Thrombolysis

Ideally, thrombolytic treatment should be given at the first opportunity, by the first qualified person to see the patient, whether this be before or after hospital admission. Personnel providing prehospital thrombolysis should be trained in all aspects of the diagnosis and treatment of myocardial infarction. Physicians giving thrombolysis may be cardiologists, internists, emergency physicians, intensivists from a hospital base, or community based general practitioners. In countries that do not have doctors on ambulances, nonphysician personnel giving thrombolysis prehospital may include paramedics and nurses trained in coronary care, but only if appreciable delay will be averted thereby, and then only for cases in whom indications are unequivocal. It is axiomatic — yet still needs to be stressed — that the final responsibility for vicarious judgements on thrombolysis must remain with the physicians responsible for ambulance care, and that all implications be carefully considered in the light of local needs, practice, and sentiment.

According to the extent of their experience and training, qualified physicians do routinely exercise clinical judgement in the many cases of suspected acute myocardial infarction where the diagnosis is uncertain or relative contraindications are present. The existence of conventional protocols for thrombolytic therapy should not necessarily override a physician's decision in these difficult cases. Due allowance must always be made for clinical skills; indeed survival has been shown to be related to the experience of the physician in charge [61]. Nonmedically qualified personnel on the other hand should not carry this responsibility; for them protocols must be rigid enough effectively to replace clinical judgement.

8.5.4. Transporting Patients With Acute Coronary Syndromes to Hospital

Although little documentation exist on the subject, we make the following recommendations for the transport of patients suffering from heart attacks:

Mode of transportation

All patients with chest pain due to a possible heart attack should be treated as stretcher cases. The position on the stretcher should be determined by what is most comfortable for the patient, but we recommend 40° elevation of the head end of the stretcher as a starting point. Peripheral intravenous access should be achieved at the outset.

Speed of transportation

These patients should be transported to hospital as rapidly as prudence permits but haste must not add to discomfort or anxiety levels. All patients given prehospital thrombolysis should be handled very carefully, and it is especially important to protect the head.

Emergency equipment

In addition to appropriate ECG equipment, all emergency ambulances used for transporting patients with acute heart attacks should have a defibrillator (manual or AED) and other conventional resuscitation equipment which must be available and ready for use at all times. The personnel manning the ambulances should be competent in its use. Monitoring of the cardiac rhythm is mandatory but must not replace continuous clinical assessment. Pulse oximetry may give valuable information. Automatic monitoring of blood pressure may also be useful. All emergency ambulances must be equipped with oxygen delivering systems.

Choice of hospitals for heart attack victims

Patients suspected of having a myocardial infarction should be taken to a hospital that is adequately equipped and staffed for diagnosis, monitoring, and reperfusion therapy: it will not necessarily be the nearest. Some consideration has to be given to distance, however, because the time taken before definitive treatment is given should generally not exceed 60 min from the time the ambulance is alerted. If this time is expected to be exceeded, prehospital thrombolysis should be considered (see Section 8.6.2.1).

Report from the ambulance to the receiving hospital

Hospitals should be alerted to the impending arrival of patients with suspected myocardial infarction [63] because of the need to shorten door-to-needle time if thrombolysis has not been given in the prehospital phase or if preparations have to be made for primary angioplasty. Ambulance crews should state the expected time of arrival and also give accurate information on patients' condition including severity of pain, haemodynamic status, cardiac rhythm, and ECG findings.

Staffing of ambulances

All emergency ambulances should be manned by at least two and ideally three persons qualified to carry out the treatment recommendations.

8.5.5. The Hospital Interface for Acute Coronary Syndromes

The hospital interface must ensure continuity between the pre- and in-hospital management of patients with acute coronary syndromes. The in-hospital facilities for patients will usually dictate the nature and site of the interface. By whatever means patients are admitted, all diagnostic information obtained before presentation must be available to the receiving team to avoid unnecessary duplication of investigations and the inherent delay in therapeutic approaches.

Delays in hospital [62]

Door delays. Registration procedures should not impede triage of the patient with suspected acute myocardial infarction. It may be expedited by prior notification of the patient's arrival. Door-

to-needle time may be shortened if i.v. cannulation and recording the ECG have already been carried out, and ECG monitoring electrodes have been attached before the patient reaches hospital but no advantage is gained if door-to-needle time is reduced at a cost of a commensurate increase in patient-to-door time.

DATA DELAYS

A standing order should ensure that if an initial or follow up ECG is required, it can be recorded without individual permission being sought. An electrocardiograph and a competent operator should be available at all times. The result should be drawn to the attention of the physician in charge of the case immediately.

DECISION DELAYS

Protracted delays in reaching a therapeutic decision may occur if the patient's history is atypical, or if the ECG shows nonspecific abnormalities, bundle branch block, or evidence of previous myocardial infarction. Much depends on the experience of the physician. Seeking a second opinion from a cardiologist may cause further delay. Some doubts can be resolved more rapidly by serial ECG recordings. Expert opinion is needed, however, if a choice is to be make between thrombolysis and primary angioplasty.

DRUG DELAYS

Thrombolytic therapy should be stored, prepared, and when appropriate initiated in the emergency department (see below).

The admission of all patients with chest pain directly to a CCU or ICU for evaluation is the preferred option. It is, however, beyond the practical capability of many units. Some patients are assessed in specific chest pain assessment areas, but most hospitals initially receive patients in an ED and subsequently arrange admission and transfer if appropriate. The time difference in achieving reperfusion therapy comparing admission to an ED with direct admission to a CCU/ICU may be as long as 45 min [63], but this is unnecessary and inexcusable. Patients should be moved from the ED to a dedicated cardiac care area within 20 min of arrival unless initiation of thrombolysis or other urgent treatment will be delayed thereby. The diagnostic and therapeutic resources of a CCU or ICU must always be immediately available to ensure smooth and rapid access to whatever procedures are needed and to avoid administrative delays.

All areas receiving patients with acute heart attacks must have a dedicated resuscitation room immediately available, with medical and nursing staff skilled in BLS and ALS. Availability of full resuscitation equipment and immediate defibrillation is mandatory. Appropriate treatment for pain, serious acute complications such as acute heart failure, and life-threatening arrhythmias must be at hand and ready for immediate use. External pacing should be available but the limitations of the technique must be recognised by all with access to it [64].

The potential role of an ED in "protecting" CCU/ICU and in-patient facilities by screening and triaging patients with undiagnosed chest pain must be acknowledged. Over half of all patients presenting to an ED with chest pain may be discharged appropriately [65]. Many inner-city EDs see very large numbers of patients every day with a wide variety of emergency conditions. As a consequence patients requiring specific treatment such as thrombolysis may experience delay [66]. These delays are principally related to the time for triage, for obtaining and correctly interpreting the 12-lead ECG, and for obtaining cardiological or specialist involvement when this is required [34,67]. Where these problems exist, they must be recognised and steps taken to counteract the delays as effectively as possible. Methods must be in place for audit of performance and regular rehearsal sessions.

For patients who do not have the advantage of prehospital thrombolysis, hospital delays may be of crucial importance especially if the interval from onset of symptoms to hospital presentation is short. "Fast tracking" systems can be effective in reducing "door-to-needle time" for patients who can be identified rapidly and unequivocally as being suitable for thrombolysis. These patients will have a clear cut clinical history and ECG changes diagnostic of acute infarction [68]. Selection of suitable patients without contraindications can be made reliably and with acceptable safety without specialist involvement or knowledge using a small set of prepared questions [69]. If immediate transfer to the CCU/ICU is not possible and PTCA is not an option, then thrombolysis can be initiated in the ED by specialist teams or in the absence of contraindications by ED staff working to agreed protocols. Bolus administration of thrombolytic agents can simplify procedures in these situations, but irrespective of the system used, a "door-to-needle time" of less than 30 min is a realistic target. If the average time is longer for patients without important contraindications the system should be examined and improved.

Unfortunately, not all patients with infarction fall into a fast-track category that gives no diagnostic difficulty. Clinical algorithms to improve diagnostic accuracy in doubtful cases have, however, proven unreliable and unwieldy [70–72]. The single most useful screening investigation remains a good quality 12-lead ECG, but its limitations must be recognised. Whilst about 80% of patients with acute infarction have an ECG at presentation that is clearly abnormal [73], in a proportion the changes are subtle and nondiagnostic. Confirmation of the diagnosis may require time, but where suspicion is high, repeat ECGs should be taken at intervals of no more than 10 min for the first 30 min. For the minority of cases in which junior medical staff experience difficulty in the interpretation of an ECG, direct transmission by electronic means for specialist interpretation can help. Fax machines may be useful for this purpose in the absence of a dedicated system [74]. Such measures are appropriate when there is a fear of clinical error; but measures to seek other opinions take time and must be avoided as far as possible.

8.6. TREATMENT OF ACUTE CORONARY SYNDROMES IN THE PREHOSPITAL PHASE

8.6.1. General Measures for Patients Without Overt Complications

8.6.1.1. Pain relief

Pain should be relieved as quickly as possible. This is a priority because pain will increase anxiety and the resulting sympathetic stimulation will aggravate myocardial ischaemia. Pain should therefore be controlled adequately as soon as possible. Opioids such as morphine (or diamorphine where its use is permitted) should be administered intravenously and titrated until pain is adequately relieved. Subcutaneous and intramuscular injections should be avoided. Nitrates and intravenous β blockers that may be given for other reasons can contribute to pain relief by improving the underlying ischaemia. Anxiolytics – in particular benzodiazepines – may be given if anxiety is perceived as a major component of the patient's distress, although in most cases the euphoriant effect of an opioid will make this unnecessary.

8.6.1.2. Treatment of early nausea, vomiting, hypotension, and bradycardia

These common features of the initial phase of acute heart attacks may be due to excess vagal tone and/or the side effects of analgesics, nitrates, and β-blockers. Antiemetic drugs such as metoclopramide may be used to counter nausea and vomiting. Bradycardia (with or without hypotension) despite the relief of pain and nausea may be improved by the administration of atropine. Persisting hypotension is likely to reflect severe myocardial damage (see 8.6.3.3).

8.6.1.3. Aspirin administration

Aspirin significantly improves the prognosis of patients with suspected acute myocardial infarction or unstable angina [75]. The efficacy of aspirin in reducing cardiovascular death seems to be similar in patients treated early and late [76]. Thus aspirin (150 to 300 mg, preferably) should be given to all patients with acute coronary syndromes in the absence of clear contraindications irrespective of the delay between presumed onset of symptoms and first evaluation. Since antiplatelet activity may be obtained within 30 min [77] antithrombotic protection should not be delayed until arrival in hospital. Aspirin is simple to administer, it does not require specific monitoring, and as a single dose it is well tolerated. The additive effect of aspirin and fibrinolytics on cardiovascular mortality and the preventive effect of aspirin on the "excess" of recurrence of myocardial infarction with thrombolysis was observed when aspirin was given immediately before the infusion of fibrinolytic agents [76]. If fibrinolytic therapy is given in the prehospital phase aspirin should be administered concomitantly to help prevent early reocclusions.

8.6.1.4. Heparin administration

Before the widespread use of fibrinolytics and aspirin, heparin was the reference antithrombotic treatment for the acute phase of myocardial infarction. A meta-analysis [78] reviewed the results of studies comparing heparin with control. In the absence of aspirin, results in favour of heparin were observed with respect to mortality, stroke, pulmonary embolism, and reinfarction. But the review of those trials in which heparin was evaluated in the presence of aspirin showed at best a modest effect for these endpoints with no benefit on stroke. Moreover, the risk of major bleeding was significantly increased by 50%. Heparin as an adjunctive treatment to streptokinase and aspirin has not been shown to improve mortality in two large trials but it did increase the risk of bleeding [79,80]. Urokinase, tPA, and rPA are more effective in the presence of heparin which is usually recommended as an adjuvant for these agents, but at present no convincing evidence exists for starting heparin in the prehospital phase even when fibrinolytics are prescribed, and caution is advised unless or until any added risk of intracerebral bleeding has been quantified.

8.6.1.5. Prehospital β-blockade

The efficacy of β-blocking agents in preventing death and reinfarction after myocardial infarction is well-established. Many trials and meta-analyses [81–84] have assessed the value of starting intravenous β-blockade early after the onset of symptoms. A meta-analysis of the trials available to early 1985 [84] showed a 13% reduction in total short term mortality ($p < 0.02$), a 20% reduction in reinfarction ($p < 0.02$), and a 15% reduction in ventricular fibrillation or cardiac arrest ($p < 0.05$) and the two subsequent large trials [81,82] were consistent with this evidence. In addition, intravenous β-blockade reduces ischaemic pain and tachyarrhythmias. Despite these results, experience of β-blockade in the early phase of myocardial infarction is limited. No evidence of a mortality benefit from early β-blockade as compared with delayed β-blockade was seen in one randomised trial [85], but the study was not powered for showing differences in mortality. A significant reduction in reinfarction was observed, however. In general, use of the drugs with thrombolytics seems to be safe, and it is also feasible in the prehospital context [86]. They may be considered for tachyarrhythmia or hypertension and as adjunctive therapy for pain relief. For routine use, however, the balance between potential benefit and possible side effects such as hypotension and bradycardia in patients who are also receiving fibrinolytics and/or nitrates should be considered very carefully. The task force consider there is no strong indication for systematic use of β-blockade before hospital admission.

8.6.1.6. Prophylactic use of oral or intravenous nitrates

More than 80,000 patients with acute myocardial infarction have been involved in 22 studies comparing early intravenous or oral nitrates with control groups. Two large studies, GISSI-3 [87] and ISIS 4 [88], contributed most of the patients and reported no mortality benefit. A meta-analysis [88] showed only a 5.5% reduction of mortality (p = 0.03). This translates into a saving of 3.8 deaths per 1,000 treated. Whether this benefit is sufficient to justify routine use of nitrates is debatable, particularly with the added uncertainties of the prehospital phase. Nitrates may be deleterious in cases of right ventricular ischaemia or infarction which may complicate inferior left ventricular changes [89]. Persistent pain or the presence of heart failure may of course be valid indications for their use for patients with these specific conditions, but they are not at present recommended for routine administration.

8.6.1.7. Prophylactic use of ACE inhibitors

Long-term use of ACE inhibitors started a few days after myocardial infarction has been established as an effective treatment to reduce mortality and reinfarction in patients with clinical signs of heart failure or with an impaired ejection fraction [90]. Early treatment with ACE inhibitors is considered relatively safe [91] although it increases the risk of hypotension, cardiogenic shock, and renal dysfunction [88]. Because of these side effects and of the lack of information on the early prehospital phase, the Task Force members cannot recommend the prophylactic prehospital use of ACE inhibitors.

8.6.1.8. Prophylactic use of antiarrhythmic therapy

Lidocaine has been advocated to prevent ventricular fibrillation in patients with acute myocardial infarction. Several studies have been performed to test the efficacy of prophylactic lidocaine for this indication. Meta-analyses [92–94] have shown a reduction of approximately 35% in the incidence of ventricular fibrillation but also a nonsignificant trend to an increase in mortality. Studies restricted to the prehospital phase have included data on 7,386 patients, but these have not provided any evidence for a reduction in mortality as a result of prophylactic antiarrhythmic therapy. One important point must be made. Under the conditions of the trials, defibrillation was immediately available so that the reduction in the incidence of ventricular fibrillation would not have been expected to have been translated into a mortality benefit. Ventricular fibrillation that was not associated with lethal haemodynamic compromise should have been promptly reversed. No advantage could therefore be gained to balance any deleterious drug effects. This would not always be so in the prehospital phase: we have, however, no direct evidence of the benefit of prophylactic lidocaine when defibrillation is not an immediate therapeutic option. With current knowledge routine use of lidocaine or other prophylactic anti-arrhythmics in the prehospital phase cannot be recommended.

8.6.2. Reperfusion Therapy

8.6.2.1. Thrombolysis

Thrombolytic therapy is beneficial by restoring patency of the infarct-related artery and improving the remodelling process, but the clinical benefit depends largely on how quickly and completely reperfusion is achieved.

Hospital trials

The Fibrinolytic Therapy Trialists' (FTT) Colla-

borative Group has reported an overview of nine randomised trials each of at least 1,000 patients with suspected acute myocardial infarction in which fibrinolytic therapy has been compared with control or placebo [95]. For patients presenting with ST elevation or bundle branch block the mortality benefit was 30/1,000 for those randomised 0–6 h, and 20/1,000 for those randomised 7–12 h from onset. This treatment has been widely assimilated into hospital practice and its use over the past decade has been associated with a fall in hospital mortality [6]. The FTT overview, while confirming that earlier treatment is associated with greater benefit, suggested that the benefit of reducing delays to thrombolysis is relatively modest. The relationship between absolute mortality reduction and time of randomisation was represented by a straight line with a negative slope of 1.6/1,000/h and an intercept of 35/1,000. The complex relationship between mortality reduction and time of administration of thrombolytic therapy may not, however, be represented accurately by a straight line [96]. A meta-analysis of 22 randomised trials of thrombolytic therapy with more than 100 patients has shown that a nonlinear benefit/time regression line provides the best fit to the data (Fig. 2) [13]. The beginning of the benefit/time regres-

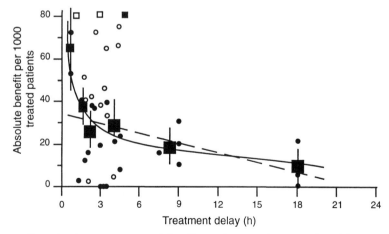

FIG. 2. Absolute 35-day mortality reduction vs. treatment delay. Regression equation reproduced from Boersma et al. [13]. The linear regression line (dotted) and nonlinear (continuous) regression line are fitted to the data. The nonlinear line provides the best fit. Small closed dots: information from trials included in FTT analysis. Open dots: information from additional trials. Small squares: data beyond scale of x\y cross. Black squares: average effects in six time-to-treatment groups.

sion line is very steep, but there is a marked inflection at about 2 h. Both of these results were drawn from a post hoc analysis of nonrandomised groups with different characteristics (e.g., age and severity of symptoms) and a reliable estimate of benefit as a function of delay cannot be established by this means. But there is no doubt that to reap the full benefit of thrombolytic therapy it has to be given as early as possible, i.e., at the first opportunity in the community.

Prehospital trials

Retrospective analyses of placebo controlled trials of thrombolytic therapy given in hospital cannot tell us by how much the mortality rate would have been reduced had the same patients been given the treatment earlier. Neither can the additional benefit of prehospital thrombolysis be inferred from the gradient of the graph shown in Fig. 2. The benefit of earlier thrombolysis can be quantified only with a trial design in which patients are randomly allocated to receive thrombolytic therapy either on presentation in the community or alternatively after admission to hospital. The three largest randomised trials comparing prehospital with hospital thrombolysis are EMIP [57] (*n* = 5469), MITI [97] (*n* = 360), and GREAT [56] (*n* = 311). It should be noted that EMIP was terminated prematurely because of lack of funds, and neither MITI nor GREAT were designed as trials with a mortality endpoint. None of the trials of prehospital thrombolysis has individually shown a statistically significant mortality difference at one month by intention to treat analysis, but as well as being small there are practical and ethical constraints on the design and conduct of such trials which reduce their ability to achieve a statistically significant result. A meta-analysis of the three major prehospital trials with additional data from five smaller ones has, however, shown a significant mortality reduction with prehospital compared with hospital thrombolysis (*p* = 0.002), with a benefit/time gradient at 35 days of 21($\pm$SE 6)/1,000/h [13]. This is the best available estimate we have of the

magnitude of the benefit of earlier thrombolysis, being derived from intention-to-treat analyses of appropriately designed trials. Early mortality is not the only consideration. Myocardial salvage and an important effect on remodelling may also reduce the tendency to subsequent heart failure. Follow-up of GREAT showed substantial deferred mortality benefit additional to that seen within the 1st month [98] whereas in MITI [99] prehospital thrombolysis showed no further influence on long-term mortality. With or without late benefit, the evidence from randomised clinical trials of prehospital thrombolysis is fully consistent with the large body of theoretical, experimental, and clinical evidence in favour of early thrombolysis.

Implications of the benefit/time gradient of thrombolysis

In terms of its potential for saving life, initiating thrombolytic therapy is as urgent as the treatment of cardiac arrest [100]. Although time is more critical in the latter situation, similar mortality benefits may be expected if both strategies were optimised. As a general policy, treatment should be initiated on site if practicable, and by the first qualified person to see the patient. Thus, thrombolytic treatment should be given ideally in the prehospital phase. Where ambulance staffing arrangements have made this policy difficult to implement (e.g., in countries that do not regularly have doctors in ambulances) strategies should be sought urgently that will allow prehospital thrombolysis if the combined journey time and in-hospital delay is more than 60 min, or if the journey time is 30 min or more. In the latter case the overall time saving will usually be in excess of an hour because in-hospital delay, seldom less than 30 min, is also obviated. If thrombolytic therapy is not given prehospital, the goal should be to reperfuse the occluded artery as quickly as possible in hospital. In the absence of contraindications, any delay to the start of definitive therapy of more than 30 min calls for a critical examination of the system.

Choice of thrombolytic agent for use prehospital

Where prehospital thrombolysis is provided by hospital physicians travelling into the community in a mobile coronary care unit, the same drugs may be used as are given in hospital. The medical staff will have daily familiarity with their doses and administration. But where domiciliary thrombolysis is to be provided by general practitioners, each using this treatment only 3—4 times a year, convenience of administration and storage are important. For most general practitioners, the need for thrombolytic agents or heparin to be administered by slow infusion precludes their use in the community, and one of the agents that can be given by bolus injection deserve consideration.

8.6.2.2. Primary angioplasty

Coronary flow is restored only after a delay following the administration of thrombolytic therapy, and in a substantial minority of patients flow may not be restored at all. Delays in achieving coronary reperfusion following drug therapy may be circumvented by the use of primary angioplasty, which may also be used for patients in whom thrombolytic therapy is contraindicated. Primary angioplasty yields higher coronary patency rates than thrombolytic therapy, and full patency is achieved immediately the angioplasty balloon is deflated following successful dilatation. But primary angioplasty is clearly a hospital procedure, and there is an unavoidable preliminary "door-to-balloon" time. Clinical trials comparing primary angioplasty with hospital thrombolysis are encouraging [101], but the full benefits of angioplasty may not be well-sustained [102]. To date, the only available evidence comparing prehospital thrombolysis with primary angioplasty has not shown any advantage with the interventionalist strategy [103] and there are no randomised trials. Early "rescue" angioplasty has a role where reperfusion by thrombolysis has failed, [104] but is often unsuccessful [105]. In localities where both prehospital thrombolysis and angioplasty are available,

local policies for the early management of patients with acute myocardial infarction should be followed.

8.6.3. Management of Complications of Acute Coronary Syndromes

8.6.3.1. Arrhythmias

Sustained arrhythmias occurring in the context of a myocardial infarction may have immediate or longer term prognostic implications. Not only should immediate treatment be considered, but adequate documentation should be achieved whenever it is possible to do so. Therefore a full 12-lead ECG should be recorded if facilities are available and if delay caused by registration will not compromise the safety of the patient. The European Resuscitation Council, after consultation with the European Society of Cardiology, has produced guidelines for the treatment of peri-arrest arrhythmias [106,107] that are potentially malignant but have not caused clinical circulatory arrest. The guidelines are presented as three algorithms: for bradyarrhythmias, for broad complex tachycardias which can be equated under emergency conditions to ventricular tachycardia unless there is good evidence to the contrary, and to narrow complex tachycardia which can be equated with supraventricular tachycardia including atrial fibrillation (Fig. 3). These guidelines are not intended to override expert assessment of situations that may be complex, but provide advice applicable for most situations.

Bradyarrhythmias

Generally the same principles apply for sinus bradycardia and for atrioventricular block. If a recognisable prelude to asystole is present (such as Mobitz II A-V block, complete heart block with a wide QRS complex, or pauses of longer than 3 s) transvenous pacing is indicated. This is unlikely to be available in the prehospital phase but the perceived need may hasten hospital admission and lead meanwhile to the consideration of the use of atropine, chronotropic catecholamines, or

EMERGENCY TREATMENT

PERIARREST ARRYTHMIAS
If not already done, give oxygen and establish i.v. access

Doses based on adult of average body weight

BRADYCARDIA

Risk of asystole ?
- History of asystole
- Mobitz II AV block
- Any pause ≥ 3 s
- Complete heart block, wide QRS

Yes → Atropine i.v. 500 μg initially to max. 3 mg and

Seek expert help

Transvenous pacing

Consider as interim measures
- External pacing
- i.v. isoprenaline or orciprenaline

No

Adverse signs?
- Clinical evidence of low cardiac output
- Hypotension: Systolic AP ≤ 90 mmHg
- Heart failure
- Rate < 40 beat min⁻¹
- Presence of ventricular arrhythmias requiring suppression

Yes → Atropine i.v. 500 μg initially to max. 3 mg → Seek expert help

Satisfactory response ?

No → Seek expert help

Yes

No

Observe

BROAD COMPLEX TACHYCARDIA
(Sustained ventricular tachycardia)

Pulse ? No → Use VF protocol

Yes

Adverse signs ?
- Systolic AP ≤ 90 mm Hg
- Chest pain
- Heart failure
- Rate ≥ 150 beat min⁻¹

Yes → Seek expert help

Sedation
Synchronized DC shock
100 J: 200 J: 360 J

Start
- Lignocaine +/–
- Magnesium and potassium *as opposite*

Further cardioversion as necessary

For refractory cases consider other pharmacological agents: amiodarone, procainamide, flecainide or bretylium; or overdrive pacing.

No →

If potassium known to be low
- Give potassium chloride up to 60 mmol, max. rate 30 mmol h⁻¹
- Give magnesium sulphate i.v. 10 ml 50% in 1 h

- Lignocaine i.v. 50 mg over 2 min repeated every 5 min to total dose of 200 mg
- Start infusion 2 mg min⁻¹ after first bolus dose

Seek expert help

Sedation
Synchronized DC shock
100 J: 200 J: 360 J

Amiodarone 300 mg over 5–15 min preferably by central line, then 300 mg over 1 h

---

NARROW COMPLEX TACHYCARDIA
(Supraventricular tachycardia)

Vagal manoeuvres (caution possible digitalis toxicity, acute ischaemia or presence of carotid bruit)

Adenosine 3 mg by bolus injection repeat if necessary every 1–2 min using 6 mg then 12 mg then 12 mg (ATP is an alternative)

Atrial fibrillation (more than 130 beat min⁻¹)

Seek expert help

Adverse signs ?
- Hypotension: Systolic AP ≤ 90 mmHg
- Chest pain
- Heart failure
- Impaired consciousness
- Rate ≥ 200 beat min⁻¹

Yes → Sedation

Synchronized cardioversion
100 J: 200 J: 360 J

Amiodarone 300 mg over 15 min then 300 mg over 1 h if necessary, preferably by central line and repeat cardioversion.

No → Choose from:
- Esmolol: 40 mg over 1 min + infusion 4 mg min⁻¹ (i.v. injection can be repeated with increments of infusion to 12 mg min⁻¹)
- Digoxin: max. dose 500 μg over 30 min × 2
- Verapamil 5–10 mg i.v.
- Amiodarone 300 mg over 1 h, may be repeated once if necessary
- Overdrive pacing (not AF)

FIG. 3. The ERC algorithm for the treatment of periarrest arrythmias updated in 1998 [108,109].

external pacing if this is available. In the absence of any immediate threat of asystole, a heart rate that is unacceptably slow in absolute terms or too slow for the haemodynamic state of the patient (which may occur either as a complication of the infarction or as a side effect of drug treatment) will usually respond to atropine in a dose of 500 µg to 3 mg. Sinus bradycardia or A-V nodal block complicating inferior myocardial infarction may best be left untreated if well tolerated, and may even be advantageous in terms of tolerance to myocardial ischaemia. Bradycardia in the acute phase of chest pain may also respond to effective analgesia which can counteract excess vagal tone.

Broad complex tachycardias

Single premature ventricular beats generally require no treatment. Some prolonged or complex arrhythmias such as couplets, or runs of ventricular beats at a relatively slow rate are usually well tolerated and likewise do not require treatment. But if arrhythmias are severe enough to cause or exacerbate pain, hypotension, or heart failure, or are judged to be a possible prelude to ventricular fibrillation, they should be treated initially with lidocaine using an intravenous dose of 50 mg over 2 min repeated to a total dose of 200 mg. One important point should be made: complex ventricular arrhythmias complicating bradycardia should be treated by measures – such as atropine – designed to increase the basic rate, and not by antiarrhythmics. Suitable second line antiarrhythmics of class I or III depend in part on local availability and custom. Repeated administration of one or several antiarrhythmics should, however, be avoided as far as possible to avoid uncontrollable (and unforeseeable) unwanted effects such as depression of the myocardium or conducting system. Where several doses are needed, drugs with a short half-life such as lidocaine or ajmaline may involve less hazard. Cardioversion in the absence of circulatory arrest is rarely indicated in the prehospital phase but severe haemodynamic compromise from rapid ventricular tachycardia

should be treated by prompt electrical cardioversion after appropriate sedation.

Narrow complex tachycardia

Patients with well-tolerated sinus tachycardia and normal or high blood pressure may not require specific treatment in the prehospital phase though β blockers should be considered (see Section 8.6.1.5.). Continuing pain or early heart failure must be excluded as a cause of sinus tachycardia. The most common narrow complex tachyarrhythmia after infarction is atrial fibrillation. Urgent cardioversion is indicated In the presence of severe haemodynamic compromise and a heart rate exceeding about 130/min. In other cases, intravenous β blockade (preferably with a short acting agent such as esmolol) may be useful. Diltiazem or amiodarone also have a role, but caution is needed in the presence of hypotension. Intravenous digoxin is likely to act too slowly to be appropriate in the prehospital phase. Paroxysmal supraventricular tachycardia is unusual as a complication of acute myocardial ischaemia, but if necessary adenosine as a bolus dose of 6 to 12 mg may be tried. Verapamil, diltiazem, or β blockers are second line options.

8.6.3.2. Acute heart failure

All patients with left ventricular failure should receive oxygen by mask or intranasally. In these patients the following treatments can be considered either separately or in combination depending on the response of symptoms: diuretics such as intravenous furosemide, intravenous glyceryl trinitrate or isosorbide dinitrate [108], or oral nitrates at doses sufficiently high to produce a vasodilating effect. These treatments may induce or potentiate hypotension and should be titrated accordingly. This is especially true for patients with higher degree AV block and/or right ventricular infarction. In refractory pulmonary oedema intubation and respirator treatment with positive end-expiratory airway pressure may be life-saving.

8.6.3.3. Cardiogenic shock

True cardiogenic shock should not be diagnosed until any important brady- or tachyarrhythmias or hypovolaemia that might be contributing to hypotension have been treated effectively. In patients with cardiogenic shock due to right ventricular infarction, volume augmentation is indicated using a test infusion limited to 200 ml of colloid. For other causes of cardiogenic shock, dopamine (2.5–5 µg/kg/min) or dobutamine (4–20 µg/kg/min) may be used alone or in combination with norepinephrine/noradrenaline (0.5–20 µg/min) or epinephrine/adrenaline (0.5–20 µg/min). (Note that the doses of epinephrine/adrenaline and norepinephrine/noradrenaline are not quoted in relation to body weight.) Dopamine in higher doses transiently increases blood pressure at the cost of a rise in left atrial pressure and a fall in cardiac output [109].

8.6.4. Cardiac arrest

Most cardiac arrests occur in the home with a relative within sight or sound. Rehabilitation programs, sports groups for coronary patients, and self-help groups can help to train the families of heart attack victims who are at risk of further episodes, but motivation is often lacking. The partners of patients affected are often elderly, a group which is least likely to accept training [110]. Younger individuals, athletes, students, and members of organized groups are much more willing to learn BLS techniques. The focus for offering training should therefore be directed to schools and other learning facilities, sports clubs, companies, or specific occupational groups, such as policemen, railway personnel, and public service drivers. Transport workers have a higher probability than most of witnessing a cardiac emergency. A "cascade" principle will help those with most aptitude become trainers and instruct an appreciable proportion of the population. In some countries a first-aid course with BLS training is required for obtaining a driver's license, a practice strongly recommended.

Guidelines for BLS have been published by the major resuscitation councils including the ERC [111]. A central problem in the performance of BLS is the aesthetic acceptability of mouth-to-mouth ventilation. The perception of risk of infection poses another barrier to acceptability. Until recently, the only other option was the mouth-to-nose method, which has similar aesthetic problems. BLS courses participants should be informed that the cardiac arrests they are most likely to witness will be in a close relative within the home. Mouth-to-mouth ventilation would almost always be acceptable in such cases.

Mouth-to-mouth ventilation is "unphysiological" since the victim is ventilated with a hypoxic/hypercarbic gas mixture [112]. In addition it is often performed badly [113] but even then it may not be fruitless [43]. Sudden cardiac arrest is initiated by malignant ventricular arrhythmias in 80–90% of patients. In such cases there will be residual oxygen in the lungs and arterial system: a circulation may then help to support life for several critical minutes. Thus chest compression alone may increase the chance of survival even if ventilation is not performed. Animal experiments support this concept [114]. Without losing sight of the goal of optimum resuscitation [115], it should be made clear in BLS teaching that even incomplete measures can contribute to the patient's survival chances [115]. This may be of special importance in communities where there is reluctance to use mouth-to-mouth ventilation because of the risk of infection [116,117].

In some cases, the patient requires not only BLS and early defibrillation but also additional measures summarized under the term advanced life support (ALS). Standard guidelines on ALS have been set up and published by the ERC the AHA and other resuscitation councils (Fig. 4) [118]. There are four major components as follows:

8.6.4.1. Defibrillation

Defibrillation is the single most important intervention producing a successful outcome from sudden cardiac arrest. There are few studies on the optimal energies or waveform to use

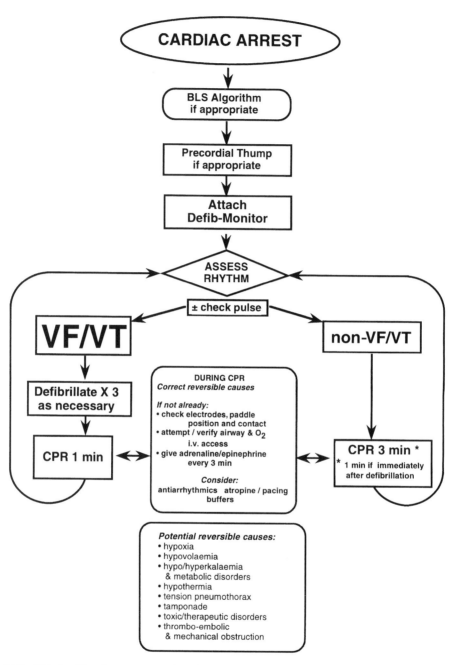

FIG. 4. The 1998 ERC algorithm for treatment of cardiac arrest [120].

[119,120]. Current recommendations are for DC shocks with a conventional damped sinusoidal waveform to be given with energies of 200 J for the first two shocks, and further ones at 360 J [118]. Emphasis on correct technique during defibrillation is crucial to maximise the chances of success [121]. Preliminary investigations with other waveforms such as biphasic rectangular and

sinusoidal shocks have shown similar results with lower energies [122]. They offer potential advantages including reducing the myocardial injury produced by a defibrillating shock and the development of smaller, lighter, and less expensive defibrillators [123], and will be acceptable for routine use if shown to be of equal or greater efficacy and safety compared with conventional shocks. Automated external defibrillators (AEDs) enable less qualified persons in multitiered rescue systems to perform defibrillation [48,124] (see section 6.4.5).

8.6.4.2. Airway management

The primary function of simple adjuncts in mouth-to-mouth ventilation is as a hygienic barrier. Complete protection from infection cannot be achieved with cloths and filters. Ventilation masks provide more effective protection but may require a second helper and therefore have only limited applicability. The basic ALS adjunct is a ventilation mask connected to a self-inflating bag with an external oxygen source. It does not protect against aspiration and makes the use of positive end-expiratory pressure (PEEP) impossible. A cuffed tracheal tube is the "gold standard" for airway protection, but requires considerable expertise and regular practice in the technique [125]. The laryngeal mask, oesophageal obturator airway, and the "Combitube" are second-line alternatives [125].

8.6.4.3. Drug therapy and delivery

The optimal route of drug delivery in cardiac arrest is pervenous. Central venous access provides the most efficient and rapid access to the circulation, but the technique is time consuming and necessitates considerable expertise and has potentially fatal hazards in relation to puncture of a noncompressible artery (a particular problem if thrombolysis may be needed subsequently) [126]. The peripheral route is usually easier, but drug delivery to the central circulation is slow; the tracheal route is a second line choice, because of impaired absorption and unpredict-able pharmacodynamics [126,127]. The drugs which can be administered by this route are limited to lidocaine, epinephrine/adrenaline, and atropine; they should be diluted in 10 ml of saline or Ringer's solution to hasten absorption.

Epinephrine/adrenaline remains the most commonly used drug in CPR. It is given in a dose of 1 mg i.v. for asystole or EMD, and after three DC shocks have been unsuccessful in terminating VF. Further doses are given at up to 3-min intervals. High dose adrenaline has not been shown to improve overall survival [128]. Recent studies suggest that other vasopressors such as vasopressin might have comparable or even more beneficial effects [129,130] but so far there is inadequate information on clinical effects and outcome.

Buffer therapy is no longer a primary component of drug therapy in resuscitation. The most widely used agent is sodium bicarbonate, and it is suggested that its use in judicious amounts (50 ml of 8.4% solution) is limited to situations of severe acidosis (arterial pH < 7.1 and base deficit > -10) [131]. Further doses should be administered under guidance of repeated arterial blood gas analysis.

Atropine is recommended for asystole, using a single intravenous 3-mg dose [107], although clear evidence of efficacy is limited. For VF persisting after $6-12$ shocks, an antiarrhythmic agent may be considered: the ERC guidelines suggest an i.v. bolus of 100 mg lidocaine [118]. Patients developing VF during acute myocardial infarction may have low plasma concentrations of potassium and magnesium. It has been assumed that magnesium supplements may be useful in the treatment and prophylaxis of resistant VF, but this has not been confirmed [88]. Magnesium is, however, highly effective in treating torsades de pointes [132]. A long QT syndrome or an iatrogenic effect of antiarrhythmic drugs is often the underlying cause of this specific arrhythmic morphology. β Blockers have been recommended in therapy-resistant malignant arrhythmias [133]. Their efficacy in the acute and convalescent phases after infarction is clear, but their effectiveness in cardiopulmonary resuscitation has not been confirmed.

The brain is the organ most sensitive to cardiac arrest and deterioration of cerebral blood flow and oxygenation. Even after restoration of circulation the processes of vascular dysfunction and inadequate regional blood flow may lead to continued damage, with leucocytes playing a prominent role in the "no-reflow" phenomenon [134]. Calcium flux changes are also believed to be important in the process of neuronal damage: they induce a cascade of deleterious biochemical processes [135]. Neither calcium antagonists, nor any other agents, have been shown to exhibit beneficial effects on outcomes [136]. These aspects reinforce the need to optimize the basic aspects of post resuscitation care with the maintenance of normal cerebral and myocardial perfusion and oxygenation and blood chemistry.

8.6.4.4. Mechanical resuscitation measures

Within limits, higher frequencies of chest compression increase cardiac output and coronary blood flow. Disadvantages are that the rescuer becomes exhausted more rapidly and a greater risk of injury to the patient [137]. The recommended chest compression frequency is 100/min [111]. Other techniques such as interposed abdominal compression, active compression/decompression (ACD), a combination of both techniques (Lifestick), and vest CPR have been shown to improve various haemodynamic aspects of CPR, but no study has shown evidence for an improved eventual outcome. Among monitoring aids, end-tidal CO_2 measuring devices are the most valuable. End-tidal CO_2 measurement during CPR provides a measure of cardiac output and is useful in quantifying the efficacy of mechanical resuscitation measures and providing a prognostic role [138].

8.6.4.5. Ethics of prehospital resuscitation from cardiac arrest

The moral aspects of any medical intervention can be defined according to the following principles [139,140]:

- The principle of beneficence – to do net good.
- The principle of nonmaleficence – to do no harm.
- The principle of respect for the patient's autonomy.
- The principle of justice.

The principles of beneficence and nonmaleficence can be considered together in this instance. CPR should in general be used only if it has a some chance of producing net benefit for the patient or victim. CPR is not harmless – it can be a violent, damaging, painful, alarming, and an undignified intervention. In situations where CPR is deemed to be futile, or if a patient has expressed an informed wish not to have CPR resuscitation, it should not be attempted. This information is, however, only exceptionally available outside the hospital.

The basis for do not attempt resuscitate (DNAR) orders falls into three categories [141,142]:

- CPR cannot be successful.
- The quality of life after CPR is likely to be poor.
- The patients informed and expressed wishes.

Where resuscitation is not appropriate, calls to the emergency services may not be made. But in any case, decisions should ideally take into consideration advice from relatives or friends: this may be possible even in the prehospital phase, because the majority of collapses occur in the patients home with relatives or carers close-by. If the patient was known to have expressed a view before his collapse with respect to resuscitation, this should weigh heavily on the doctor's decision though such advance directives are not always made in the light of real knowledge. In the absence of relevant information resuscitation should proceed.

Once resuscitation has been started, it should be discontinued only for well-defined reasons [118]. New information may become available on the approximate duration of cardiac arrest or on underlying disease and its prognosis. In the absence of definite indications for cessation, attempt at resuscitation should continue as long as the waveform of ventricular fibrillation is present. Nevertheless, asystole which has lasted for 15 min or more is evidence of futility. Exceptions to this advice relate to the special situations of children, drowning, hypothermia, and drug intoxication.

8.6.5. Psychological Aspects of Prehospital Care

The need for psychological support for a victim of a heart attack is clear. The topic, however, has been poorly assessed in guidelines and textbooks, whilst physicians and nurses who are overloaded by the need for giving clinical care tend to neglect this essential facet. Every individual needs to feel secure. This need is undermined by any illness that is perceived as posing a major threat. Although the chest pain of a coronary heart attack may not be severe, it is usually identified correctly as being of cardiac origin [143] whether or not the victim is prepared to accept this recognition to the extend of calling for aid. Once help is available the patient is moved into an unfamiliar vehicle, then into an often overcrowded and fraught emergency department, followed by a unit characterised by intimidating high technology. Many procedures follow, executed by a succession of strangers working in an atmosphere of extreme urgency. All of this poses a considerable psychological challenge and leaves little time for adequate communication [144–146]. Relatives or other bystanders also need support, particularly if they were involved in a resuscitation attempt, whether or not this was successful.

Consequences of psychological stress

The uncertainty, fear, anxiety, and stress felt by the patient are unpleasant experiences and likely to be an adverse factor in the evolution of myocardial ischaemia. Heightened sympathetic activity may induce changes in heart rate, arterial pressure, and myocardial oxygen consumption that may be equivalent to reasonably strenuous physical exertion. In addition there may be adverse changes in coronary vascular resistance particularly in atherosclerotic segments, increases

in platelet aggregation, and antifibrinolytic factors that can all interfere with coronary flow. It is axiomatic that the management of anxiety and stress should play an important part in the treatment of acute ischaemic attacks.

Pharmacological approach

Drugs such as opioids and benzodiazepines play an important role in the relief of anxiety. Opioids themselves may suffice, but anxiety can often outlive pain: for some cases therefore, anxiolytic agents may be needed when indications for opioids are no longer present.

Psychological support

This should be provided continually using plain language that can be understood by the patient, given that their mental state may be obtunded by illness and drugs. "There is perhaps no other situation in medicine in which the words of a physician bear as much potential for good or evil as in the management of myocardial infarction" [147]. Psychological support is required throughout the illness and into the convalescent phase, but this should be started at the earliest opportunity. Ideally patients should be told in advance of what is in store for them: a description of a coronary care unit can mitigate the anxiety of the patients first experience.

The rights of the patients

Patients have a right to be kept well informed. They should understand the origins of their illness and what is being done to help. The hospital mortality of acute ischaemic syndromes is now low enough to permit an optimistic appraisal, and clearly emphasis on a good prognosis is more helpful than undue discussion on risk. Whilst truth should never be compromised, the wise physician will couch it in terms that are likely to be acceptable to the patient. Optimism can also be boosted by discussions about the future, including early plans for rehabilitation and return to work.

Consent for standard therapy

Many have suggested the need to discuss with patients the risks of fibrinolytic therapy. Whilst different European countries might vary in convention and legal requirement, the point should be made that full information presented thoughtlessly may well frighten the patient and thereby increase risk: this must be a questionable procedure in terms of good medical practice and ethics. It should be sufficient to explain to a patient (who will be anxious or under the influence of sedation or both) that the treatment to be given will improve the chances of a good recovery. In this particular emergency situation full information may protect the doctor but not the patient. In this case appropriate partial disclosure should be supported universally by informed medical opinion.

8.7. PRINCIPAL RECOMMENDATIONS

Large differences exist between and also within countries with regard to access to care for victims of acute cardiac emergencies. The arrangements for the prehospital management of heart attack victims also varies greatly between countries. The preferred option of doctors on emergency ambulances is not a practical possibility within the foreseeable future in some European countries, but the principles of triage and arrangements for care are similar for all systems. We recommend minimum requirements for the organisation and implementation of emergency care that should exist in all European countries now ("basic") and also for more advanced strategies that should be adopted when it is practicable to do so ("optimal"). We also give a step-by-step guide to prehospital management of acute heart attacks.

Access to Care

Public education

*   Basic: Widespread knowledge of symptoms of acute heart attack.

*   Basic: Access to a central emergency number and free calls to an ambulance dispatching centre.
*   Optimal: Public media campaigns to teach symptoms of heart attacks, how to respond, and the reasons for community involvement.
*   Optimal: Community wide knowledge of and training in Basic Life Support.
*   Optimal: Use of the agreed common European emergency number (112) more widely implemented.

Ambulance dispatch

*   Basic: Strategic positioning of ambulances in order to minimise ambulance delay.
*   Basic: Trained dispatchers using priority based systems.
*   Optimal: Dispatch controlled by physicians.
*   Optimal: Telephone assisted CPR.

Prehospital resuscitation for cardiac arrest

*   Optimal: Early defibrillation by introduction of semiautomated defibrillators activated by trained disciplined groups, following ERC guidelines.
*   Basic: All emergency ambulances with defibrillators and ECG monitors and operators competent in their use.
*   Basic: All emergency ambulances with the means of delivering high concentrations of oxygen.
*   Basic: Licence for ambulance personnel to perform basic life support and defibrillation according to ERC guidelines.

Prehospital triage and arrangements for care for acute coronary syndromes

*   Basic: Ambulances staffed by at least two and preferably three people qualified to carry out all appropriate recommendations.
*   Optimal: All emergency ambulances equipped to record an ECG with staff trained in its use. Interpretation immediately available by a phy-

sician on the ambulance, by appropriately trained nurses or paramedics in countries without ambulance physicians, by a computerised ECG algorithm, or by use of telephone or radio transmission.

* Optimal: Prehospital administration of thrombolysis by physicians especially when the time saved is likely to be more than 60 min (strongly recommended).
* Optimal: Consideration of prehospital initiation of thrombolytic therapy by medically trained and certified non physician personnel if any other strategy leads to considerable delays. Any such system must be under strict medical control, use stringent inclusion and exclusion criteria, and should be subject to continuing medical audit.
* Basic: Hospitals should be notified of the impending arrival of possible heart attack victims to facilitate immediate continuity of care.
* Optimal: Direct admission to CCU or appropriate dedicated area for immediate reperfusion therapy, based on advanced information from ambulance (preferred option for in-hospital treatment).
* Basic: Registration procedures for heart attack victims should not impede triage nor delay urgent treatment.

Early in-hospital management

* Basic: Triaged admission to Emergency Department if direct transfer to CCU or other dedicated area not possible.
* Basic: Electrocardiography must be immediately available in all Emergency Departments with operators skilled in their use.
* Basic: Suitability for thrombolysis to be assessed by first receiving physician without routine doctor-to-doctor referral.
* Basic: Thrombolysis not delayed by transfer of patients to CCU. Those not treated prehospital and not admitted directly to CCU should have treatment initiated in the Emergency Department using a fast-track system for those without contraindications and having immediate advice available for those with uncertain indi-

cations (if necessary with use of fax machine, telephone, or other electronic method for ECG transmission).

Prehospital treatment of acute coronary syndromes

The management of acute coronary syndromes in hospital is broadly agreed, but circumstances when the victim is first seen in the community demand some differences in the approach. The following steps are offered as a step-by-step guide to management in this different environment, but it is recognised that other traditions or variations in the availability of facilities or drugs must necessitate some regional modifications in practice.

A. Management of noncomplicated chest pain of presumed cardiac origin

1. Take brief relevant history.
2. Make brief assessment of vital signs (including BP and HR).
3. Establish ECG monitoring.
4. Ensure resuscitation equipment is available or coming.
5. Give short acting nitrate if pain is still present and SBP > 90 and no bradycardia.
6. Take 12-lead ECG.
7. Give oxygen: 3–5 l/min via a face mask (unless this causes undue patient distress).
8. Establish i.v. access.
9. Give aspirin 150–300 mg orally (or i.v. if available) unless contraindicated.
10. If no pain relief obtained with a nitrate, give morphine i.v. starting with 5 mg (or equivalent dose if other opioid used) titrated up to a maximum prehospital dose of 20 mg for acceptable pain control.
11. Give antiemetic such as metoclopramide 20 mg i.v. if necessary.
12. If patient remains anxious despite opioid give benzodiazepine.
13. If indications are present for thrombolysis (and in the absence of contraindications or arrangements for primary angioplasty) initiate

thrombolysis if appropriate in the prehospital phase (recommended especially if journey time may be more than 30 min or the delay or call-to-needle time for in-hospital thrombolysis may exceed 60 min).

14. If indications for thrombolysis are not present, but the ECG shows evidence of ischaemia, a bolus of heparin should be given. This will not preclude subsequent thrombolysis or primary PTCA in the hospital.

B. Management of respiratory distress of presumed cardiac origin, in addition to any relevant measures shown above

1. Give oxygen: nasopharyngeal catheter or face mask 6–8 l/min.
2. Rapidly increase nitrate i.v. up to 150 µg/kg/min according to blood pressure tolerance. Buccal nitrate is a more convenient preparation for prehospital use and can provide rapid and useful nitrate concentrations.
3. Give furosemide (frusemide) 40–80 mg i.v.
4. Give morphine 5 mg i.v. (or equivalent) if not already administered. Titrate using increments of half the original dose until adequate pain relief obtained.
5. In the absence of obvious improvement consider continuous positive airway pressure (CPAP) if available.
6. If the patient's condition remains or becomes critical, immediate oral endotracheal intubation is mandatory, followed by mechanical ventilation with positive airway pressure (PAP) titrated according to blood pressure and oxygenation.
7. If an arrhythmia has contributed to the development of pulmonary oedema it should be treated, if possible to do so, before hospital admission.

C. Management of left ventricular failure presenting as cardiogenic shock:

1. If there is no clinical pulmonary oedema careful volume loading. Test with 100–200 ml of colloid.

2. Give dobutamine 4–20 µg/kg/min.
3. Consider vasopressor if patient remains or becomes critical.

D. Management of symptomatic arrhythmias

For symptomatic sinus tachycardia:

1. If sinus tachycardia more than 120 beats per minute without overt heart failure, give metoprolol or atenolol 5 mg slowly i.v. Can be repeated up to total dose of 15 mg i.v. (three doses with 2-min intervals).

For bradyarrhythmias and tachycardia:

1. Ensure pain relief is adequate.
2. Consider need for blood pressure control.
3. Follow algorithm for bradyarrhythmias, broad complex tachycardias, and narrow complex tachycardias shown in Fig. 3.

E. Management of cardiac arrest:

1. Use precordial thump for witnessed event.
2. Administer 100% oxygen and CPR if defibrillator not available for immediate use. Defibrillator made ready.
3. Follow algorithm for VF/VT and non-VF/VT rhythms shown in Fig. 4.

ACKNOWLEDGEMENTS

The work of the Task Force was supported by grants from Astra Hässle AB; Bayer plc.; Boehringer Ingelheim; Heartstream Inc.; Knoll AG; Laerdal, Monmouth Pharmaceuticals; Serono Laboratories; Ortivus AB; Zeneca Pharma; Zoll Medical UK Ltd.

8.8. REFERENCES

1. The Task Force on the Management of Acute Myocardial Infarction of the European Society of Cardiology. Acute myocardial infarction: pre-hospital and in-hospital management. Eur Heart J 1996;17:43–63.
2. Chambless L, Keil U, Dobson A, Mähönen M, Kuulasmaa K, Rajakangas A-M, Löwel H, Tunstall-Pedoe

H, for the WHO MONICA Project. Population versus clinical view of case fatality from acute coronary heart disease: Results from the WHO MONICA Project 1985–1990. Circulation 1997;96:3849–3859.

3. Sans S, Kesteloot H, Kromhout D on behalf of the Task Force. The burden of cardiovascular mortality in Europe. Task Force of the European Society of Cardiology on Cardiovascular Mortality and Morbidity Statistics in Europe. Eur Heart J 1997;18:1231–1248.

4. Norris RM on behalf of The United Kingdom Heart Attack Study Collaborative Group. Fatality outside hospital from acute coronary events in three British health districts: 1994–1995. Br Med J 1998;316: 1065–1070.

5. Löwel H, Lewis M, Hörmann A. Prognostic significance of the pre-hospital phase in acute myocardial infaction: results of the Augsburg infarct register, 1985–1988 (in German). Dtsch Med Wschr 1991; 116:729–733.

6. Dellborg M, Eriksson P, Riha M, Swedberg K. Declining hospital mortality in acute myocardial infarction. Eur Heart J 1994;15:5–9.

7. Koenig W, Löwel H, Lewis M, Hörmann A. Long-term survival after myocardial infarction: relationship with thrombolysis and discharge medication. Results of the Augsburg myocardial infarction follow-up study 1985 to 1993. Eur Heart J 1996;17:1199–1206.

8. Löwel H, Lewis M, Keil U, Hörmann A, Bolte H-D, Willich S, Gostomzyk J. Time trends of acute myocardial infarction morbidity, mortality, 28-day-case-fatality and acute medical care: results of the Augsburg myocardial infarction register from 1985 to 1992 (in German). Z Kardiol 1995;84:596–605.

9. Tunstall-Pedoe H, Morrison C, Woodward M, Fitzpatrick B, Watt G. Sex differences in myocardial infarction and coronary deaths in the Scottish MONICA population of Glasgow 1985 to 1991. Presentation, diagnosis, treatment, and 28-day case fatality of 3991 events in men and 1551 events in women. Circulation 1996;93:1981–1992.

10. Ambrose JA, Tannenbaum MA, Alexopoulos D, Hjemdahl-Monson CE, Leavy J, Weiss M, Borrico S, Gorlin R, Fuster V. Angiographic progression of coronary artery disease and the development of myocardial infarction. J Am Coll Cardiol 1988;12:56–62.

11. Reimer KA, Lowe JE, Rasmussen MM, Jennings RB. The wavefront phenomenon of ischemic cell death. 1. Myocardial infarct size vs duration of coronary occlusion in dogs. Circulation 1977;56:786–94.

12. Weaver WD. Time to thrombolytic treatment: factors affecting delay and their influence on outcome. J Am Coll Cardiol 1995;25(Suppl):3S–9S.

13. Boersma E, Maas ACP, Deckers JW, Simoons ML. Early thrombolytic treatment in acute myocardial infarction: reappraisal of the golden hour. Lancet

1996;348:771–775.

14. Charney R, Cohen M. The role of the coronary circulation in limiting myocardial ischemia and infarct size. Am Heart J 1993;126:937–945.

15. Rentrop KP. Thrombolytic therapy in patients with acute myocardial infarction. Circulation 1985;71: 627–631.

16. Rogers WJ, Hood WP, Mantle JA, Baxley WA, Kirklin JK, Zorn GL, Nath HP. Return of left ventricular function after reperfusion in patients with myocardial infarction: importance of subtotal stenoses or intact collaterals. Circulation 1984;69:338–349.

17. Anzai T, Yoshikawa T, Asakura Y, Abe S, Akaishi M, Mitamura H, Handa S, Ogawa S. Preinfarction angina as a major predictor of left ventricular function an long-term prognosis after a first Q wave myocardial infarction. J Am Coll Cardiol 1995;26:319–327.

18. Lesnefsky EJ, Lundergan CF, Hodgson JMcB, Nair R, Reiner JS, Greenhouse SW, Califf RM, Ross AM. Increased left ventricular dysfuntion in elderly patients despite successful thrombolysis: the GUSTO-I angiographic experience. J Am Coll Cardiol 1996:28;331–337.

19. Haider AW, Andreotti F, Hackett DR, Tousoulis D, Kluft C, Maseri A, Davies GJ. Early spontaneous intermittent myocardial reperfusion during acute myocardial infarction is associated with augmented thrombogenic activity and less myocardial damage. J Am Coll Cardiol 1995;26:662–667.

20. Kannel WB, Thomas HE. Sudden coronary death: the Framingham study. Ann NY Acad Sci 1982;382:3–21.

21. Wennerblom B, Holmberg S. Death outside hospital with special reference to heart disease. Eur Heart J 1984;5:266–274.

22. O'Doherty M, Taylor DI, Quinn E, Vincent R, Chamberlain DA. Five hundred patients with myocardial infarction monitored within one hour of symptoms. Br Med J 1983;286:1405–1408.

23. Campbell RWF, Murray A, Julian DG. Ventricular arrhythmias in first 12 hours of acute myocardial infarction. Natural history study. Br Heart J 1981;46: 351–357.

24. Viskin S, Belahassen B. Idiopathic ventricular fibrillation. Am Heart J 1990;120:661–671.

25. Schaffer WA, Cobb LA. Recurrent ventricular fibrillation and modes of death in survivors of out-of-hospital ventricular fibrillation. N Engl J Med 1975;293:259–262.

26. Blohm MB, Hartford M, Karlson BW, Luepker RV, Herlitz J. An evaluation of the results of media and educational campaigns designed to shorten the time taken by patients with acute myocardial infarction to decide to go to hospital. Heart 1996;76:430–434.

27. Meischke H, Ho MT, Eisenberg MS, Schaeffer SM,

Larsen MP. Reasons patients with chest pain delay or do not call 911. Ann Emerg Med 1995;25:193– 197.

28. Hackett TP, Cassem NH. Factors contributing to delay in responding to the signs and symptoms of acute myocardial infarction. Am J Cardiol 1969;24:651–658.

29. Gilchrist IC. Patient delay before treatment of myocardial infarction. Br Med J 1973;I:535–537.

30. Rawles JM, Metcalfe MJ, Shirreffs C, Jennings K, Kenmure ACF. Association of patient delay with symptoms, cardiac enzymes, and outcome in acute myocardial infarction. Eur Heart J 1990;11:643–648.

31. Kenyon LW, Ketterer MW, Gheorghiade M, Goldstein S. Psychological factors related to prehospital delay during acute myocardial infarction. Circulation 1991; 84:1969–1976.

32. Trent RJ, Rose EL, Adams JN, Jennings KP, Rawles JM. Delay between the onset of symptoms of acute myocardial infarction and seeking medical assistance is influenced by left ventricular function at presentation. Br Heart J 1995;73:125–128.

33. Rawles J, Sinclair C, Waugh N. Call-to-needle times in Grampian: the pivotal role of the general practitioner in achieving early thrombolysis. Heart 1996;75(Suppl 1):63 (Abstract).

34. Birkhead JS on behalf of the joint audit committee of the British Cardiac Society and cardiology committee of the Royal College of Physicians of London. Time delays in provision of thrombolytic treatment in six district hospitals. Br Med J 1992;305:445–448.

35. Bleeker JK, Simoons ML, Erdman RAM, Leenders CM, Kruyssen HACM, Lamers LM, van der Does E. Patient and doctor delay in acute myocardial infarction: a study in Rotterdam, The Netherlands. Br J Gen Pract 1995;45:181–184.

36. Leprohon J, Patel VL. Decision-making strategies for telephone triage in emergency medical services. Med Decis Making 1995;15:240–253.

37. Sramek M, Post W, Koster RW. Telephone triage of cardiac emergency calls by dispatchers. A prospective study of 1386 emergency calls. Br Heart J 1994;71: 440–445.

38. Culley LL, Henwood DK, Clark JJ, Eisenberg MS, Horton C. Increasing the efficiency of emergency medical services by using criteria based dispatch. Ann Emerg Med 1994;24:867–872.

39. Ahnefeld FW. Die Wiederbelebung bei Kreislaufstillstand. Verhandlungen Deutsche Gesellschaft für Innere Medizin 1968;74:279–287.

40. Cummins R, Ornato JP, Thies WH, Pepe PE. Improving survival from sudden cardiac arrest: the "chain of survival" concept. A statement for health professionals from the Advanced Cardiac Life Support Subcommittee and the Emergency Cardiac Care Committee, American Heart Association. Circulation 1991;83:

1832–1847.

41. The Council of the European Communities: Council decision of 29/7/91 on the introduction of a single European emergency call number (91/396/EEC). OJ 1991;L217:6.08.1991.

42. Herlitz J, Ekstrom L, Wennerblom B, Axelsson Å, Bång A, Holmberg S. Effect of bystander initiated cardiopulmonary resuscitation on ventricular fibrillation and survival after witnessed cardiac arrest outside hospital. Br Heart J 1994;72:408–412.

43. Bossaert L, Van Hoeyweghen R, and Cerebral Resuscitation Study Group. Bystander cardiopulmonary resuscitation (CPR) in out-of-hospital cardiac arrest. Resuscitation 1989;17(Suppl):S55–S69.

44. Stults KR, Brown DD, Schug VL, Bean JA. Prehospital defibrillation performed by emergency medical technicians in rural communities. N Engl J Med 1984; 310:219–223.

45. European Resuscitation Council AED Taskforce. Position statement on the use of automated external defibrillation. Resuscitation 1998;(In press).

46. Weaver WD, Hill D, Fahrenbruch CE, Copass MK, Martin JS, Cobb LA, Hallstrom AP. Use of the automatic external defibrillator in the management of out-of-hospital cardiac arrest. N Engl J Med 1988;319: 661–666.

47. White RD, Asplin BR, Bugliosi TF, Hankins DG. High discharge survival rate after out-of-hospital ventricular fibrillation with rapid defibrillation by police and paramedics. Ann Emerg Med 1996;28:480–485.

48. O'Rourke MF. Donaldson E, Geddes JS. An airline cardiac arrest program. Circulation 1997;96:2849–2853.

49. Bossaert L, Callanan V, Cummins RO. Early defibrillation. An advisory statement by the Advanced Life Support Working Group of the International Liaison Committee on Resuscitation. Resuscitation 1997;34:113–115.

50. Jaggarao NSV, Heber M, Grainger R, Vincent R, Chamberlain DA. Use of an automated external defibrillator by ambulance staff. Lancet 1982;ii:73–75.

51. Eisenberg MS, Horwood BT, Cummins RO, Reynolds-Haertle R, Hearne TR. Cardiac arrest and resuscitation: a tale of 29 cities. Ann Emerg Med 1990;19: 179–186.

52. Het Belgisch Staatsblad, 1 January 1961; Article 422 bis-ter.

53. Capone RJ, Visco J, Curwen E, VanEvery S. The effect of early prehospital transtelephonic coronary intervention on morbidity and mortality: experience with 284 post myocardial infarction patients in a pilot program. Am Heart J 1984;107:1153–1160.

54. Culley LL, Clark JJ, Eisenberg MS, Larsen MP. Dispatcher-assisted telephone CPR: common delays and time standards for delivery. Ann Emerg Med 1991;

20:362–366.

55. Eisenberg MS, Hallstrom AP, Carter WB, Cummins RO, Bergner L, Pierce J. Emergency CPR instructions via the telephone. Am J Pub Health 1985;75:47–50.

56. GREAT Group. Feasibility, safety, and efficacy of domiciliary thrombolysis by general practitioners: Grampian region early anistreplase trial. Br Med J 1992;305:548–553.

57. The European Myocardial Infarction Project Group. Prehospital thrombolytic therapy in patients with suspected acute myocardial infarction. N Engl J Med 1993;329:383–389.

58. Grijseels EWM, Deckers JW, Hoes AW, Boersma E, Hartman JAM, van der Does E, Simoons ML. Implementation of a pre-hospital decision rule in general practice. Triage of patients with suspected myocardial infarction. Eur Heart J 1996;17:89–95.

59. Karagounis L, Ipsen SK, Jessop MR, Gilmore KM, Valenti DA, Clawson JJ, Teichman S, Anderson JL. Impact of field-transmitted electrocardiography on time to in-hospital thrombolytic therapy in acute myocardial infarction. Am J Cardiol 1990;66:786–791.

60. Assanelli D, Zywietz C, Mertins V, Canclini S, Giovanni G, Vignali S. Digital ECG transmission from ambulance cars with application of the European standard communications protocol Scp-Ecg. Eur Heart J 1996;17(Suppl):579.

61. Jollis JG, DeLong ER, Peterson ED, Muhlbaier LH, Fortin DF, Califf RM, Mark DB. Outcome of acute myocardial infarction according to the specialty of the admitting physician. N Engl J Med 1996;335:1880–1887.

62. National heart attack alert program coordinating committee 60 minutes to treatment working group. Emergency department: rapid identification and treatment of patients with acute myocardial infarction. US Department of Health and Human Services, National Institutes of Health, 1993.

63. Burns JMA, Hogg KJ, Rae AP, Hillis WS, Dann FG. Impact of a policy of direct admission to a coronary care unit on use of thrombolysis treatment. Br Heart J 1989;61:322–325.

64. Rosenthal E, Thomas N, Quinn E, Chamberlain D, Vincent R. Transcutaneous pacing for cardiac emergencies. Pace 1988;11:2160–2167.

65. Tachakra SS, Pawsey S, Beckett M, Potts D, Idowu A. Outcome of patients with chest pain discharged from an accident and emergency department. Br Med J 1991;302:504–505.

66. Pell ACH, Miller HC. Delays in admission of patients with myocardial infarction to coronary care: implications for thrombolysis. Health Bull 1990;48:225–230.

67. Emerson PA, Russell NJ, Wyatt J, Crichton N, Pantin CF, Morgan AD, Fleming PR. An audit of doctor's management of patients with chest pain in the accident and emergency department. Q J Med 1989;263:213–220.

68. Pell ACH, Miller HC, Robertson C E, Fox KAA. Effect of "fast track" admission for acute myocardial infarction on delay to thrombolysis. Br Med J 1992;304:83–87.

69. More R, Moore K, Quinn E, Perez Avila C, Davidson C, Vincent R, Chamberlain D. Delay times in the administration of thrombolytic therapy: the Brighton experience. Int J Cardiol 1995;49(Suppl):S39–S46.

70. Goldman L, Cook EF, Brand DA, Lee TH, Rouan GW, Weisberg MC, Acampora D, Stasiulewicz C, Walshon J, Terranova G, Gottlieb L, Kobernick M, Goldstein-Wayne B, Copen D, Daley K, Brandt AA, Jones D, Mellors J, Jakubowski R. A computer protocol to predict myocardial infarction in emergency department patients with chest pain. N Engl J Med 1988;318:797–803.

71. Pozen MW, d'Agostino RB, Mitchell JB, Rosenfeld DM, Guglielmino JT, Schwartz ML, Teebagy N, Valentine JM, Hood WB. The usefulness of a predictive instrument to reduce inappropriate admissions to the coronary care unit. Ann Int Med 1980;92:238–242.

72. Tierney WM, Roth BJ, Psaty B, McHenry R, Fitzgerald J, Stump DL, Anderson FK, Ryder KW, McDonald CJ, Smith DM. Predictors of myocardial infarction in emergency room patients. Crit Care Med 1985;13:526–531.

73. Adams J, Trent R, Rawles J, on behalf of the GREAT Group. Earliest electrocardiographic evidence of myocardial infarction: implications for thombolytic treatment. Br Med J 1993;307:409–413.

74. Srikanthan VS, Pell AC, Prasad N, Tait GW, Rae AP, Hogg KJ, Dunn FG. Use of fax facility improves decision making regarding thrombolysis in acute myocardial infarction. Heart 1997;78:198–200.

75. Antiplatelet Trialists' Collaboration. Collaborative overview of randomised trials of antiplatelet therapy-I: prevention of death, myocardial infarction, and stroke by prolonged antiplatelet therapy in various categories of patients. Br Med J 1994;308:81-1-6.

76. ISIS-2 (Second International Study of Infarct Survival) Collaborative Group. Randomised trial of intravenous streptokinase, oral aspirin, both, or neither among 17 187 cases of suspected acute myocardial infarction: ISIS-2. Lancet 1998:349–360.

77. Reilly IA, Fitzgerald GA. Inhibition of thromboxane formation in vivo and ex vivo: implications for therapy with platelet inhibitory drugs. Blood 1987;69:180–186.

78. Collins R, MacMahon S, Flather M, Baigent C, Remvig L, Mortensen S, Appleby P, Godwin J, Yusuf S, Peto R. Clinical effects of anticoagulant therapy in suspected acute myocardial infarction: systematic over-

view of randomised trials. Br Med J 1996;313: 652–659.

79. ISIS-3 (Third International Study of Infarct Survival) Collaborative Group. ISIS-3: a randomised comparison of streptokinase vs tissue plasminogen activator vs anistreplase and of aspirin plus heparin vs aspirin alone among 41 299 cases of suspected acute myocardial infarction. Lancet 1992;339:753–770.

80. Gruppo Italiano per lo Studio della Sopravvivenza nell'Infarto miocardico. GISSI-2: a factorial randomised trial of alteplase versus streptokinase and heparin versus no heparin among 12 490 patients with acute myocardial infarction. Lancet 1990;336:65–71.

81. ISIS-I (First International Study of Infarct Survival) Collaborative Group. Randomised trial of intravenous atenolol among 16 027 cases of suspected acute myocardial infarction: ISIS-I. Lancet 1986;ii:57–66.

82. The MIAMI Trial Research Group. Metoprolol in acute myocardial infarction (MIAMI). A randomised placebo-controlled international trial. Eur Heart J 1985;6: 199–226.

83. Borzak S, Gheorghiade M. Early intravenous beta-blocker combined with thrombolytic therapy for acute myocardial infarction: the thrombolysis in myocardial infarction (TIMI-2) trial. Prog Cardiovasc Dis 1993; 36:261–266.

84. Yusuf S, Peto R, Lewis J, Collins R, Sleight P. Beta blockade during and after myocardial infarction: an overview of the randomized trials. Prog Cardiovasc Dis 1985;27:335–371.

85. The TIMI Study Group. Comparison of invasive and conservative strategies after treatment with intravenous tissue plasminogen activator in acute myocardial infarction. Results of the thrombolysis in myocardial infarction (TIMI) phase II trial. N Engl J Med 1989; 320:618–627.

86. Leizorovicz A, Teppe J-P, Payen C, Haugh MC, Boissel J-P, for EMIP-BB Pilot Study Group. Pre-hospital treatment of patients with suspected acute myocardial using a beta-blocking agent : a double-blind feasibility study. Clin Trials and Meta-Analysis 1994;29:125–138.

87. Gruppo Italiano per lo Studio della Sopravvivenza nell'Infarto miocardico. GISSI-3: effects of lisinopril and transdermal glyceryl trinitrate singly and together on 6-week mortality and ventricular function after acute myocardial infarction. Lancet 1994;343:1115–1122.

88. ISIS-4 (Fourth International Study of Infarct Survival) Collaborative Group. ISIS-4: a randomised factorial trial assessing early oral captopril, oral mononitrate, and intravenous magnesium sulphate in 58,050 patients with suspected acute myocardial infarction. Lancet 1995;345:669–685.

89. Ferguson JJ, Diver DJ, Boldt M, Pasternak RC. Significance of nitroglycerin-induced hypotension with inferior wall acute myocardial infarction. Am J Cardiol 1989;64:311–314.

90. Rutherford JD, Pfeffer MA, Moyé LE, Davis BR, Flaker GC, Kowey PR, Lamas GA, Miller HS, Packer M, Rouleau JL, Braunwald E, on behalf of the SAVE Investigators. Effects of captopril on ischemic events after myocardial infarction: results of the survival and ventricular enlargement trial. Circulation 1994;90: 1731–1738.

91. Pfeffer MA, Greaves SC, Arnold MO, Glynn RJ, LaMotte FS, Lee RT, Menapace FJ, Rapaport ER, Ridker PM, Rouleau J-L, Solomon SD, Hennekens CH for the Healing and Early Afterload Reducing Therapy (HEART) Trial Investigators. Early versus delayed angiotensin-converting enzyme inhibition therapy in acute myocardial infarction. The healing and early afterload reducing therapy trial. Circulation 1997; 95:2643–2651.

92. MacMahon S, Collins R, Peto R, Koster RW, Yusuf S. Effects of prophylactic lidocaine in suspected acute myocardial infarction: an overview of results from the randomized, controlled trials. JAMA 1988;260: 1910–1916.

93. Hine LK, Laird N, Hewitt P, Chalmers TC. Meta-analytic evidence against prophylactic use of lidocaine in acute myocardial infarction. Arch Int Med 1989; 149:2694–2698.

94. Teo KK, Yusuf S, Furberg SD. Effects of prophylactic antiarrhythmic drug therapy in acute myocardial infarction: an overview of results from randomized controlled trials. JAMA 1993;270:1589–1595.

95. Fibrinolytic Therapy Trialists' Collaborative Group. Indications for fibrinolytic therapy in suspected acute myocardial infarction: collaborative overview of early mortality and major morbidity results from all randomised trials of more than 1000 patients. Lancet 1994;343:311–322.

96. Rawles J. What is the likely benefit of earlier thrombolysis? Eur Heart J 1996;17:991–995.

97. Weaver WD, Cerqueira M, Hallström AP, Litwin PE, Martin JS, Kudenchuk PJ, Eisenberg M, for the Myocardial infarction Triage and Intervention Project Group. Pre-hospital-initiated vs hospital-initiated thrombolytic therapy. JAMA 1993;270:1211–1216.

98. Rawles J. Quantification of the benefit of earlier thrombolic therapy: 5-year results of the Grampian early anistreplase trial (GREAT). J Am Coll Cardiol 1997;30:1181–1186.

99. Brouwer MA, Martin JS, Maynard JS, Wirkus M, Litwin PE, Verheugt FWA, Weaver WD, for the MITI Project Investigators. Influence of early pre-hospital thrombolysis on mortality and event-free survival (The Myocardial Infarction Triage and Intervention [MITI] randomized trial). Am J Cardiol 1996;78:

497–502.

100. Cannon CP, Antman EM, Walls R, Braunwald E. Time as an adjunctive agent to thrombolytic therapy. J Thrombosis Thrombolysis 1994;1:27–34.

101. Stone GW, Grines CL, Rothbaum D, Browne KF, O'Keefe J, Overlie PA, Donohue BC, Chelliah N, Vlietstra R, Catlin T, O'Neill WW, for the PAMI Trial Investigators. Analysis of the relative costs and effectiveness of primary angioplasty versus tissue-type plasminogen activator: the primary angioplasty in myocardial infarction(PAMI) trial. J Am Coll Cardiol 1997;29: 901–907.

102. The Global Use of Strategies to Open Occluded Coronary Arteries in Acute Coronary Syndromes (GUSTO IIb) Angioplasty Substudy Investigators. A clinical trial comparing primary coronary angioplasty with tissue plasminogen activator for acute myocardial infarction. N Engl J Med 1997;336:1621–1628.

103. Every NR, Parsons LS, Hlaty M, Martin JS, Weaver D, for the Myocardal Infarction Triage and Intervention Investigators. A comparison of thrombolytic therapy with primary coronary angioplasty for acute myocardial infarction. N Engl J Med 1996;335:1253–1260.

104. Ellis SG, da Silva ER, Heydricks G et al. For the RESCUE-Investegators. Randomized comparison of rescue angioplasty with conservative management of patients wit early failure of thrombolysis for acute anterior myocardial infarction. Circulation 1994;20:2280–2284.

105. McKendall GR, Forman S, Sopko G, Braunwald E, Williams DO, and the Thrombolysis in Myocardial Infarction Investigators. Value of rescue percutaneous transluminal coronary angioplasty following unsuccessful thrombolytic therapy in patients with acute myocardial infarction. Am J Cardiol 1995;76:1108–1111.

106. A statement for the Advanced Cardiac Life Support Committee of the European Resuscitation Council, 1994. Management of peri-arrest arrhythmias. Resuscitation 1994;28:151–159. (Update: Resuscitation 1996;31:281.)

107. A statement for the Advanced Cardiac Life Support Committee of the European Resuscitation Council, 1994. Management of peri-arrest arrhythmias. Resuscitation 1998 (Update: see Chapter 7, pp. 159–167).

108. Cotter G, Metzkor E, Kaluski E. Faigenberg Z, Miller R, Simovitz A, Shaham O, Marghitay D, Koren M, Blatt A, Moshkovitz Y, Zaidenstein R, Golik A. Randomised trial of high-dose isosorbide dinitrate plus low-dose furosemide versus high-dose furosemide plus low-dose isosorbide dinitrate in severe pulmonary oedema. Lancet 1998;351:389–393.

109. Timmis AD, Fowler MB, Chamberlain DA. Comparison of haemodynamic responses to dopamine and salbutamol in severe cardiogenic shock complicating acute myocardial infarction. Br Med J 1981;282:7–9.

110. Dracup K, Heany DM, Taylor SE, Guzy PM, Breu C. Can family members of high-risk cardiac patients learn cardiopulmonary resuscitation? Arch Int Med 1989;149:61–64.

111. A Statement by the Basic Life Support Working Party of the European Resuscitation Council, 1998. Guidelines for basic life support. Resuscitation (In press).

112. Wenzel V, Idris AH, Banner MJ, Fuerst RS, Tucker KJ. The composition of gas given by mouth-to-mouth ventilation during CPR. Chest 1994;106:1806–1810.

113. Moser DK, Coleman S. Cardiopulmonary resuscitation: recommendations for improving cardiopulmonary resuscitation skills retention. Heart Lung 1992; 32:372–380.

114. Berg RA, Kern KB, Hilwig RW, Berg MK, Sanders AB, Otto CW, Ewy GA. Assisted ventilation does not improve outcome in a porcine model of single-rescuer bystander cardiopulmonary resuscitation. Circulation 1997;95:1635–1641.

115. Van Hoeyweghen R J, Bossaert LL, Mullie A, Calle P, Martens P, Buylaert WA, Delooz H, Belgium Cerebral Resuscitation Study Group. Quality and efficency of bystander CPR. Resuscitation 1993;26:47–52.

116. Ornato JP. Should bystanders perform mouth-to-mouth ventilation during resuscitation. Chest 1994; 106:1641–1642.

117. Locke CJ, Berg RA, Sanders AB, Davis MF, Milander MM, Kern KB, Ewy GA. Bystander cardiopulmonary resuscitation: concerns about mouth-to-mouth contact. Arch Int Med 1995;155:938–943.

118. A Statement by the Advanced Life Support Working Group of the European Resuscitation Council, 1998. Guidelines for advanced life support. Resuscitation 1998;17(2):(In press) (See also this volume Chapter 3.1, pp. 36–47).

119. Jakobsson J, Rehnqvist N, Nyquist O. Energy requirement for early defibrillation. Eur Heart J 1989;10: 551–554.

120. Weaver WD, Cobb LA, Copass MK, Hallstrom AP. Ventricular defibrillation: a comparative trial using 175 J and 320 J shocks. N Engl J Med 1982;307: 1101–1106.

121. Kern K, Ewy G. Clinical defibrillation: optimal transthoracic and open chest techniques. In: Tacker W (ed) Defibrillation of the Heart. Mosby, 1994.

122. Bardy GH, Gliner BE, Kudenchuk PJ, Poole JE, Dolack GL, Jones GK, Anderson J, Troutman C, Johnson G. Truncated biphasic pulses for transthoracic defibrillation. Circulation 1995;91:1768–1774.

123. Reddy R, Gleva MJ, Glina BE, Dolack GR, Kudenchuk PJ, Poole JE, Bardy GH. Biphasic transthoracic defibrillation causes fewer ECG ST-segment changes after shock. Ann Emerg Med 1997;30:127–134.

124. Weisfeldt ML, Kerber RE, McGoldrick P, Moss AJ,

Nichol G, Ornato JP, Palmer DG, Riegel B, Smith SC. Public access defibrillation: A Statement for Healthcare Professionals from the American Heart Associaton Task Force on Automatic External Defibrillation. Circulation 1995;92:2763.

125. A Statement by the Airway and Ventilation Management Working Group of the European Resuscitation Council. Guidelines for the advanced management of the airway and ventilation during resuscitation. Resuscitation 1996;31:201–230.

126. Hapnes SA, Robertson C. CPR – drug delivery routes and systems. Resuscitation 1992;24:137–142.

127. Aitkenhead AR. Drug administration during CPR: what route? Resuscitation 1991;22:191–195.

128. Callaham M, Madsen CD, Barton CW, Saunders CE, Pointer J. A randomized clinical trial of high-dose epinephrine and norepinephrine vs standard-dose epinephrine in pre-hospital cardiac arrest. JAMA 1992; 268:2667–2672.

129. Lindner KH, Prengel AW, Pfenninger EG, Lindner IM, Strohmenger H-U, Georgieff M, Lurie KG. Vasopressin improves vital organ blood flow during closed-chest cardiopulmonary resuscitation in pigs. Circulation 1995;91:215–221.

130. Lindner KH, Dirks B, Strohmenger H-U, Prengel AW, Lindner IM, Lurie KG. Randomised comparison of epinephrine and vasopressin in patients with out-of-hospital ventricular fibrillation. Lancet 1997;349: 535–537.

131. Koster R, Carli P. Acid-base management. A statement for the Advanced Life Support Working Party of the European Resuscitation Council. Resuscitation 1992; 24:143–146.

132. Tzivoni D, Banai S, Schuger C, Benhorn J, Keren A, Gottlieb S, Stern S. Treatment of torsade de pointes with magnesium sulfate. Circulation 1988;77:392–397.

133. Wiesfeld ACP, Crijns JGM, Tuininga YS, Lie KI. Beta adrenergic blockade in the treatment of sustained ventricular tachycardia or ventricular fibrillation. Pace 1996;19:1026–1035.

134. Kochanek PM, Hallenbeck JM. Polymorphonuclear leukocytes and monocytes/macrophages in the pathogenesis of cerebral ischemia and stroke. Stroke 1992;23:1367–1379.

135. Siesjö BK. Historical overview: calcium, ischemia and death of brain cells. Ann NY Acad Sci 1988;522: 638–661.

136. Gustafson I, Edgren E, Hulting J. Brain-oriented intensive care after resuscitation from cardiac arrest. Resuscitation 1992;24:245–261.

137. Kern KB, Sanders AB, Raife J, Milander MM, Otto CW, Ewy GA. A study of chest compression rates during cardiopulmonary resuscitation in humans. Arch Int Med 1992;152:145–149.

138. Trillo G, von Planta M, Kette F. ETCO2 monitoring during low flow states: clinical aims and limits. Resuscitation 1994;27t1-8.

139. Beauchamp TL, Chindress JF. Principles of biomedical ethics. Oxford: Oxford University Press, 1989.

140. Gillon, R. Philosophical Medical Ethics. Chichester: John Wiley & Sons, 1985.

141. Tomlinson, T, Brody H. Ethics and communication in do-not-resuscitate orders. N Engl J Med 1988;318: 43–46.

142. Florin D. Do not resuscitate orders: the need for the policy. J Royal Coll Phys 1993;27:1358.

143. Hartford M, Karlson BW, Sjolin M, Holmberg S, Herlitz J. Symptoms, thoughts, and environmental factors in suspected acute myocardial infarction. Heart-Lung 1993;22:64–70.

144. Dellipiani AW, Cay EL, Phillip AE, Vetter NJ, Colling WA, Donaldson RJ, McCormack P. Anxiety after a heart attack. Br Heart J 1976;38:752–757.

145. Vetter NJ, Cay EL, Phillip AE, Strange RC. Anxiety on admission to a coronary care unit. J Psychosomatic Res 1977;21:73–78.

146. Thompson DR, Cordle CJ, Sutton TW. Anxiety in coronary patients. Int Rehab Med 1982;4:161-4.7.

147. Harrison TR, Reeves TJ. Ischemic Heart Disease. Chicago: Year Book, 1968;295.

9. Ethical Considerations in Resuscitation

CONTENTS:

9.1. Ethical Principles in Out-of-Hospital Cardiopulmonary Resuscitation

"You can treat and must not kill, but do not try to bring a dead soul to life."

"Anyone, anywhere, can now initiate cardiac resuscitative procedures. All that is needed are two hands."

These two statements by Pindar [1] and Kouwenhoven et al. [2] point to the ethical challenge of cardiopulmonary resuscitation: the span between fatalistic acceptance of death and the enthusiastic technical approach. Modern resuscitation techniques have made it possible to bring dead patients back to life, but at the same time have lead to questions and uncertainties, mainly since in most cases the emergency situation requires prompt action while prognostic factors are widely unknown. In the same way that fatal circumstances may create the ultimate tragedy in a survivor – severe brain damage [3] – another case which primarily had been judged as hopeless may end in *restitutio ad integrum*.

The situation in which out-of-hospital cardiopulmonary resuscitation is required focusses literally on ethical problems, not at least since, in view of technologic progress in medicine and different values in society today in contrast to earlier eras, there are no obligatory rules defining one behaviour as the only correct one. The problem is not the end of life but the possibility of reacting differently in view of death and dying. So the conditions in this special field are also determined by societal characteristics and by the discussions and uncertainties of our cultural framework [4].

Ethics in out-of-hospital emergency medicine, especially in resuscitation, do not mean special ethics, but ethics in special situations which are characterized by limitations: limited time, limited diagnostic knowledge, limited therapeutic possibilities [5], and limitations in the relationship between patient and health care provider. The special features of emergency medical practice might lead to the assumption that emergency medicine represents an area free of ethics, with ethical considerations being displaced by various obligations, i.e., the obligation to act immediately. Such an assumption would fail to appreciate two aspects:

1) emergency medicine is understood as part of in-hospital intensive care medicine (instrumentality of the ICU), and with this is subject to the same general ethical principles;

2) ethical considerations remain useless if reflected on in the emergency situation for the first time – they should and have to be nurtured through advance preparation and training [6].

There is no simple, single way to answer ethical questions, but a variety of theories and sources for moral guidance of which one approach, however, has come to the fore during recent years: the biomedical ethics by Beauchamp and Childress [7]. The authors suggest four principles for acceptance as action guides in medicine:

- the principle of beneficence,
- the principle of nonmaleficence,
- the principle of respect for autonomy,
- the principle of justice.

Beneficence

The principle of beneficence includes the fundamental objects of medicine: preservation of life, restoration of health, relief of suffering, and restoration or maintenance of function [8]. Modern CPR techniques, citizen CPR training programmes and growing effectiveness of EMS systems have saved numerous victims from sudden cardiac death. Attempts have been made to identify favourable factors as far as outcome after out-of-hospital CPR is concerned to provide criteria helping in the decision of whether or not resuscitation attempts should be initiated, withheld or discontinued [9,10]. The highest survival rates have been reported in cases of observed, primarily cardiac, arrest with ventricular fibrillation, CPR initiated by bystanders and short response intervals of the EMS system [10]. However, survival between the point of out-of-hospital cardiac arrest and hospital discharge is poor with rates ranging from 0 to 20%. But on the other hand we know from interviews that the majority of survivors value their experience positively and would choose to be resuscitated again should the situation arise [11,12].

Nonmaleficence

Whereas beneficence means the performance of positive acts in favour of the patient to promote **good** [7], the principle of nonmaleficence implies avoiding anything having possible negative consequences. In most cases CPR attempts remain unsuccessful; outcome studies show that in about 50% there is no return to spontaneous circulation and that another 30% die in hospital after admission [13]. Thus, resuscitation means for many patients an extension of the dying process, considerable suffering for the patient and his relatives, and a heavy burden for all involved, including hospital staff. About 20–50% of the survivors suffer from neurologic disabilities [14], ranging from slight disturbances of cognitive functions to persistent vegetative state.

Evaluation of survivors of cardiac arrest revealed a decrease in functional status caused by the fear of another arrest as well as a reduced capacity to perform daily life activities [11,15]. Altered social contacts and social isolation were common after cardiac arrest [15].

The poor survival rates after traumatic arrest even in physician-staffed EMS systems have led to discussions on futility in resuscitation; resuscitation should be withheld or discontinued when there is no doubt that the attempt would be futile [16]. The initiation of a resuscitation attempt is obviously not indicated when there are signs of death, such as postmortem lividity, rigor mortis or decomposition, but the aspect of futility should also be considered in absence of these signs when the success of the attempt may be doubtful. For a treatment to be judged futile it must be ascertained that it has no benefit, with the benefit depending on the outcome of the intervention, the probability of that outcome, and the patient's perception of that outcome [17]. Thus, a physician's decision to withhold or discontinue resuscitation may be justified:

- in patients whose vital functions deteriorate despite optimal treatment and maximal therapy (e.g., in progressive cardiogenic shock),
- in patients where appropriate therapy has been attempted for adequate time without return of spontaneous circulation, and
- in conditions where scientific studies have clearly demonstrated that resuscitation attempts would be ineffective [16].

Respect for Autonomy

Health care workers do not have the right to treat patients without their consent; the informed consent of the patient has to be obtained before undertaking any invasive procedure. An informed consent includes the components: 1) competence, 2) disclosure of information, 3) understanding of information, 4) voluntariness, and 5) authorization [7]. It is important to notice the elements of information and understanding as prerequisites for an informed consent, as studies have shown that, especially in elderly people, the anticipated acceptance of resuscitation attempts decreased significantly after information on the procedure of resuscitation and the prognostic implications was given [18]. From an ethical point of view informed consent includes the patient's autonomy and dignity which have to be considered by the physician, the patient himself and society; so it would be more precise to talk of a moral, legal and free informed consent [19].

In a situation requiring resuscitation the patient normally is unconscious. Although still autonomous since autonomy is, like dignity, an inseparable part of man, he cannot express the rights and obligations arising from his autonomy [20]; he has lost the decision-making capacity, the ability of communicating his treatment preferences, and the possibility to accept or refuse treatment. On the other hand the circumstances require the initiation of a resuscitation attempt urgently if it is to be of any success. This situation leads to burdensome but avoidable ethical conflicts in health care workers, bystanders and the society, and one might ask if it is ethically acceptable that most people do not take measures in advance regarding possible emergency situations and document their preferences when they are still able to do so [20]. This problem with its societal and cultural roots requires further debate.

However, the discussion about do-not-resuscitate (DNR) or do-not-attempt-resuscitation (DNAR) orders shows that there is a way to express ones preferences in advance. Such orders, written by patients or their physicians in a moment when the patient still is capable of making informed decisions, have been established to provide a mechanism for withholding specific treatments in case of cardiac arrest. But in an out-of-hospital emergency situation there is little time to look for written advance directives or to verify personal statements of relatives, add to this that the position of such policies is rarely defined sufficiently in the legislature of most European countries [3].

Hence, in the prehospital setting the decision to start CPR is usually made without involvement of the patient, presuming that resuscitation is in the patient's best interest and that he would have agreed to the treatment if he had been able to do so. Since in most situations cause and consequences of the arrest cannot be assessed adequately there is nothing left but the criterion of caution in form of a crisis intervention [21]. How-

ever, from this must not follow an automatism of treatment. While performing CPR the physician should try to get additional indications of the patient's presumed wishes as well as further medical information regarding possible termination of the attempt. Initiation of resuscitation does not justify an automatic sequence of therapeutic steps defined by technology which is reconsidered only after admission to hospital. Medical and ethical considerations are continuously necessary during any stage of resuscitation. Both emergency medical treatment based only on technical feasibility and termination of resuscitation based only on medical futility are ethically deficit, since in both cases the patient's interests as decisive criterion are neglected [20].

Justice

This principle affecting priorities in the allocation of resources may be defined as giving each person that which is due, and which can be claimed legitimately [7]. Performing an inappropriate or futile CPR attempt may delay or prevent emergency treatment in other patients with better chances of survival [13]. Although every citizen should have the right to receive CPR it has been shown that in some places race and socioeconomic factors influence the probability of CPR being attempted, of admission to hospital, and of survival [22,23]; in other countries, however, such differences could not be demonstrated [24].

The aspect of organ donation has been a subject of discussion in connection with resuscitation. In nearly all countries there is a serious shortage of organs for transplantation, so the appropriateness of initiating or maintaining resuscitation procedures only for this purpose has to be questioned. This aspect surely needs further consideration.

Conclusions

The out-of-hospital emergency situation requiring resuscitation is characterized by uncertainties, not allowing the initiation of CPR procedures only in those patients who have a potential chance of long-term survival. Thus, if there is any doubt about the appropriateness of withholding a resuscitation attempt CPR should be started. If the patient's wishes and preferences remain unclear, as it will be the case in the majority of these emergencies, the principle *in dubio pro CPR* represents an ethically acceptable solution.

REFERENCES

1. Pindar, 5th century B.C., cit. from Negovsky VA. Death, dying and revival: ethical aspects. Resuscitation 1993;25:99–107.

2. Kouwenhoven WB, Jude JR, Knickerbocker GG. Closed-chest cardiac massage. J Am Med Assoc 1960;173:1064–1067.

3. Baskett PJF. Ethics in cardiopulmonary resuscitation. Resuscitation 1993;25:1–8.

4. Illhardt FJ. Medizinische Ethik: Ein Arbeitsbuch. Berlin, Heidelberg, New York, Tokyo: Springer, 1985.

5. von Engelhardt D. Zur Begründung ethischer Prinzipien in der Notfallmedizin. In: Mohr M, Kettler D (eds) Ethik in der Notfallmedizin: Präklinische Herz-Lungen-Wiederbelebung. Berlin, Heidelberg, New York: Springer, 1997.

6. American College of Emergency Physicians. Policy statement: code of ethics for emergency physicians. Dallas, 1997.

7. Beauchamp TL, Childress JF. Principles of biomedical ethics, 4th edn. New York: Oxford University Press, 1994.

8. Snider GL. The do-not-resuscitate order. Ethical and legal imperative or medical decision? Am Rev Resp Dis 1991;143:665–674.

9. Bonin MJ, Pepe PE, Kimball KT, Clark PS. Distinct criteria for termination of resuscitation in the out-of-hospital setting. J Am Med Assoc 1993;270:1457–1462.

10. Eisenberg MS, Cummins RO, Larsen MP. Numerators, denominators and survival rates: reporting survival from out-of-hospital cardiac arrest. Am J Emerg Med 1991;9:544–546.

11. Bedell SE, Delbano TL, Cook EF, Epstein FH. Survival after cardiopulmonary resuscitation in the hospital. N Engl J Med 1983;309:569–576.

12. Röwer N, Klöss T, Püschel K. Langzeiterfolg und Lebensqualität nach präklinischer kardiopulmonaler Reanimation. Anästhesiol Intensivmed Notfallmed Schmerzther 1985;20:244–250.

13. Mohr M, Kettler D. Ethical aspects of resuscitation. Br J Anaesth 1997;79:253–259.

14. Eleff SM, Hanley DF. Postresuscitation prognostication and declaration of brain death. In: Paradis NA, Halperin HR, Nowak RM (eds) Cardiac Arrest: The Science and Practice of Resuscitation Medicine. Baltimore: Williams and Wilkins, 1996.

15. Sunnerhagen KS, Johansson O, Herlitz J, Grimby G. Life after cardiac arrest; a retrospective study. Resuscitation 1996;31:135–140.

16. Holmberg S. Ethics and practicalities of resuscitation. Resuscitation 1992;24:239–244.

17. Crimmins TJ. Ethical issues in adult resuscitation. Ann Emerg Med 1993;22:495–501.

18. Murphy DJ, Burrows D, Santilli S, Kemp AW, Tenner S, Kreiling B, Teno J. The influence of the probability of survival on patients' preferences regarding cardiopulmonary resuscitation. N Engl J Med 1994;330:545–549.

19. von Engelhardt D. Zur Systematik und Geschichte der Medizinischen Ethik. In: von Engelhardt D (ed) Ethik im Alltag der Medizin. Spektrum der Medizinischen Disziplinen. Berlin, Heidelberg: Springer, 1989.

20. Beckmann JP. Zur Frage der ethischen Legitimation von Handeln und Unterlassen angesichts des Todes. In: Mohr M, Kettler D (eds) Ethik in der Notfallmedizin: Präklinische Herz-Lungen-Wiederbelebung. Berlin, Heidelberg, New York: Springer, 1997.

21. Irrgang B. Grundriß der medizinischen Ethik. München Basel: Reinhardt, 1995.

22. Becker LB, Han BH, Meyer PM, Weight FA, Rhodes KV, Smith DW, Barrett J and the CPR Chicago Project. Racial differences in the incidence of cardiac arrest and subsequent survival. N Engl J Med 1993;329:600–606.

23. Hallstrom A, Boutin P, Cobb L, Johnson E. Socioeconomic status and prediction of ventricular fibrillation survival. Am J Pub Health 1993;83:245–248.

24. Naess AC, Steen E, Steen PA. Ethics in treatment decisions during out-of-hospital resuscitation. Resuscitation 1997;33:245–256.

9.2. The Ethics of Resuscitation in Clinical Practice

A Statement on behalf of the European Resuscitation Council, 1994

Present day knowledge, skill, pharmacy, and technology have proved effective in prolonging active life for many patients. Countless thousands have good reason to be thankful for cardiopulmonary resuscitation, and the numbers rise daily. Yet, in the wake of this advance, there is a small but important shadow of bizarre and distressing problems. These problems must be freely and openly addressed if we are to avoid criticism from others and from our own consciences.

Resuscitation attempts in the mortally ill do not enhance the dignity and serenity that we hope for our relatives and ourselves when we die. All too often resuscitation is begun in patients already destined for life as cardiac or respiratory cripples or who are suffering the terminal misery of untreatable cancer. From time to time, but fortunately rarely, resuscitation efforts may help to create the ultimate tragedy — the human vegetable — as the heart is more tolerant than the brain to the insult of hypoxia.

Merely Prolonging the Process of Dying

The reasons for these apparent errors of judgement are several. In a high proportion of cases, particularly those occurring outside hospital, the victim and his circumstances are unknown to the rescuer, who may well not be competent to assess whether resuscitation is appropriate or not in the particularly individual. Sadly, through lack of communication, this state of affairs also occurs from time to time in hospital practice. A junior ward nurse, unless explicitly instructed not to do so, feels, not unreasonably, obliged to call

the resuscitation team to any patients with cardiorespiratory arrest. She is not qualified to certify death. The team is often unaware of the patient's condition and prognosis and, because of the urgency of the situation, begins treatment first and asks questions afterwards.

Ideally, resuscitation should be attempted only in patients who have a very high chance of successful revival for a comfortable and contented existence. A study of published reports containing results of series of resuscitation attempts shows that this ideal is far from being attained. Typical figures include a 12% survival rate for 1 month in 1972 [1], a 14% discharge rate [2], and, more recently, a discharge rate of 14% in 1982 [3], and 21.3% in 1984 [4]. De Bard, reviewing published studies in 1981, reported an overall discharge rate of 17% [5]. More recent works [6–10] still put overall survival rates in the general wards of hospitals at around 15%. In each of these series a substantial number — usually about 50–60% — failed to respond to the initial resuscitation attempts. In many of these, particularly the younger patients, effort was clearly justified initially. The cause of the arrest was apparently myocardial ischaemia, and the outcome cannot be confidently predicted in any individual patient. However, some of the papers drew attention to the large proportion of patients in whom resuscitative efforts were inappropriate and unjustified. Sowden et al. reported an incidence of 25% of cases in which resuscitation merely prolonged the process of dying.

A 32-year-old woman was admitted in a quadriplegic state due to a spinal injury incurred when she had thrown herself from the Clifton Suspension Bridge. She had made 18 previous attempts at suicide over the previous 5 years, sometimes by taking an overdose of tablets of various kinds and sometimes by cutting her wrists. She had been injecting herself with heroin for the past 7 years and had no close relationships with her family and no close friends. During her stay of 2 days in the intensive care unit she developed pneumonia and died. A conscious decision not to provide artificial ventilation and resuscitation had been made beforehand.

Though assessments are undoubtedly easier in retrospect, there are clearly many cases in which the decision not to resuscitate might have been made before the event. As the number of deaths in hospital always exceeds the number of calls for resuscitation, a decision not to resuscitate is clearly being made in many instances. There is, however, much room for improvement.

The matter has been addressed by national authorities in the USA [11] by the European Resuscitation Council [12,13] and by the Resuscitation Council (UK) in their Advanced Life Support Manual [14]. Clearly national differences exist dictated by legal, economic and social variables [15] but it is apparent that noncoercive guidelines can be set out to reduce the number of futile resuscitation attempts and to offer advice as to when resuscitation should be discontinued in the unresponding patient.

Selection of Patients "Not for Resuscitation"

Two situations may be envisaged:
- The unexpected cardiorespiratory arrest with no other obvious underlying disease. In this situation resuscitation should be attempted without question or delay.
- The unexpected cardiorespiratory arrest in a patient with serious underlying disease. It is patients in this group who should be assessed beforehand as to whether a resuscitation attempt is considered appropriate or not.

The decision not to resuscitate revolves around many factors — the patient's own wishes which may include a "Living Will", the patient's prognosis both immediate and long-term, the views of relatives and friends who may be reporting the known wishes of a patient who cannot communicate and the patient's perceived ability to cope with disablement in the environment for which he or she is destined. The decision should not revolve around doctor pride.

The examples in italics may serve as food for thought as to whether the value judgement was right or wrong.

Decisions on whether or not to resuscitate a patient are generally made on an individual basis, in the atmosphere of close clinical supervision prevalent in critical care units, and the decision is then communicated to the resident medical and nursing staff. In the general wards, however, the potential situation in specific patients may not actually be considered, and inappropriate resuscitation occurs by default. There has been a reluctance to label a mentally alert patient, who is nevertheless terminally ill, "Not for resuscitation." There are, sadly, doctors who refuse to acknowledge that the patient has reached end stage disease, perhaps because they have spent so much time and effort in treating them. There are those who, having spent their career in hospital practice, cannot comprehend the difficulties for the severely disabled of an existence without adequate help in a poor and miserable social environment. There are those who fear medico-legal sanctions if they put their name to an instruction not to resuscitate.

Fortunately, the climate of opinion is now changing and there are now few members of the public or professionals who disagree with the concept of selection of patients **not for** resuscitation.

The decision maker should be the senior doctor in charge of the patient's management. That senior doctor, however, will usually want to take cognisance of the opinions and wishes of the patient, the relatives and the views of the junior doctors, family practitioner and nurses who have cared for the patient, before arriving at the decision.

Once the decision not to resuscitate has been made, it should be clearly communicated to the medical and nursing staff on duty and recorded in the patient's notes. Because circumstances may change, the decision must be reviewed at intervals which may range from a few hours to weeks depending on the stability of the patient's condition.

A Hospital Ethical Resuscitation Policy

Do not resuscitate policies have been introduced in Canada [16,17] and the USA [18]. They tend to be very formal affairs with a strict protocol to be followed.

Nevertheless, to minimise tragedies and to improve success rates associated with resuscitation, it is helpful to establish an agreed noncoercive hospital ethical policy based on the principles of resuscitation for all except where contraindicated. The promulgation of such guidelines serve as a reminder that the decision must be faced and made.

The guidelines for such a policy should be that:
- The decision not to resuscitate should be made by a senior doctor who should consult others as appropriate;
- The decision should be communicated to medical and nursing staff recorded in the patient's notes and reviewed at appropriate intervals;
- The decision should also be shared with the patient's relatives except in a few cases where this would be decreed inappropriate;
- Other appropriate treatment and care should be continued.

Below is an extract from the guidelines approved by the medical staff committee at Frenchay Hospital, Bristol, which has been in use for the past 12 years.

There can be no rules, every case must be considered individually and this decision should be reviewed as appropriate – this may be on a weekly, daily, or hourly basis.

The decision should be made before it is needed and in many patients this will be on admission.

"A decision to 'DO NOT RESUSCITATE', IS ABSOLUTELY COMPATIBLE WITH CONTINUING MAXIMUM THERAPEUTIC AND NURSING CARE.

1) Where the patient is competent (i.e., mentally fit and conscious), the decision 'DO NOT RESUSCITATE' should be discussed where possible with the patient. This will not always be appropriate but, particularly in those patients with a slow progressive deterioration, it is important to consider it.
2) If the patient is not competent to make such decisions, the appropriate family members should be consulted.
3) Factors which may influence the decision to be made should include:

a) Quality of life prior to this illness (highly subjective and only truly known to the patient himself).

b) Expected quality of life (medical and social) assuming recovery from this particular illness.

c) Likelihood of resuscitation being successful.

If at any time patients or their relatives request an attempt at resuscitation contrary to medical opinion – this should be carried out.

The decision to 'DO NOT RESUSCITATE' should be recorded clearly in medical and nursing notes, signed, dated, and should be reviewed at appropriate intervals."

During the period of clinical use there have been no objections to the guidelines from either the medical or nursing staff.

A 62-year-old woman had a cardiac arrest in a thoracic ward 2 days after undergoing pneumonectomy for respectable lung cancer. Her remaining lung was clearly fibrotic and malfunctioning and her cardiac arrest was probably hypoxic and hypercarbic in origin. Because no instructions had been given to the contrary, she was resuscitated by the hospital resuscitation team and spontaneous cardiac rhythm restarted after 20 min. She required continuous artificial ventilation and was unconscious for 1 week.

Over the next 6 weeks she gradually regained consciousness but could not be weaned from the ventilator. She was tetraplegic – presumably as a result of spinal cord damage from hypoxia – but regained some weak finger movements over 2 months. At 3 months her improvement had tailed off and she was virtually paralysed in all four limbs and dependent on the ventilator. She died 5 months after the cardiac arrest. She was supported throughout her illness by her devoted and intelligent husband, who left his work to be with her and continued to hope for a spontaneous cure until very near the end.

The Termination of Resuscitation Attempts

If resuscitation does not result in a relatively early return of a spontaneous circulation then one of two options must be considered: i) termination of further resuscitation efforts, or ii) support of the circulation by mechanical means such as cardiac pacing, balloon pumping or cardiopulmonary bypass.

The decision to terminate resuscitative efforts will depend on a number of factors:

- The environment and access to Emergency Medical Services (EMS).

Cardiac arrest occurring in remote sites when access to EMS is impossible or very delayed is not associated with a favourable outcome.

- The interval between the onset of arrest and the application of Basic Life Support (BLS).

This is crucial in determining outcome with intact neurological function. Generally speaking, if the interval is greater than 5 min the prognosis is poor unless there are mitigating factors such as hypothermia or prior sedative drug intake. Children also tend to be more tolerant of delay in some cases.

- The interval between BLS and the application of Advanced Life Support measures.

Survival is rare if defibrillation and/or drug therapy is unavailable within 20 min of arrest. Each case must be judged on individual merit taking into account evidence of cardiac death, cerebral damage and the ultimate prognosis.

- Evidence of cardiac death.

Persistent ventricular fibrillation should be actively treated until established asystole or electromechanical dissociation (pulseless electrical activity) supervenes. Patients with asystole who are unresponsive to adrenaline and fluid replacement are unlikely to survive unless there are extenuating circumstances and resuscitation should be abandoned after 15 min.

- Evidence of cerebral damage.

Persistent fixed and dilated pupils unrelated to previous drug therapy are usually, but not invariably, an indication of serious cerebral damage and consideration should be given to abandoning resuscitation in the absence of mitigating factors. If the measurement system is in place intracranial pressure values greater than 30 mmHg are a poor prognostic sign.

- Potential prognosis and underlying disease process.

Resuscitation should be abandoned early in patients with a poor ultimate prognosis and end stage disease. Prolonged attempts in such patients are rarely successful and are associated with a high index of cerebral damage.

- Age

Age in itself has less effect on outcome than the underlying disease process [7] or the presenting rhythm [4]. Nevertheless patients in their 70s and 80s do not have good survival rates compared to their younger fellow citizens, generally because of underlying disease [19] and earlier curtailment of resuscitative efforts is indicated. By contrast young children on occasion appear to be tolerant of hypoxia and resuscitation should be continued for longer than in adults.

- Temperature

Hypothermia confers protection against the effects of hypoxia and therefore resuscitation efforts should be continued for much longer than in normothermic patients. Cases have been reported of survival with good neurological function after more than 45 min submersion in water. Resuscitation should be continued in hypothermic patients during active rewarming using cardiopulmonary bypass if available and appropriate.

- Drug intake prior to cardiac arrest.

Sedative, hypnotic or narcotic drugs taken prior to cardiac arrest also provide a degree of cerebral protection against the effects of hypoxia and resuscitative efforts should be prolonged accordingly.

- Remediable precipitating factors.

Resuscitation should continue while potentially remedial conditions giving rise to the arrest are treated. Such conditions include tension pneumothorax and cardiac tamponade. Outcome after arrest due to haemorrhagic hypovolaemia is notoriously poor. Factors to be taken into account include the immediate availability of very skilled surgery and very rapid transfusion facilities. Even under optimal conditions survival rates are poor and early termination of resuscitation is generally indicated if bleeding cannot be immediately controlled.

Other Resuscitation Procedures

- Use of cardiac pacing

Cardiac pacing (internal or transthoracic) has little application in cardiac arrest. Pacing should be reserved for those with residual P wave activity or with very slow rhythms.

- Balloon pump and cardiopulmonary bypass

Clearly the use of this equipment depends on the immediate availability of the apparatus and skilled staff to operate it.

Such intervention should be reserved for patients with a potentially good prognosis, i.e., cases of hypothermia, drug overdose and those with conditions amenable to immediate cardiac, thoracic or abdominal surgery.

Legal Aspects

Doctors, nurses and paramedical persons functioning in their official capacity have an obligation to perform CPR when medically indicated and in the absence of a "do not resuscitate" decision.

Many countries apply "Good Samaritan" laws in relation to CPR to protect lay rescuers acting in good faith provided they are not guilty of gross negligence. In other countries the law may not be specifically written down but the "Good Samaritan" principle is applied by the judiciary. Such arrangements are essential for the creation and continuance of a community and hospital CPR policy. At the time of writing, the author does not know of any case in which a lay person who has attempted CPR reasonably has been successfully sued. Similar protection applies to teachers and trainers of citizen CPR programmes.

Health care professionals performing CPR outside their place of work and acting as a bystanding citizen are expected to perform basic CPR within the limitations of the environment and facilities available to them on the occasion.

When acting in an official capacity, health care professionals are expected to be able to perform BLS and all doctors are expected additionally to provide the major elements of Advanced Life Support including airway management, ventilation with oxygen, defibrillation, i.v. cannulation and appropriate drug therapy. Hospitals are expected to provide the appropriate resuscitation equipment and facilities. With increasing expectation of higher standards, it is likely that these requirements will extend to family medical and dental practices, leisure, sports and travel centres, trains, planes and ships and major work places in the future.

The position of "do not resuscitate" policies is rarely defined precisely in the legislature of most European countries. The majority of the judiciary, however, accept in practice a decision not to resuscitate carefully arrived at and based on the guidelines outlined above.

Infection Hazards During Resuscitation

Mouth-to-mouth ventilation

Cross-infection between victim and rescuer potentially may occur during mouth-to-mouth or mouth-to-nose ventilation. The incidence is remarkably rare but isolated cases of cutaneous tuberculosis, herpes labialis, staphylococcal and streptococcal infections and meningococcal meningitis have been reported.

Of great concern to would-be rescuers at the present time is the possibility of acquiring Human Immonodeficiency Virus (HIV) during mouth-to-mouth contact. Fortunately it appears that HIV is not contained in saliva in amounts sufficient to cause infection (20) but there always remains the possibility of transmission from open oral wounds in both parties. There is, however, no record of this occurring at the time of writing and so the possibility must be considered almost negligible. The chance of infection with the Hepatitis B Virus (HBV) virus is greater, however.

On the evidence currently available, it is reasonable to encourage would-be rescuers in the community to continue to perform unprotected mouth-to-mouth ventilation in patients with cardiorespiratory arrest with the assurance that the risk of infection is negligible. Any one lay individual is unlikely to perform CPR more than 6 times in a lifetime and there is a 75% chance that the resuscitation will be given to a relative, close friend or a workmate. Nevertheless, small simple protective plastic film devices (e.g., Ambu Life Key and Laerdal Resusciade) are available to prevent direct contact and the use of these by lay bystanders is to be encouraged if they are imme-

diately available. However, resuscitation should never be delayed while the equipment is fetched.

Health care professionals have a much higher chance of being called upon to perform resuscitation and it is therefore reasonable that protective devices should be readily available in each patient area to offer protection against infection and to reduce aesthetic antagonism. The Laerdal Pocket Resuscimask is one of the most satisfactory devices for this purpose. Similar devices are made by other manufacturers.

Blood-to-blood contact

Advanced life support is frequently an invasive procedure. It is good practice for all professional rescuers to wear protective gloves throughout. Special care should be taken to minimise needle stick injuries and ampoule cuts. Sharps disposal boxes should be immediately available. Goggles should be worn particularly when patients are thought to be special risks.

Training manikins

Training manikins have not been shown, in practice, to be a source of viral infection in resuscitation students. Nevertheless, the potential for bacterial infection does exist and it is good practice to disinfect the equipment after each use accordingly to the manufacturers' instructions.

Other Ethical Problems Arising in Relation to Resuscitation

There are a number of other unsolved ethical problems arising in relation to resuscitation which require to be addressed.

The diagnosis of death

Traditionally, death is pronounced by medical practitioners. However, the question arises as to the wisdom and practicality of death being determined by nonmedical health care professionals such as nurses and ambulance men in some cases.

Such a policy might obviate the need for futile or excessively prolonged resuscitation attempts. Certainly there would be no argument in straightforward cases such as decapitation, incineration, very prolonged submersion and massive mutilation. However, the question also arises in cases of extreme senility and terminal illness where no previous medical instructions have been given and in patients who are unresponsive to prolonged resuscitation attempts outside hospital. This subject is currently under debate by authorities in the United Kingdom and other countries.

The Involvement of Relatives and Close Friends

Bystanders are encouraged to undertake immediate Basic Life Support in the event of cardiorespiratory arrest. In many cases the bystander will be a close relative. Traditionally relatives will be escorted away from the victim when the health care professionals arrive. However, it is clear that some relatives do not wish to be isolated from their loved ones at this time and are deeply hurt if this is insisted upon. Aspects of this debate have been published [21] with contributions from a relative and members of the medical profession and opinion confirms the need to identify and respect relatives' wishes to remain with the patient. Clearly care and consideration of the relative in these stressful situations becomes of increasing concern as the invasiveness of the resuscitation escalates from basic life support to defibrillation and venous access and perhaps to chest drainage, cricothyrotomy and even open chest cardiac massage.

The Use of the Recently Dead for Training in Practical Skills

Opportunities for hands-on training in the practical skills required for resuscitation are limited. It is clear that tracheal intubation cannot be taught to everyone attending a cardiac arrest. While the laryngeal mask may offer an alternative option for airway management in the short term, the introduction of that device on a widespread scale into anaesthetic practice has reduced the opportu-

nities for tracheal intubation training in the anaesthetic room. Mannekin training offers an alternative, though most would agree that training on patients is required to amplify mannekin experience. Training in tracheal intubation on the recently dead has engendered a sharp debate and, while supported by some doctors, has met with strong opposition from members of the nursing profession. Informed consent is difficult to obtain at the very sensitive and emotional time of bereavement and approaches might be construed as coercion. Proceeding without consent might be thought of as an assault.

The dilemma does not stop with tracheal intubation and other techniques such as fibreoptic intubation, central venous access, surgical cut down venous access, chest drain insertion, surgical cricothyrotomy, etc., should be considered.

Modern medicine brings problems and ethical dilemmas. Public expectations have changed and will continue to change. More and more, doctors' actions are questioned in the media and in the Courts of Law. We need to formulate answers and be more open with the public to explain how our actions are related entirely to their well-being. Only in this way will we keep **in tune** with society and practice the science of resuscitation with art and compassion.

REFERENCES

1. Wildsmith JAW, Denyson WG, Myers KW. Results of resuscitation following cardiac arrest. Br J Anaesth 1972;44:716–719.
2. Eltringham RJ, Baskett PJF. Experience with a hospital resuscitation service including an analysis of 258 calls to patients with cardiorespiratory arrest. Resuscitation 1973;2:57–68.
3. Hershey CO, Fisher L. Why outcome of cardiopulmonary resuscitation in general wards is so poor. Lancet 1982;ii:32.
4. Sowden GR, Baskett PJF, Robins DW. Factors associated with survival and eventual cerebral status following cardiac arrest. Anaesthesia 1984;39:1.
5. De Bard ML. Cardiopulmonary resuscitation: analysis of six years experience and review of the literature. Ann Emerg Med 1981;10:408–416.
6. Council on Ethical and Judicial Affairs, American Heart Association. Guidelines for the appropriate use of do-not-resuscitate orders. J Am Med Ass 1991;265:

1968–1971.

7. Bedell SE, Delbanco TL, Cook EF, Epstein FH. Survival after cardiopulmonary resuscitation in hospital. N Engl J Med 1983;309:569–576.

8. Evans AL, Brody BA. The do not resuscitate order in teaching hospitals. J Am Med Ass 1985;253:2236–2239.

9. Moss AH. Informing the patient about cardiopulmonary resuscitation: when the risks outweigh the benefits. J Gen Int Med 1989;4:349–355.

10. Tunstall Pedoe H, Bailey L, Chamberlain DA, Marsden AK, Ward ME, Ziderman DA. Survey of 3765 cardiopulmonary resuscitations in British Hospitals. The BRESUS study: Methods and Overall Results. Br Med J 1992;304:1347–1351.

11. American Heart Association; Emergency Cardiac Care Committee. Guidelines for Cardiopulmonary Resuscitation and Emergency Cardiac Care. Ethical Considerations in Resuscitation. J Am Med Ass 1992;268:2282–2288.

12. Baskett PJF. Ethics in Cardiopulmonary Resuscitation (Invited Editorial). Resuscitation 1993;25:1–8.

13. Holmberg S, Ekstrom L. Ethics and practicalities of resuscitation. Resuscitation 1992;24:239–244.

14. Resuscitation Council UK. Advanced Life Support Manual. Ed Handley A J. 1992; Pub. Resuscitation Council U.K. c/o British Cardiac Society. Fitzroy Square, London.

15. Bossaert L. Ethical issues in resuscitation. In: Vincent JL (ed) Yearbook of Intensive Care and Emergency Medicine. Springer-Verlag, 1994;408–415.

16. McPhail A, Moore S, O'Connor J, Woodward C. One hospital's experience with a "Do not resuscitate" policy. Can Med Assoc J 1981;125:830–836.

17. Canadian Medical Association. Proceedings of the annual meeting including the transactions of the General Medical Association, 1974.

18. Lo B, Steinbrook RL. Deciding whether to resuscitate. Arch Int Med 1983;143:1561–1563.

19. Ritter G, Wolfe RA, Goldstein S, Landis JR, Vash CM, Acheson A, Leighton R, Medendrop SV. The effect of bystander CPR on survival of out of hospital cardiac arrest victims. Am Heart J 1985;110:932–937.

20. Center for Disease Control Update: universal precautions for prevention of transmission of human immunodeficiency virus, hepatitis B virus and other blood borne pathogens in health care settings. Morbid Mortal Weekly Rep 1988;37:377–388.

21. Adams S, Whitlock M, Higgs R, Bloomfield P, Baskett PJF. Should relatives be allowed to watch resuscitation. Br Med J 1994;308:1687–1689.